R. Erbel H. J. Nesser J. Drozdz (Eds.)

Atlas of Tissue Doppler Echocardiography – TDE

With 130 Figures, Most in Color

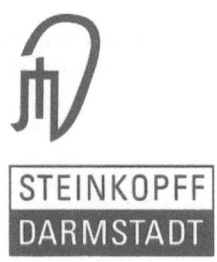

STEINKOPFF
DARMSTADT

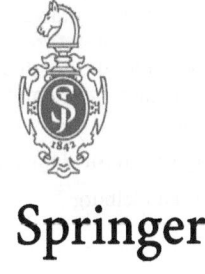

Springer

Raimund Erbel, MD, FESC, FACC
Dept. of Cardiology, University-GHS Essen
Hufelandstrasse 55, D-45122 Essen, Germany

H. Joachim Nesser, MD
Division of Cardiology, K. d. Elisabethinen
Fadingerstrasse 1, A-4010 Linz, Austria

Jaroslaw Drozdz, MD
Dept. of Cardiology, University of Lodz
Jonscher Hospital, Milionowa 14
Lodz, 93-113, Poland

ISBN-13: 978-3-642-47069-1   e-ISBN-13: 978-3-642-47067-7
DOI: 10.1007/978-3-642-47067-7

Die Deutsche Bibliothek – CIP-Einheitsaufnahme
Atlas of tissue doppler echocardiography: TDE / R. Erbel ...
(ed.). – Darmstadt : Steinkopff, 1995

NE: Erbel, Raimund [Hrsg.]; TDE

Medical Editor: Sabine Ibkendanz – English Editor: James C. Willis

Produktion Editing: PRO EDIT GmbH, Heidelberg

Printing on acid free paper

Preface

This is the first book to present an overview of the exciting new cardiac imaging technique of tissue Doppler echocardiography (TDE).

In order to understand the background of this technique, it is necessary to compare the physical properties of blood, which reflects ultrasound poorly but moves with high velocity (up to 150 cm/s) with those of the myocardium, which reflects ultrasound strongly but moves with low velocity (less than 10 cm/s). In tissue Doppler imaging, existing Doppler technology has been modified to bypass the high-pass filter and enhance calculation of low velocities, thus enabling selective visualization of the myocardium rather than of the blood. Because the color Doppler tissue images are superimposed on the conventional two-dimensional ultrasound images, this technique is known as TDE.

Following a brief introduction, the history of ultrasound and Doppler imaging is presented. It is now about 150 years since the death of Christian Doppler, who described the "Doppler" effect, and more than 100 years since Pierre Curie discovered the piezoelectric effects of crystals.

TDE was developed by Nobuo Yamazaki and Yoshitaka Mine at the Medical Engineering Laboratory, Toshiba Corporation, Tochigi, Japan. Engineers involved in the development of the technique have provided important technical information, which the reader will find an invaluable background to potential applications of TDE.

An extensive chapter summarizes the normal features of TDE, which is an important introduction to some of the pathological conditions described later. In order to properly appreciate the rapid changes in the magnitude and direction of tissue velocities, TDE requires digital cineloop archiving and frame-by-frame analysis. TDE is strongly angle dependent and is influenced by total heart movement, a new aspect for echocardiography.

Successive chapters document TDE images obtained in patients with coronary artery disease and with hypertrophic, dilated, and restrictive cardiomyopathies. The enhancement of structure identification by TDE is explained, with particular reference to the measurement of right ventricular wall thickness. Adjacent thoracic and pericardial structures are not color coded, in contrast to the right ventricular myocardium, thus allowing precise delineation.

The potential use of TDE to assess regional systolic and diastolic function is then discussed. M-mode TDE affords the possibility of measuring global and regional systolic and diastolic time intervals (STI/DTI) of both the left and right ventricles.

The final chapters explain how TDE may be useful in the assessment and understanding of disturbances of cardiac rhythm and document experience with a variety of subjects, including tumors and spontaneous echo contrast.

Our first book on echocardiography, *Fortschritte der Echokardiographie*[1], which was published 10 years ago, included transesophageal and color Doppler imaging; it was followed in 1989 by *Transesophageal Echocardiography – A New Window to the Heart*[2]. We hope that this new book, *Tissue Doppler Echocardiography*, will demonstrate that a further chapter has been opened in the history of echocardiography.

We wish to thank our collaborating authors for their intensive work. Particular praise must go to Thomas Buck for organizing the publication; David R. Wallbridge for his editorial assistance; Petra Merz for her secretarial work; Christiane Plato for her work in the echocardiographic laboratory; and Ilse Scharein for her photographic work. The close cooperation of the publishing staff, particularly Sabine Ibkendanz, is also acknowledged.

The pictures presented in this book would not have been possible without the support of Toshiba Medical Systems. Mr. K. Machida (Europe), Mr. U. Stöcker, and Mr. W. Randhan (Germany) have been most generous in their assistance.

R. Erbel   H. J. Nesser   J. Drozdz

The work was supported by the Herz-Kreislaufzentrum Essen, Gesellschaft für Herz-Kreislaufforschung e. V.

References

1. Erbel R, Meyer J, Brennecke R (eds) (1985) Fortschritte der Echokardiographie. Springer, Berlin Heidelberg New York
2. Erbel R, Khandheria D, Brennecke R, Meyer J, Seward JP, Tajik A (eds) (1989) Transesophageal echocardiography – a new window to the heart. Springer, Berlin Heidelberg New York

List of Contents

List of Contributors

Thomas Buck, MD
Dept. of Cardiology
University-GHS Essen
Hufelandstrasse 55
D-45112 Essen – Germany

Frank Schön, MD
Schwarzenbergstrasse 25 a
D-45472 Mülheim an der Ruhr
Germany

Hans Ulrich Stöcker
Toshiba Medical Systems
(Germany)
Hellersbergstrasse 4
D-41460 Neuss – Germany

David R. Wallbridge, MD
Dept. of Cardiology/Pathophysiology
University-GHS Essen
Hufelandstrasse 55
D-45112 Essen – Germany

Nobuo Yamazaki
Toshiba Corporation
Medical Engineering Laboratory
1385, Shimoishigami
Otawara-Shi, Toshigi-Ken
324 Japan

José Zamorano, MD
Servicio de Cardiologia
Hospital Clinico
Plaza de Cristo Rey
E-28040 Madrid – Spain

Chapter 1 **Introduction**

R. Erbel

Echocardiography has become the diagnostic workhorse in cardiology and has evolved to a method enabling cardiovascular hemodynamics to be analyzed. Ventricular function frequently needs to be assessed in the echocardiographic laboratory, and both global and regional indices are currently derived from two-dimensional echocardiography. Guidelines for the analysis of left ventricular volume and ejection fraction have been published by the American Society of Echocardiography [1], but similar standards have yet to be established for the right ventricle and the atria. Regional wall motion is determined either semiquantitatively, by dividing the left ventricle into 16 segments and scoring the degree of abnormality in each of these, or quantitatively, using the centerline, radiant, and trajectory methods. The limitations of these methods, due to cardiac motion, rotation of the heart, and changes in the centre of gravity of the left ventricle, become more important after myocardial infarction or cardiac surgery or in subjects with cardiomyopathy.

While global diastolic function can be relatively easily assessed by analyzing the transmitral and pulmonary venous flow patterns, measurement of regional diastolic function by echocardiography is more problematic. Research in this field is called *diastology*. Regional impairment of diastolic and systolic function may precede changes in more global indices of function due to compensatory hyperactivity of healthy tissue.

The pioneering work of Gibson in the 1970s highlighted the importance of ventricular asynchrony in cardiac disease. Using frame-by-frame analysis of ventricular angiograms, he demonstrated that abnormalities of early diastolic filling were present in subjects with coronary artery disease [2] (Figs. 1.1, 1.2) and hypertrophic cardiomyopathy [3]. Echocardiographic methods that include only end-diastolic and end-systolic frames are unable to determine such changes.

With the development of M-mode echocardiography, attention was directed toward the quantifica-

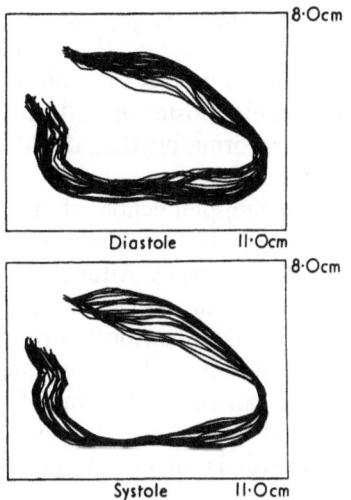

Fig. 1.1. Successive cavity outlines from the left ventriculogram showing inferior akinesia and an area of abnormal movement of the anterior wall during diastole. (From [2])

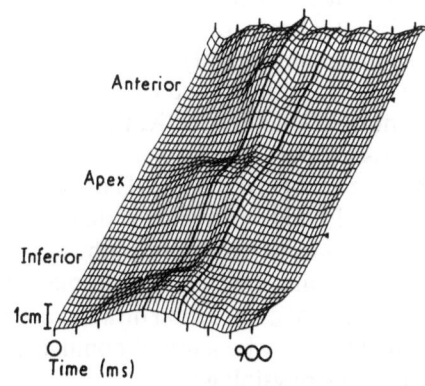

Fig. 1.2. Plots of regional wall movement against time from the left ventriculogram of a patient with coronary artery disease. During isovolumic relaxation, indicated by the two *bold lines*, there is outward movement along the anterior border and inward movement along the inferior border. (From [2])

tion of the excursion of the left ventricular posterior wall. In retrospect, it is perhaps easy to understand why neither endocardial nor epicardial posterior wall velocities provided an accurate measure of total left ventricular performance in patients with coronary artery disease [4]. Nevertheless, interesting observations were made, such as the fact that exercise-induced angina was accompanied by the development of abnormal diastolic velocities in the presence of preserved systolic function [5]. Somewhat later, Isaaz [6] showed that conventional pulsed Doppler imaging can be used for the direct analysis of the left ventricular posterior wall and that it appears to be more informative than the M-mode technique for systolic measurements.

Tissue Doppler echocardiography (TDE) displays color-coded tissue velocities as an overlay on conventional images. After a short period of experimental validation, clinical applications continue to emerge. The distribution of velocities across the myocardium can be observed and transmural gradients calculated. This may facilitate the study of subendocardial function as an early indicator of myocardial ischemia or as a marker of viable myocardium.

The ability of TDE to demonstrate ventricular asynchrony with high temporal resolution is an exciting step forward. This may prove very useful for assessing global and regional left ventricular function, but it must take into account the whole heart motion, a completely new area for echocardiography. The color interfaces of M-mode TDE can be used to measure the duration of the different phases of the cardiac cycle, including regional systolic (STI) and diastolic time intervals (DTI), for both left and right ventricles.

Abnormal electrical activation of the heart, by an accessory pathway or ventricular ectopic focus, may be recognized by TDE contraction patterns. It has already been shown that TDE can detect the position of accessory pathways in Wolff-Parkinson-White (WPW) syndrome and that the early signs of contraction disappear after ablation. Thus TDE may be a useful noninvasive technique for electrophysiology.

TDE shows potential in the assessment of abnormalities of ventricular function in patients with cardiomyopathies. Analysis of the patterns of myocardial velocities may be helpful to distinguish between amyloidosis and hypertrophic cardiomyopathy. Whether differences exist between TDE patterns in hypertrophic cardiomyopathy and arterial hypertension remains to be established.

The role of TDE in the evaluation of cardiac tumors, thrombi, and vegetations requires further evaluation. Measurements of wall thickness are improved, particularly for the right ventricle. The aorta is also easily studied by TDE, with the possibility of new insights into altered aortic compliance in systemic hypertension.

It is hoped that the various chapters of the book will give the reader a first insight into the emerging technique of TDE.

References

1. Schiller NB, Shah PM, Crawford M, DeMaria A, Devereux R, Feigenbaum H, Gutgesell H, Reichek N, Sahn D, Schnittger J, Silverman AH, Tajik AJ (1989) Recommendations for quantification of the left ventricle by two-dimensional echocardiography. J Am Soc Echocardiogr 2:358–367
2. Gibson DG, Prewitt TA, Brown DJ (1976) Analysis of left ventricular wall movement during isovolumic relaxation and its relation to coronary artery disease. Br Heart J 38:1010–1019
3. Sanderson JE, Gibson DG, Brown DJ, Goodwin JF (1977) Left ventricular filling in hyertrophic cardiomyopathy. An angiographic study. Br Heart J 39:661–670
4. Ludbrook P, Karliner JS, London A, Peterson KL, Leopold GR, O'Rourke RA (1974) Posterior wall velocity: an unreliable index of total left ventricular performance in patients with coronary artery disease. Am J Cardiol 33:475–482
5. Fogelman AM, Abbasi AS, Pearce ML, Kattus AA (1972) Echocardiographic study of the abnormal motion of the posterior left ventricular wall during angina pectoris. Circulation 46:905–913
6. Isaaz K, Thompson A, Ethevenot G, Cloez JL, Brembilla B, Pernot C (1989) Doppler echocardiographic measurement of low velocity motion of the left ventricular posterior wall. Am J Cardiol 64:66–75

Chapter 2　Milestones in Cardiovascular Ultrasound

H. J. Nesser

The engineering aspects using ultrasound for diagnostic purposes date far back, to the year 1883, when *Galton* developed a pipe producing vibrations as high as 25000 cycles per second.

During the First World War, *Langevin* made experiments generating ultrasound waves by quartz crystals. The intensity of the waves was sufficient enough to kill fish in a water tank. The first to describe an ultrasound technique to localize flaws in metals was *Sokolov* [67] in 1929. During the Second World War, ultrasound was particularly used to fix the position of underwater objects and was a goal of military research. It was *Firestone* [26], who again initiated the technique for non destructive testing.

One of the first to register reflected ultrasonic waves from cardiac structures was *Keidel* in 1950, who measured cardiac volumes [43].

In 1954, the term "ultrasonic cardiogram" was created by *Hertz* and *Edler*. Their early works included descriptions of the left ventricular posterior wall and the anterior mitral leaflet [14]. During the late 1950s *Edler* was engaged, with using the technique to analyze valve diseases such as mitral valve stenosis [15, 16]. A left atrial thrombus was reported by him [17] in 1955, and by *Effert* [19] a left atrial myxoma in 1959.

In 1957, *Reid* and *Wild* were the first in the United States to use medical ultrasound to examine excised hearts [82]. *Reid* and *Joyner* [40] worked together to start the first clinical applications of cardiac ultrasound in the USA. Their article dealing with mitral valve disease was published in *Circulation* in 1963.

Feigenbaum and associates at Indiana University began to work with cardiac ultrasound in 1963. In this year pericardial effusion was first detected in his laboratory with the use of ultrasound [22]. Measurements of myocardial wall thickness [23], left ventricular dimensions [24] and left ventricular stroke volume [25] were also first reported by the same group.

In 1969, a very important contribution to the development of cardiac ultrasound was provided by *Gramiak* creating the contrast echo technique [30].

It may be of interest that the term "Echocardiography" was introduced by the American Institute of Ultrasound in accordance with the term "Echoencephalography".

Two-dimensional Echocardiography

Whereas M-mode echocardiography only produced small detailed images of the heart, two-dimensional sector scanning developed in the mid 1970s, allowed real-time tomographic images of cardiac morphology and function [1, 81].

Ultrasonic two-dimensional imaging was primarily used in radiological and obstetric applications [81]. *Asberg* described the first scanner operating at seven frames per second already in 1967 [1]. Five years later, in 1972, *King* demonstrated two-dimensional imagings with a static contact B-scanner [45]. Eventually, this technique achieved clinical importance, when *Bom* [4] and coworkers constructed the linear array system. In 1974, the mechanical real-time sector scanner was introduced by *Griffith* and *Henry* [31]. The electronic phased array sector scanner was developed by *Somer* [68] in 1968, but it was not until 1974 that *Thurstone* and von *Ramm* [76] took the next steps to non invasively diagnose heart diseases with this technology in the USA.

Because of the increased diagnostic safety, myocardial infarction, cardiomyopathies and coronary artery disease were analyzed with the new technique [39, 71]. At present three-dimensional echocardiography, clinically initiated by *Wollschläger* and coworkers [83], is one of the endpoints of a long history of imaging cardiac structures and function. Today, it is still under clinical investigation.

Three-dimensional Echocardiography

A system for ultrasonical imaging of the human heart in three dimensions was already introduced independently by *Dekker* [10] and *Moritz* [56] in 1974. Most of the following reports [8, 29, 50] dealt with three-dimensional reconstruction of the left ventricle. In 1989, *Wollschläger* [83, 84] set the next step with the development of transesophageal echo computer tomography, which allows dynamic 3-D imaging of heart chambers, valve structures and function. On-line three-dimensional echocardiography is expected to become available in the near future.

Transesophageal Echocardiography

In 1971, *Side* and *Gosling* [66] combined for the first time a standard gastroscope with CW-Doppler to measure blood velocities. *Olson* and *Shelton* could show pulsatile changes of the diameter of the thoracic aorta in 1972 [57]. *Duck* [13] was the first to use pulsed Doppler wave interrogation in 1972, and *Frazin* [28], who introduced transesophageal M-mode echocardiography, improved this technique. Cross-sectional real-time imaging was first reported in 1977 by *Hisanaga* [36] and intra-operative monitoring of left ventricular performance by *Matsumoto* [48] in 1980.

Also in 1980, *Di Magno* [11] from the Stanford Research Institute produced images of intraabdominal anatomy with a 10-MHz side-viewing linear array endoscopic device, whereas *Souquet* used an electronic phased array transducer [69] and introduced the biplane transesophageal probe in 1982 [70].

Initial clinical results in regard to ventricular performance, based on the monoplane approach, were represented by *Hanrath* in 1981 [32] and with the biplane probe in 1982 [33], which was modified by the biplane phased array matrix allowing orthogonal biplane scanning [58]. Later on, the clinical utility was described, by among others, *Erbel* and coworkers, e.g., for aortic dissection [20, 21]. A further step forward was the development of a multiplane imaging system as proposed by *Harui* and *Souquet* in 1985 [34], which turned out to be optimal for three-dimensional reconstruction.

Stress Echocardiography

Since the introduction of dipyridamole stress electrocardiography by *Tauchert* et al. in 1976 [74], exercise echocardiography by *Wann* et al. in 1979 [80], and dobutamine stress and dipyridamol echocardiography by *Mazeika* [51], *Picano* [62] and *Segar* [65] in 1992, these techniques have achieved clinical acceptance.

Doppler Echocardiography

The Doppler effect for light was first described in detail by *Christian Johann Doppler* in 1842 [12]. Doctor *Doppler*, an Austrian professor of mathematics and geometry, lived from 1803 to 1853. The concept he developed has since been used in astronomy. Later, Doctor *Bays Bellot* applied this principle to sound. In 1956, *Satomura* [64] was the first to study blood flow velocities with the Doppler technique, whereas *Lindstrom* and *Edler* showed the Doppler frequency spectrum for mitral flow a decade later [18]. For these measurements a continuous wave instrument was used.

In 1969, *Peronneau* et al. [61] and *Baker* [2] introduced the pulsed ultrasonic Doppler instrument, by which the velocity in a small-range cell could be studied. The first commercial pulsed Doppler was combined with an M-mode locator system and released in 1975. *Stevenson* and associates used time interval histography to differentiate shunt lesions from valvular regurgitation [73].

In 1976, *Holen* and coworkers published a Doppler technique by which the pressure drop across a flow obstruction could be estimated using the Bernoulli equation [38]. Recording of velocities in combination with two-dimensional imaging were already performed by *Baker* and coworkers in 1970 [2]. With *Gessert*'s application of fast Fourier transform (SST) to spectral display, linear analysis of velocity curve profiles has become possible.

Complementary to two-dimensional echocardiography the Doppler techniques provide valuable information in regard to valvular obstruction, regurgitations and shunt lesions.

It is a credit to *Hatle* and *Angelson* that continuous wave Doppler echocardiography has achieved an outstanding role in non-invasive quantitative diagnosis of cardiac diseases [7, 35].

Color Doppler Echocardiography

This multigated pulsed-Doppler method was developed by *Fish*, *Kanaka*, *Rienemann*, *Brandestini* and *Matsuo* in the 1970s [6, 27, 41, 49, 63]. The shortcomings of their technique were that only velocity profiles along the M-mode beam could be defined. "Real-time two-dimensional Doppler echocardiography" or "2-D Doppler", based on the pulsed Doppler concept was introduced into clinical application by *Omoto* [59] in the mid 1980s. This was a break-through for visualizing flow non-invasively, which revolutionized echocardiographic examinations. Autocorrelation improved the technique, which has become indispensable in echocardiographic diagnosis [42].
Today, "Color Doppler" or "Color Doppler Flow Imaging" is the generally used term for this technique. At present the combination of Color Doppler and three-dimensional echocardiography is in an experimental phase.

Two-dimensional Intravascular Ultrasound

First attempts to develop catheter-based ultrasound images date back to 1960, and were primarily designed for intracardiac investigation [5, 9, 44]. Initial clinical studies with the use of intravascular ultrasound have been published in 1988 [37, 60, 86]. Intravascular ultrasound shows details of arterial wall structure and atherosclerotic plaque composition and reveals the shortcomings of contrast angiography. Its potential as a new method for guiding interventional vascular procedures was established in the early 1990s [77].

Ultrasonic Backscatter

Ultrasonic characterization of myocardium with integrated backscatter provides functional and structural information by quantifying tissue acoustic properties through analysis of unprocessed radiofrequency data [53, 79]. Laboratory research dates back to the 1970s and faced particularly ischemia, infarctions [46, 54] and later also cardiomyopathies [47, 75, 78]. Despite new imaging systems and integration of cyclic variation this technique has not achieved importance for routine clinical use up to now.
It seems to be that the technique of Tissue Doppler Echocardiography introduced by *McDicken* [52] in 1992, *Steward* [72], *Miyatake* et al. [55] and

Yamazaki et al. [85] in 1993 will change the future of analyzing function and structure of myocardial tissue by means of a new concept.

References

1. Asberg, A (1969) Ultrasonics 5:113–117
2. Baker, DW (1970) Pulsed ultrasonic Doppler blood-flow sensing. IEEE Trans on S and US SU-17:170–185
3. Barker FE, Baker DW, Nation AW, Strandness DE Jr., Reid JM (1974) Ultrasonic duplex echo Doppler scanner. IEEE Trans Biomed Eng BME 21(2):109
4. Bom N, Lancee CT, van Zwieten G, Kloster FE, Roelandt J (1973) Multiscan echocardiography: Technical description. Circulation 48:1066–1075
5. Bom N, Lancee CT, van Egmond FC (1972) An ultrasonic intracardiac scanner. Ultrasonics 10:72–76
6. Brandestini MA, Howard EA, Weile EB, Stevenson JG, Eyer MK (1979) The synthesis of echo and Doppler in M-mode and sectorscan paper. Proceedings of Annual Meeting of AIUM No. 704:125
7. Brubakk AO, Angelson BAJ, Hatle L (1977) Diagnosis of valvular heart disease using transcutaneous Doppler ultrasound. Cardiovasc Res 11:461–469
8. Chandran KB, Skorton DJ, Attarwala Y, Oishansky B, Collins SM, Pandian N, Nikravesh PE, Kerber RE (1983) Three-dimensional echocardigraphic reconstruction of the intact heart: Calculation of the normal diastolic elastic properties of the canine left ventricle. Circulation 68:III-4 (abstract)
9. Cieszynski T (1960) Intracardiac method for the investigation of structure of the heart with the aid of ultrasonics. Arch Immun Ter Dosw 8:551
10. Dekker DL, Piziali RL, Dong E (1974) A system for ultrasonically imaging the human heart in three dimensions. Comput Biomed Res 7:544–553
11. Di Maggno EP, Buckston JL, Regan PT, Hattery RR, Wilson DA, Suarez JR, Green PS (1980) Ultrasound endoscope. Lancet 1:629–631
12. Doppler CJ (1842) Über das farbige Licht der Doppelsterne: Abhandlungen der Kgl. Böhmischen Gesellschaft der Wissenschaften 4:465 ff
13. Duck FA, Hodson CJ, Tomlin PJ (1972) An esophageal Doppler probe for aortic flow velocity monitoring. Ultrasound Med Biol 1:233–241
14. Edler I, Hertz CH (1954) Use of ultrasonic reflectoscope for continuous recording of movements of heart walls. Kunigl. Fysiogr. Sallad Lund Forhandl 24:5 ff
15. Edler I (1956) Ultrasound cardiogram in mitral valve disease. Acta chir scand 11:230 ff
16. Edler I, Gustavson A (1957) Ultrasonic cardiogram in mitral stenosis. Acta med scand 159:85 ff
17. Edler I (1955) The diagnostic use of ultrasound in heart disease. Acta med scand (suppl) 308:32 ff
18. Edler I, Lindstrom K (1969) Ultrasonic Doppler technique used in heart disease. I. An experimental study. In: Bock, J, Ossoinig K. Ultrasono Graphia Medica Separaum. 1st. World Congress on Ultrasonic Diagnosis in Medicine and SIDUO III. Verlag der Wiener Medizinischen Akademie Vienna pp 445–461

19. Effert S, Domanik E (1959) Diagnostik intraaurikulärer Tumoren und großer Thromben mit dem Ultraschall-Echoverfahren. Dtsch med Wschr 84:6ff

20. Erbel R, Mohr-Kahaly S, Rohmann S, Schuster S, Drexler M, Wittlich N, Pfeiffer C, Schreiner G, Meyer J (1987) Diagnostic value of transesophageal Doppler echocardiography. Herz 12:177–186

21. Erbel R, Mohr-Kahaly S, Rennollet, Brunier J, Drexder M, Wittlich N, Iversen S, Oelert H, Thelen M, Meyer J (1987) Diagnosis of aortic dissection: the value of transeophageal echocardiography. Thorac Cardiovasc Surg 35 (Special issue 2) 126–133

22. Feigenbaum H, Waldhausen JA, Hyde LP (1965) Ultrasound diagnosis of pericardial effusion. JAMA 191:107

23. Feigenbaum H, Popp RL, Chip JN, Haine CL (1968) Left ventricular wall thickness measured by ultrasound. Arch intern Med 121:391–395

24. Feigenbaum H, Wolfe SB, Popp RL, Haine CL, Dodge HT (1969) Correlation of ultrasound with angiography in measuring left ventricular diastolic volume. Amer J Cardiol 23:111ff

25. Feigenbaum H, Zaky HA, Nasser WK (1967) Use of ultrasound to measure left ventricular stroke volume. Circulation 35:1092ff

26. Firestone FA (1945) The supersonic reflectoscope, an instrument for inspection of the interior of solid parts by means of sound waves. J Accust Soc Amer 17:287ff

27. Fish PJ (1975) Multichannel, direction resolving Doppler angiography. Abstracts of 2nd European Congress of Ultrasound in Medicine 72ff

28. Frazin L, Talano JV, Stephanides L (1976) Esophageal echocardiography. Circulation 54:102–108

29. Geiser EA, Lupkiewicz SM, Christie LG, Ariet M, Conetta DA, Conti CR (1980) A framework for three-dimensional time-varying reconstruction of the human left ventricle: sources of error and estimation of their magnitude. Comput Biomed Res 13:225–241

30. Gramiak R, Shah PM, Kramer DH (1969) Ultrasound cardiography: Contrast studies in anatomy and function. Radiology 92:939–948

31. Griffith JM, Henry WL (1974) A sector scanner for real-time two-dimensional echocardiography. Circulation 49:1147–1152

32. Hanrath P, Kremer P, Langenstein BA, Matsumoto M, Bleifeld W (1981) Transoesophageale Echokardiographie: Ein neues Verfahren zur dynamischen Ventrikelfunktionsanalyse. Dtsch Med Wochenschr 106:523–525

33. Hanrath P, Schlüter M, Langenstein BA, Polster J, Engels S (1982) Transesophageal horizontal and sagittal imaging of the heart with a phased array system: Initial clinical results. In: Hanrath P, Bleifeld W, Cardiovascular Diagnosis by Ultrasound. The Hague: Martinus Nijholf Publishers pp 251–259

34. Haroui N, Souquet J (1985) Transesophageal echocardiography scanhead. United States Patent No. 4543960 Oct 1

35. Hatle L, Brubakk AO, Tromsdal A, Angelson BAJ (1978) Non-invasive assessment of pressure drop in mitral stenosis by Doppler ultrasound. Br Heart J 40:131–140

36. Hisanaga K, Hisanaga A, Nagata K, Yoshida S (1977) A new transesophageal real-time two-dimensional echocardiographic system using a flexible tube and its clinical application. Proc Jpn Soc of Ultrasonics in Med 32:43–44

37. Hodgson JMcB, Eberle MJ, Savakus AD (1988) Validation of a new real-time percutaneous intravascular ultrasound imaging catheter (Abstract). Circulation 78:2–21

38. Holen J, Aarlid R, Landmark K, Simonsen S (1976) Determimation of pressure gradient in mitral stenosis with a non-invasive ultrasound Doppler technique. Acta Med Scand 199:455–460

39. Inoue K, Amulyan H, Mookherjee S, Eich RH (1971) Ultrasonic measurement of left ventricular wall motion in acute myocardial infarction. Circulation 43:778–785

40. Joyner CR, Reid JM, Bond JP (1963) Reflected ultrasound in the assessment of mitral valve disease. Circulation 27:506ff

41. Kanaka M, Teresawa Y, Konno K, Nitta K, Kashiwagi M, Watanabe S, Meguro T, Hikichi H, Takeda H, Ebina T, Okujima M, Ohtsuki S (1976) Measurement of intracardiac blood flow velocity distribution and flow pattern by the M-sequence modulated ultrasonic Doppler method. The Japan Society of Ultrasonics in Medicine. Proceedings of the 30th Meeting, 30:231–232

42. Kasai C, Namekawa K, Koyano A, Omoto R (1980) Real time two-dimensional blood flow imaging using an autocorrelation technique. IEEE Trans Sonics Ultrason Ultrason 32:400ff

43. Keidel WD (1950) Über eine Methode zur Registrierung der Volumenänderungen des Herzens am Menschen. Zeitschr f Kreislauf 39:257ff

44. Kimoto S, Omoto R, Tsunemoto M (1964) Ultrasonic tomography of the liver and detection of heart atrial septal defect with the aid of ultrasonic intravenous probes. Ultrasonics 2:82ff

45. King DL (1972) Cardiac ultrasonography. A stop-action technique for imaging intracardiac anatomy. Radiology 103:387–392

46. Lele PP, Namery J (1974) A Computer-based system for the detection and mapping of myocardial Infarcts. Proc. San Diego Biomed Symp 13:121–132

47. Masuyama T, Nellessen U, Schnittger I, Tye TL, Haskell WL, Popp RL (1989) Ultrasonic tissue characterization with a real-time integrated backscatter imaging system in normal and aging human hearts. J Am Coll Cardiol 14:1702–1708

48. Matsumoto M, Oka Y, Strom J, et al. (1980) Application of transesophageal echocardiography to continuous intraoperative monitoring of left ventricular performance. Am J Cardiol 46:95–105

49. Matsuo H, Inoue M, Kitabatake A, Hayashi T, Asao M, Terao Y, Mishima M, Senda S, Shimazu T, Tanouchi J, Morita H, Abe H, Cihara K, Hirayama M, Inokuchi S, Sakurai Y (1978) Analysis of Doppler flow signal by WINOGRAD Fourier transform algorithm-detection of intracardiac flow dynamics by computer-based ultrasonic multigated pulsed Doppler flowmeter. The Japan Society of Ultrasonics in Medicine, Proceedings of the 34th Meeting 34:3–4

50. Maurer G, Ghosh A, Nanda NC (1981) Volume determination and three-dimensional reconstruction of echocardiographic images using rotation method. Circulation 64:IV–206 (abstract)

51. Mazeika P, Nadazdin A, Oakley CM (1992) Dobutamine Stress Echocardiography for Detection and Assessment of Coronary Artery Disease. J Am Coll Cardiol 19:1203–1211

52. McDicken WN, Sutherland GR, Moran CM, Gordon LN (1992) Color Doppler velocity imaging of the myocardium. Ultrasound Med Biol 18:651–654

53. Miller GJ, Perret JE, Sobel BE (1985) Ultrasonic characterisation of myocardium. Prog Cardiovasc Dis 28:85–110

54. Mimbs JW, Yuhas DE, Miller JG, Weiss AN, Sobel BE (1977) Detection of myocardial infarction in vitro altered attenuation of ultrasound. Circ Res 41:192–194

55. Miyatake K, Yamagishi M, Tanaka N et al. (1993) A new method for evaluation of left ventricular wall motion by color-coded tissue Doppler echocardiography: in vitro and in vivo studies (abstract). Circulation 8:I–48

56. Moritz WE, Shreve PL (1974) A microprocessor-based spatial locating system for use with diagnostic ultrasound. Proc IEEE 64:966ff

57. Olson RM, Shelton DK (1972) A non-destructive technique to measure wall displacement in the thoracic aorta. J Appl Physiol 32:147–151

58. Omoto R, Kyo S, Matsumura M, Adachi H, Maruyama M, Matsunaka T (1990) New direction of biplane transesophageal echocardiography with special emphasis on real-time biplane imaging and matrix phased array biplane transducer. Echocardiography 7:691–698

59. Omoto R, Yokote Y, Takamoto S, Kyo S, Leda K, Asano H, Namekawa K, Kasai C, Kondo Y, Koyano A (1984) The development of real-time two-dimensional echocardiography and its clinical significance in acquired valvular diseases which special references to the evaluation of valvular regurgitation. Jap Heart J 25:325–340

60. Pandian N, Kreis A, Desnoyers M et al (1988) In vivo ultrasound angioscopy m humans and animals: Intraluminal imaging of blood vessels using a new catheter-based high resolution ultrasound probe (Abstract). Circulation 78:222ff

61. Peronneau P, Deloche A, Bui-Mong-Hung, Hinglas J (1969) Debitmetrie Ultrasonore: Dévelopments et applications expérimentales. Europ Surg Res 1:147–156

62. Picano E (1992) Stress echocardiography. Springer, Berlin–Heidelberg–New York–London–Paris–Tokyo–Hongkong–Barcelona–Budapest pp 1–215

63. Rienemann RS, Hoeks A, Slot HB, Merode T (1982) The on-line recording of velocity profiles and its potential in the diagnosis of peripheral arterial lesions. In: Diethrich EB, John Wright: Non-invasive assessment of the cardiovascular system. Psg Inc

64. Salomura S (1956) A Study on examining the heart wilh ultrasonics. I. Principles; II. Instrument Jpn Circ J 20:227ff

65. Segar DS, Brown SE, Sawada SG, Ryan T, Feigenbaum H (1992) Dobutamine Stress Echocardiography: Correlation With Coronary Lesion Severity as Determined by Quantitative Angiography. J Am Coll Cardiol 19:1197–1202

66. Side CD, Gosling RG (1971) Non-surgical assessment of cardiac function. Nature 232:335–36

67. Sokolov S (1929) Elektrische Nachrichtentechnik 6:451ff

68. Somer JC (1968) Electronic sector scanning for ultrasonic diagnosis. Ultrasonics 6:153–159

69. Souquet J, Hanrath P, Zitelli L, Kremer P, Langenstein BA, Schlüter M (1982) Transesophageal phased array for imaging the heart, IEEE. Tran Biomed Eng 29:707–712

70. Souquet J (1982) Phased array transducer technology for transesophageal imaging of the heart: current status and future aspects. In: Hanrath et al.: Cardiovascular diagnosis by ultrasound. London: Martinus Nijhoff 251–259

71. Stefan G, Bing RJ (1972) Echocardiographic findings in experimental myocardial infarction of the posterior left ventricular wall. Am J Cardiol 30:629–39

72. Steward MJ, Grundstrom WE, Sutherland GR et al. (1993) Myocardial imaging by colour coded velocity mapping – a new method for the assessment of myocardial contractility (abstract). Eur Heart J 14:467

73. Stevenson JG, Kawabori I, Guntheroth WG (1977) Differentiation of ventricular septal defect from mitral regurgitation by pulsed Doppler Echocardiography. Circulation 6:14ff

74. Tauchert M, Behrenbeck DW, Hölzl J, Hilger HH (1976) Ein neuer pharmakologischer Test zur Diagnose der Koronarinsuffizienz. Dtsch Med Wschr 101:35–43

75. Thomas LJ III, Barzilai B, Perez JE, Sobel BE, Vickline SA, Miller JG (1989) Quantitative real-time imaging of myocardium based on ultrasonic integrated backscatter. IEEE Trans Ultrason Ferroeletter Frequency Control 36:466–470

76. Thurstone FL, von Ramm OT (1974) A new ultrasound imaging technique employing two-dimensional electronic beam steering. In: Green PS Acoustical holography. Vol. 5. New York: Plenum Press 149–159

77. Tobis JM, Mallery J, Gessert J et al. (1989) Intravascular ultrasound cross-sectional arterial imaging before and after ballon angioplasty in vitro. Circulation 80:873ff

78. Vered Z, Barzilai B, Mohr GA et al. (1987) Quantitative ultrasonic tissue characterisation with real-time integrated backscatter imaging in normal human subjects and in patients with dilated cardiomyopathy. Circulation 76:1067–1073

79. Vickline SA, Sobel BE (1989) Ultrasonic tissue characterization: Prospects for Clincial Cardiology. JACC 14, 7:1709–1711

80. Wann LS, Faris JV, Childress RH, Dillon JC, Weyman AE, Feigenbaum H (1979) Exercise Cross-sectional Echocardiography in Ischemic Heart Disease. Circulation 60:1300–1308

81. Wells PNT (1977) Biomedical ultrasonics. London: Academic Press 282–353

82. Wild JJ, Crawford HD, Reid JM (1957) Visualisation of the excised human heart by means of reflected ultrasound or echography. Am Heart J 54:903ff

83. Wollschläger H, Zeiher AM, Klein HP, Kasper W, Wollschläger S, Just H (1989) Transesophageal echo computer tomography: a new method for dynamic 3-D imaging of the heart. JACC 13:68 A

84. Wollschläger H, Zeiher AM, Klein HP, Geibel A, Wollschläger S (1990) Transesophageal echo computer tomography (Echo-CT): a new method for perspective views of the beating heart. Circulation 82 (suppl. III):670

85. Yamazaki N, Mine Y, Sano A et al. (1994) Analyzis of ventricular wall motion using color coded tissue Doppler imaging system. Jpn J Appl Phys 33:3141–3146

86. Yock P, Linker D, Saether O et al. (1988) Intravascular two-dimensional catheter ultrasound. Initial clinical studies (Abstract). Circulation 78:2–21

Chapter 3   Principle of Doppler Tissue Velocity Measurements

N. Yamazaki

Principle of the Tissue Doppler Method

Doppler signals from ventricular wall motion differ from signals of blood flow (moving red blood cells) in two major respects.

First, ventricular wall motion velocity is approximately 10 cm/s or less, which is significantly lower than blood-flow velocity in the ventricular cavity (approximately 10 to 100 cm/s).

Second, the amplitude of the Doppler signal from ventricular wall motion is significantly higher (approximately 40 dB higher, or 100 times greater) than that of the blood-flow signal.

In conventional color Doppler systems, Doppler signals from the cardiac walls or from valve motion are eliminated using a high-pass filter in order to obtain the blood-flow signal only (Fig. 3.1).

The tissue Doppler method, on the other hand, provides ventricular wall motion velocity based on the same color Doppler method. As shown in Fig. 3.2, in the tissue Doppler method, low-amplitude blood-flow signals are eliminated by gain adjustment to permit only high-amplitude Doppler signals from wall motion to enter the velocity calculation circuit.

System Operating Principles and Features

A tissue Doppler imaging system analyzes the Doppler signal from tissue motion using the autocorrelation method, superimposes tissue motion velocity on a two-dimensional echocardiogram in color, and permits both tissue morphology and motion to be evaluated in real-time images and static images. The autocorrelation method employed in such systems is the same type of frequency analysis (called the color Doppler method) used in blood-flow imaging systems, and has already established itself in a wide range of clini-

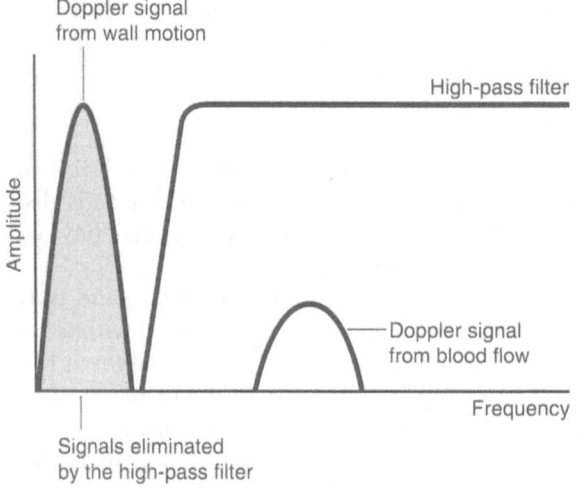

Fig. 3.1. Extracting the Doppler signal originating from blood-flow

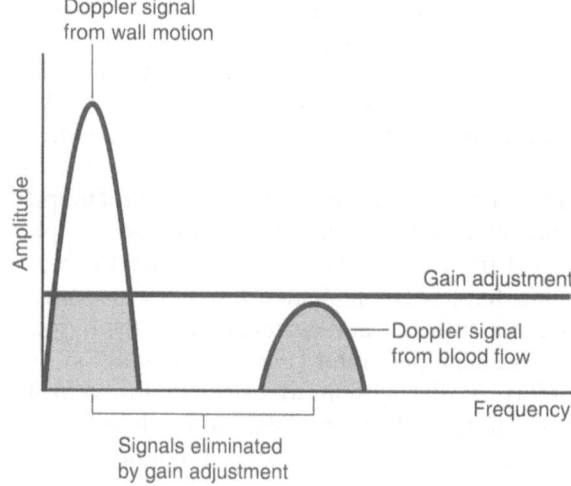

Fig. 3.2. Extracting the Doppler signal from wall motion

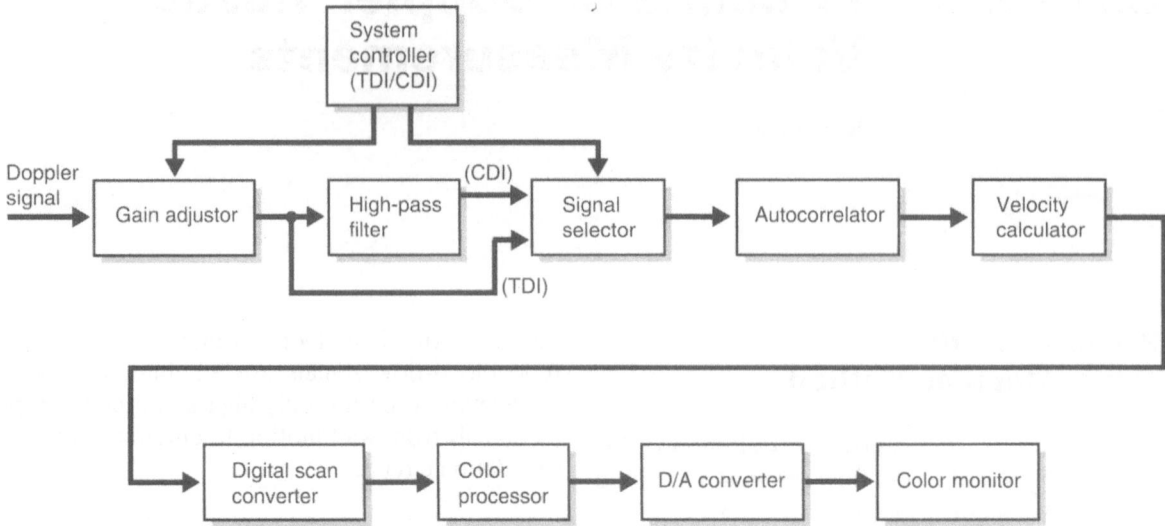

Fig. 3.3. Block diagram of a tissue Doppler imaging system. (*CDI* = color Doppler imaging, *TDI* = tissue Doppler imaging, *D/A* = Digital/Analog)

cal applications. In other words, the tissue Doppler method is basically an extension of the conventional color Doppler method.

The operating principles and features of a tissue Doppler imaging system are described below, focusing on the differences from conventional blood-flow imaging systems.

Analyzing the Doppler Signal Originating from Tissue Motion

Figure 3.3 shows a block diagram of a system incorporating a conventional blood-flow imaging system plus tissue Doppler imaging functions.

In blood-flow imaging, it is necessary to eliminate the Doppler signals originating from the cardiac walls or from valve motion using a high-pass filter in order to extract only the blood-flow signals for frequency analysis (Fig. 3.1). In a tissue Doppler imaging system, on the other hand, the Doppler signal from which the blood-flow signal components have been eliminated through gain control are put into the autocorrelator directly, bypassing the high-pass filter (Fig. 3.2). In addition, the ability of the system to calculate low-velocity flows in the velocity calculation unit is enhanced in order to measure cardiac wall motion velocity, which is significantly lower than blood-flow velocity of the heart.

Color Display Format for Enhancement of Low Velocities

In color blood-flow imaging employing the color Doppler method, the Doppler signals reflected from red blood cells are used to calculate the direction and mean velocity of blood flow, which are then displayed as variations in brightness and hue. In this technique, the maximum color brightness corresponds to the upper limit of the measurable velocity range, or the maximum value (fd_{max}) of the Doppler shift frequency (fd). In the color Doppler method, the ultrasound pulse repetition frequency (fr) is the sampling frequency. Therefore, fd_{max} is expressed as follows from the sampling theorem.

$$fd_{max} = fr/2$$

In blood-flow imaging, the range from $-fr/2$ to $+fr/2$ or the Doppler shift frequency (fd) is displayed in color. For blood flow velocities beyond this range, aliasing occurs.

In tissue Doppler imaging, on the other hand, only low-velocity components are displayed with a full scale of color brightness and hue, as shown in Fig. 3.4, by enhancing the ability of the velocity calculation unit to measure low-velocity flows.

In the examples shown in this figure, fd is displayed with a full scale in the range (1) $-fr/8$ to $+fr/8$ or (2) $-fr/16$ to $+fr/16$. In these examples, the low-velocity calculation and display precisions are enhanced by (1) 4 times and (2) 8 times,

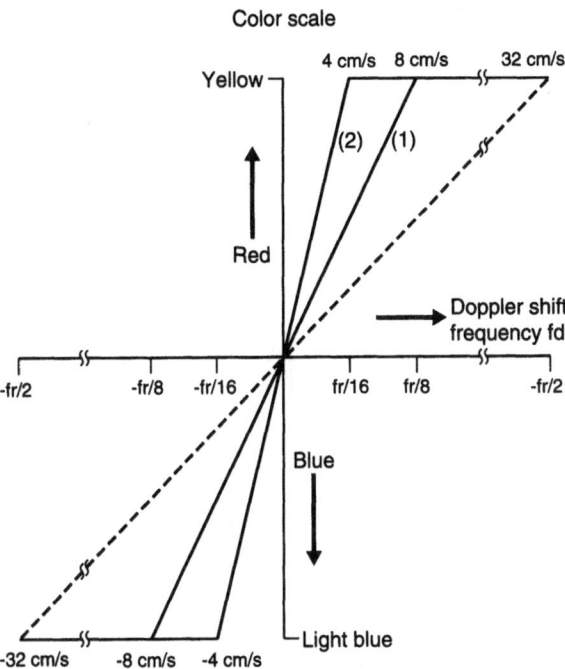

Fig. 3.4. Enhancing low-velocity components

greater than 32 cm/s, aliasing occurs (displayed in blue). When the velocity is less than -32 cm/s, on the other hand, velocity is displayed in red. Because ventricular wall motion velocity is about 10 cm/s or less, it is not likely that aliasing will occur under these conditions.

Tissue Doppler Echocardiography

In tissue Doppler imaging it is possible to detect ultralow velocities using super-high-speed scanning, making it easier to detect changes in systolic and diastolic velocity during the cardiac cycle and to assess asynchrony of the ventricular wall.

This technique differs from the basic concept of blood-flow imaging, i.e., "the frame rate must be sacrificed in order to increase low-velocity detection capabilities". Refer to "Basic Principles of the Color Doppler Method" below for an explanation of how the low-velocity detection capability can be enhanced while maintaining a high frame rate.

Basic Principles of the Color Doppler Method

(1) Changes in Echoes from Moving Objects over Time

As shown in Fig. 3.5, it is assumed that a reflective object is moving at an angle θ relative to the beam and with a velocity V.

In the pulsed Doppler method, ultrasound pulses are repeatedly transmitted to and received from one position to obtain measurements. However, if the reflective object is moving, as in this figure, the position of the received echo changes slightly for each pulse repetition. That is, in time T, the distance between the transducer and the reflective object changes by $VT \cos\theta$ and the echo changes by the ultrasound return time $2VT \cos\theta/c$ corresponding to $VT \cos\theta$.

In fact, ultrasound echoes are returned as a complex waveform because interference occurs due to the presence or multiple reflective objects along the pathway of the beam. In this situation, it is difficult to detect velocity as motion of the envelope of the echoes. For this reason, a method is often used in which velocity is detected as the phase shift of the echo or the position of the wave in the envelope. In this method, changes in echoes over time are viewed at a fixed position and the frequency of this signal corresponds to the Doppler shift frequency.

respectively, compared with blood-flow imaging using the same pulse repetition frequency (fr).

In display method (1) (Fig. 3.4), for example, fd is displayed with the maximum gradation of blue in the range $-\text{fr}/2 \leqq \text{fd} \leqq -\text{fr}/8$, while fd is displayed with the maximum gradation of red in the range $+\text{fr}/8 \leqq \text{fd} \leqq +\text{fr}/2$. In tissue Doppler imaging aliasing occurs as well (red and blue are displayed in reverse) when $\text{fd} \leqq -\text{fr}/2$ or $\text{fd} \geqq +\text{fr}/2$ only.

A concrete example follows.

Assume that the upper limit of measurable velocity is 32 cm/s based on the sampling theorem. Following this assumption, the range from -8 to $+8$ cm/s is displayed with differences in brightness and hue if the display method shown in Fig. 3.4-(1) is employed; velocities in the range from -32 to -8 cm/s are displayed with the maximum gradation of blue and velocities in the range from $+8$ to $+32$ cm/s are displayed with the maximum gradation of red. In the same manner, the range from -4 to $+4$ cm/s is displayed with differences in brightness and hue if the display in Fig. 3.4-(2) is selected; velocities in the range from -32 to -4 cm/s are displayed with the maximum gradation of blue and velocities in the range from $+4$ to $+32$ cm/s are displayed with the maximum gradation of red. In either case, when the velocity is

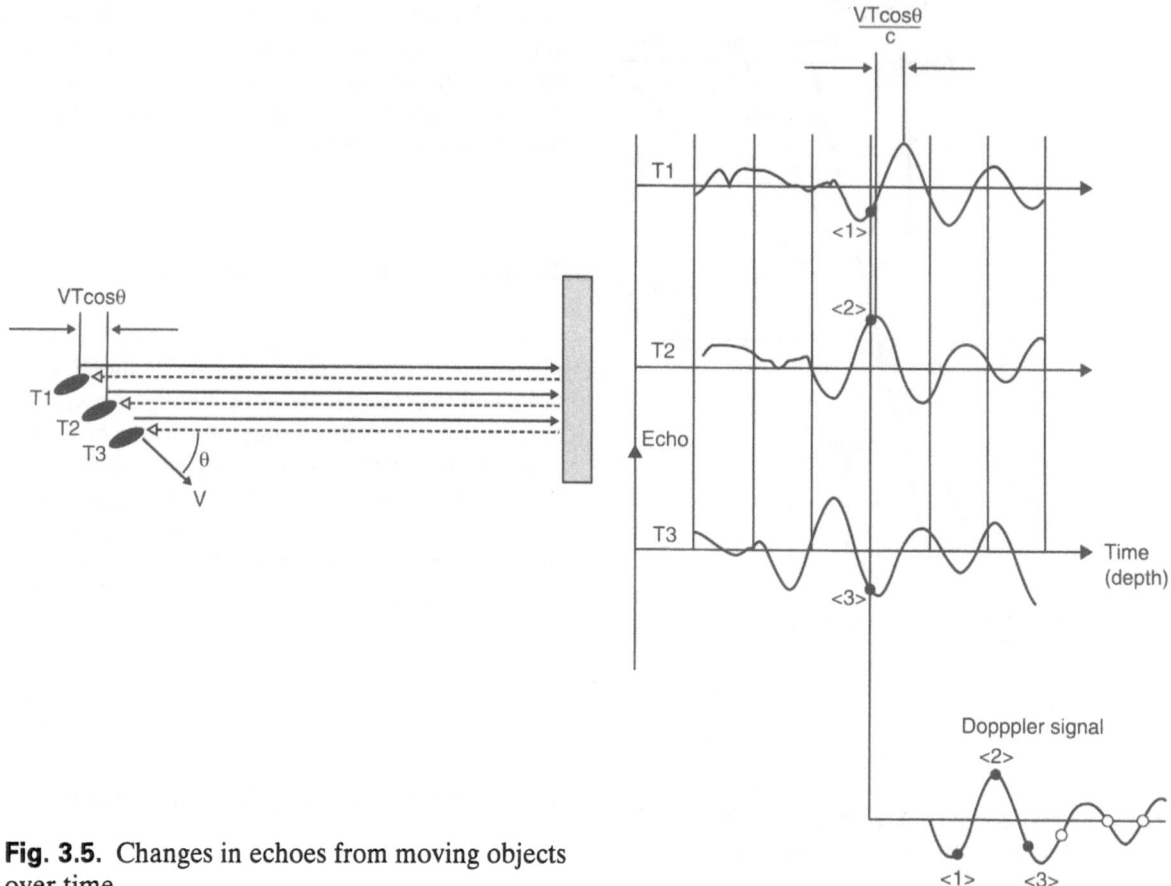

Fig. 3.5. Changes in echoes from moving objects over time

(2) Frequency Analysis

While various methods are available for frequency analysis, the tissue Doppler technique uses the autocorrelation function method, which is widely employed in the color Doppler tomographic technique.

The first-order autocorrelation function represents the correlation with the signal shifted by one sample over time. For an echo waveform representing changes in echoes at a certain position, the signal shifted by one sample is determined from the waveform and motion velocity of the echo if the echo is moving. The echo waveform has a complicated shape, called a "speckle pattern," with small changes in frequency. For this reason, the phase shift is close to the frequency of the transmitted pulse. Therefore, the phase shift after one-sample shift corresponds to motion. This phase shift can be obtained from the phase of the autocorrelation function or from the argument of the complex number (Fig. 3.6).

It should be noted that, in principle, the velocity of a moving object can be obtained through trans-

mission/reception twice if the autocorrelation method is used. The high-pass filter plays a very important role in blood-flow imaging. In order to explain the reason it is necessary to increase the number of ultrasound pulses transmitted/received in the same direction to obtain precise low-velocity measurements in blood-flow imaging.

(3) Method by which Blood Flow is Discriminated from Tissues

Normally, echoes from blood in the cardiac chambers or great vessels are not visible in ultrasound tomographic images. This is because intense echoes, such as comet tails, which occur at the rear of side lobes, from surrounding tissues or strongly reflective objects mask echoes from red blood cells. Extraneous signals from tissues are called "clutter" and must be eliminated in order to extract blood-flow information.

For this purpose, a multichannel low-cut filter that functions at two or more locations simultaneously called the MTI filter (an abbreviation of termi-

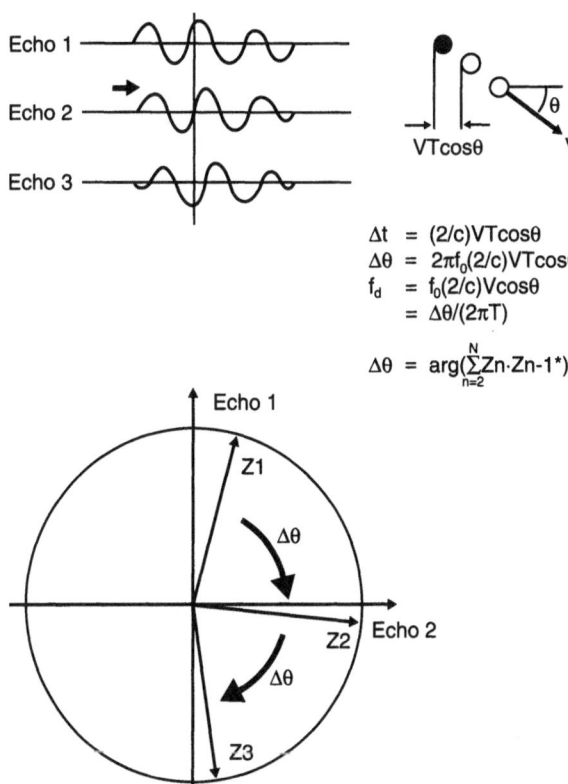

$$\Delta t = (2/c)VT\cos\theta$$
$$\Delta\theta = 2\pi f_0 (2/c)VT\cos\theta$$
$$f_d = f_0(2/c)V\cos\theta$$
$$= \Delta\theta/(2\pi T)$$

$$\Delta\theta = \arg\left(\sum_{n=2}^{N} Z_n \cdot Z_{n-1}^*\right)$$

Fig. 3.6. Frequency analysis

nology borrowed from radar technology, Moving Target Indicator) or a high-pass filter is used. This filter function eliminates slow-moving objects (objects with low Doppler shift frequencies) based on the fact that extraneous clutter signals from tissues have a high amplitude but slow movement. Figure 3.7 shows the operation of a high-pass filter consisting of digital filters.

An example of the simplest configuration for a high-pass filter is the method by which the mean value of two or more adjacent input data items, or the moving average value, is calculated as the output data are obtained by subtracting the mean value from the input data. A method for extracting only blood-flow signals from Doppler signals containing both blood-flow signals of higher frequency and clutter signals of lower frequency is considered, as shown in the figure. In this method, the number of data items used to calculate the moving average is closely related to the cut-off frequency of the filter.

When the number of data items used to calculate the moving average is set appropriately, as shown in Fig. 3.7-(2), it is possible to eliminate only

clutter signal components to extract blood-flow signals only.

However, if the number of data used to calculate the moving average is small, as shown in Fig. 3.7-(1), the cut-off frequency of the filter becomes high, eliminating blood-flow signals as well as clutter signals. On the other hand, if the number of measured items is increased, the cut-off frequency can be decreased further. However, the clutter signal cannot be eliminated completely if the cut-off frequency is too low, as shown in Fig. 3.7-(3).

With regard to the high-pass filters employed in clinically available color Doppler systems, adjacent input data items are assigned specific weighting coefficients before they are added, rather than simply calculating the average movement of the input data items. For the number of added data items (corresponding to the type of the digital filter), the weighting coefficients are changed under conditions fixed to a certain degree to vary the cut-off frequency.

As shown in this figure, however, a large number of data items is theoretically required to completely eliminate clutter signals while maintaining blood-flow signals when the cut-off frequency of the high-pass filter is reduced.

In color Doppler systems, the number of data items is closely related to the number of transmissions/receptions of ultrasound pulses in one direction (packet size or dwell time). This fact is easily understood if it is remembered that only one input data item can be obtained by one ultrasound transmission/reception because the pulsed Doppler method traces changes in echoes at a fixed position over time.

(4) Blood-Flow Imaging vs. Tissue Doppler Imaging

The preceding discussion is summarized below:

First, the autocorrelation method permits the velocity of a moving object to be calculated from signals of two transmissions/receptions in principle. In blood-flow imaging, on the other hand, it is necessary to eliminate clutter signals in advance to obtain blood-flow velocities. To do this, a high-pass filter is required. However, a large number of data is needed to eliminate clutter signals completely while maintaining blood-flow signals when the cut-off frequency of the high-pass filter is reduced. To increase the number of items, it is necessary to increase the number of ultrasound pulses transmitted/received in one direction (Fig. 3.8-1).

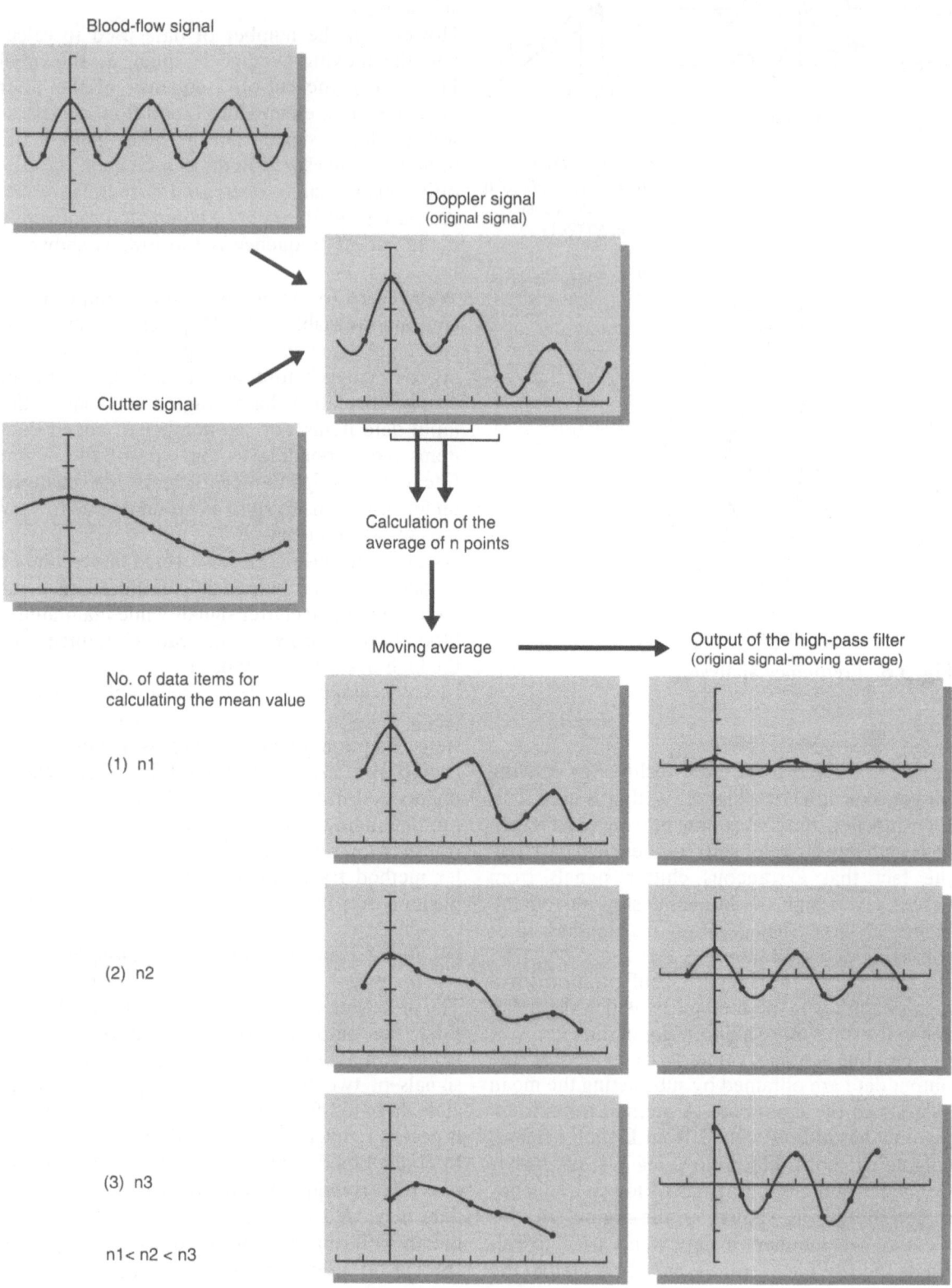

Fig. 3.7. Operation of the high-pass filter

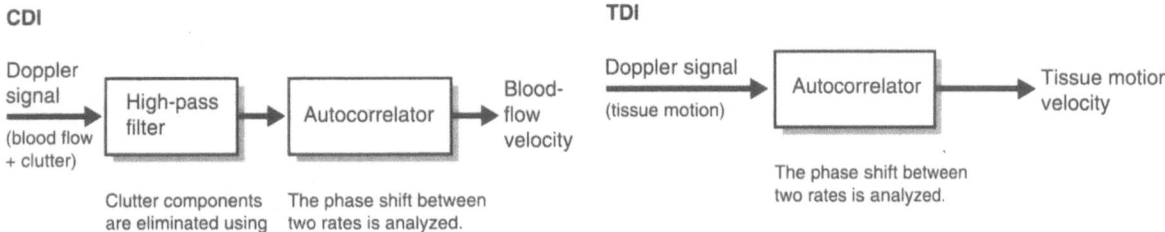

CDI

Doppler signal
(blood flow + clutter)

High-pass filter → Autocorrelator →

Blood-flow velocity

Clutter components are eliminated using continuous data of multiple rates.

The phase shift between two rates is analyzed.

Fig. 3.8-1. Blood-flow imaging (CDI)

TDI

Doppler signal
(tissue motion) → Autocorrelator →

Tissue motion velocity

The phase shift between two rates is analyzed.

Fig. 3.8-2. Tissue Doppler imaging (TDI)

Conclusion

Applying this principle to tissue Doppler imaging, the high-pass filter is eliminated and the Doppler signal directly enters the autocorrelator in order to obtain the mean frequency treated as the clutter signal in blood-flow imaging.

Therefore, the number of transmissions/receptions is determined by the number of data items required for the autocorrelation calculation; a minimum of two transmissions/receptions is sufficient (Fig. 3.8-2).

Thus, the low-velocity detection capability is not adversely affected when scanning with a high-frame rate is performed by reducing the number of transmissions/receptions in the tissue Doppler method.

Chapter 4 Image Processing

H. U. Stöcker

Introduction

The ultrasound technique has become an integral element in cardiac diagnostics.

Ultrasound application in medicine and cardiology started in the 1940s. The M-Mode technique has been applied by Edler and Hertz for motion analysis of the mitral valve 1954. In the seventies it was possible to improve the diagnostic value of cardiac ultrasound essentially by introducing the B-mode technique. The development of various Doppler techniques was undertaken in parallel. By combining both methods in the 1980s assessment of blood flow information became possible under 2D image control.

After introduction of two-dimensional Color-Doppler in the mid-1980s, progress in ultrasound technology came to a relative standstill. Quality of ultrasound devices was improved. By introduction of computer technology the assessment of myocardial wall thickening and contraction was enhanced, but quantification of myocardial wall motion abnormalities still was unsatisfactory.

Tissue Doppler Echocardiography – TDE – is a new method, which for the first time allows quantification of motion abnormalities.

In order to understand the basics of TDE better and to interpret TDE-images it is necessary to focus on some basics of ultrasound theory and parameters influencing image acquisition.

Basics: Differences between TDE Images and Conventional Ultrasound Images

The conventional ultrasound structure image is amplitude coded. Each displayed grey level represents a certain amplitude range. High amplitudes cause high grey level intensities, and low amplitudes cause low grey level intensities.

The frequency shift phenomenon (Doppler-Phenomenon) which regularly occurs in ultrasound echoes from moving structures has not yet been taken into account in ultrasound processing. TDE analyses both parameters, echo amplitude and frequency shift, i.e. the TDE image is a two-dimensional Doppler image. Its quality is dependent on the echo amplitude, the calculated frequency shift and its amplitude.

By combination of both parameters in M-mode and B-mode images two diagnostically relevant advantages result:
- In conventional amplitude images it is difficult to filter echoes caused by gas/air satisfactorily due to structure-equivalent amplitudes, however these echoes lack the shift component. Hence analysis of amplitude- and shift-component provides tissue information.
- With aid of the colour-coded tissue Doppler imaging method it is easier to assess wall motion abnormalities. The quantification of wall motion is improved.

A great amount of physical and technical parameters and individual examination circumstances make a variety of variable machine settings necessary, in order to optimize image quality and visualization of velocity changes.

Frame Rate in 2DE

Frame rate in 2DE is primarily dependent on the average sound velocity in tissue (1540 ms^{-1}), sound penetration depth and the amount of ultrasound beams. The conventional 90° sector image is composed of 120 beams.

Correlation of these parameters is given by:

Penetration depth:	20 cm
Average sound velocity:	$1540\ ms^{-1}$
Beams:	120

Frame rate $= 1540$ ms^{-1} / $2 \cdot 0.2$ m $\cdot$ 120 $= 32.08$ frames sec^{-1}

The frame rate achieved is sufficient for conventional 2D real-time image display.

When performing TDE examinations in order to qualify and quantify wall motion it is necessary to take the frame rate into account, illustrated by the following example:

Sector angle:	90°
Diff. between lateral wall and sector:	45°
Diff. between septum and sector:	45°
Penetration depth:	20 cm

Difference between t1 and t4 ≈ 0.031 s
Difference between t2 and t3 ≈ 0.016 s

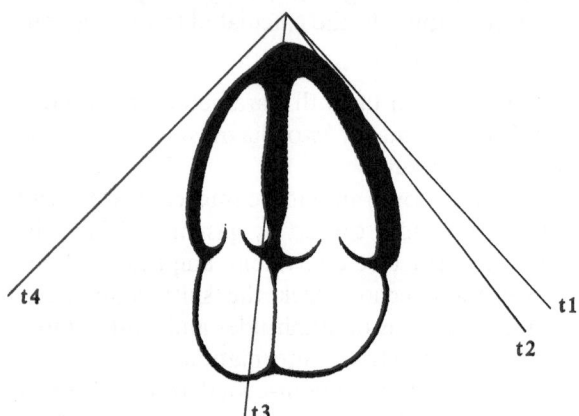

Fig. 4.1. Scheme of four chamber view

Assuming a heart rate of 90 beats per minute, a time delay of 0.023 s between t1 and t2 occurs in relation to the ECG.

Only by applying new scan techniques, for instance *High-Speed Echocardiography*, where one echo pulse is being processed twice or four times simultaneously by parallel or quad processing technology, it is possible to generate 45° sector images with 20 cm penetration depth at a rate of 158 frames per second.

Echo Amplitude

The reflected echo amplitude mainly depends upon the following factors, which are considerably important for TDE image interpretation:

– Reflection
– Absorption
– Frequency
– Scan field geometry
– Scattering
– Acoustic pressure level
– Amplification

Reflection

The influence of myocardial fiber orientation can provoke drop-out effects resulting from low reflection amplitude. Especially in short axis view reflection amplitude of tissue areas can be below the noise filter threshold.

Absorption

Sound absorption is dependent on penetration depth and correlates exponentially. Time gain dependent amplification is applied in order to compensate this effect.

Frequency

Ultrasound frequency is a proportional determinant of the absorption coefficient. In consequence the reflected echo amplitude correlates directly to the beam frequency, lower frequencies generate higher reflection amplitudes.
Resolution is inversely proportional to beam-frequency. Therefore penetration depth, applied frequency, and resolution need to be compromised.

Scan Field Geometry

Scan field geometry can be changed by adjusting the position of the beam focus, where echo amplitude is highest. Position and amount of the beam-focus points is adjustable and must be adapted to examination measures.

Scattering

Scatter is responsible for non-directional echoes which cause image artefacts. By filtering and optimizing image correlation scattering is minimized.

Acoustic Pressure Level

Increasing the acoustic pressure level results in higher echo amplitudes. High acoustic pressure level can cause biological side-effects. In diagnostic ultrasound the level of acoustic pressure applied is controlled by the FDA and other national and international (IEC) regulations, which limit the emitted acoustic pressure for safety reasons. By these means negative effects caused by diagnostic ultrasound devices are avoided.

Amplification

Depending on the individual influence of tissue absorption and reflection, it is necessary to visually optimize the received images by gain and time-gain compensation adjustments.

Doppler Shift

Tissue Doppler imaging is dependent on the same physical laws as pulsed-wave Doppler and continuous-wave Doppler.

Doppler shift is dependent on:
- Probe frequency
- Pulse repetition frequency
- Angle between ultrasound beam direction and motion vector

Especially angle dependency makes it necessary to switch between various probe positions in order to determine true tissue-velocities. Probe frequency is dependent on necessary image display depth. In addition, pulse repetition frequency is correlated to the maximum possible frame-rate achievable.

TDE Velocity Maps

In order to observe wall motion abnormalities and to quantify velocities, several velocity maps are provided by the TDE system. Depending on the diagnostic question, these maps offer improved recognition and imaging.

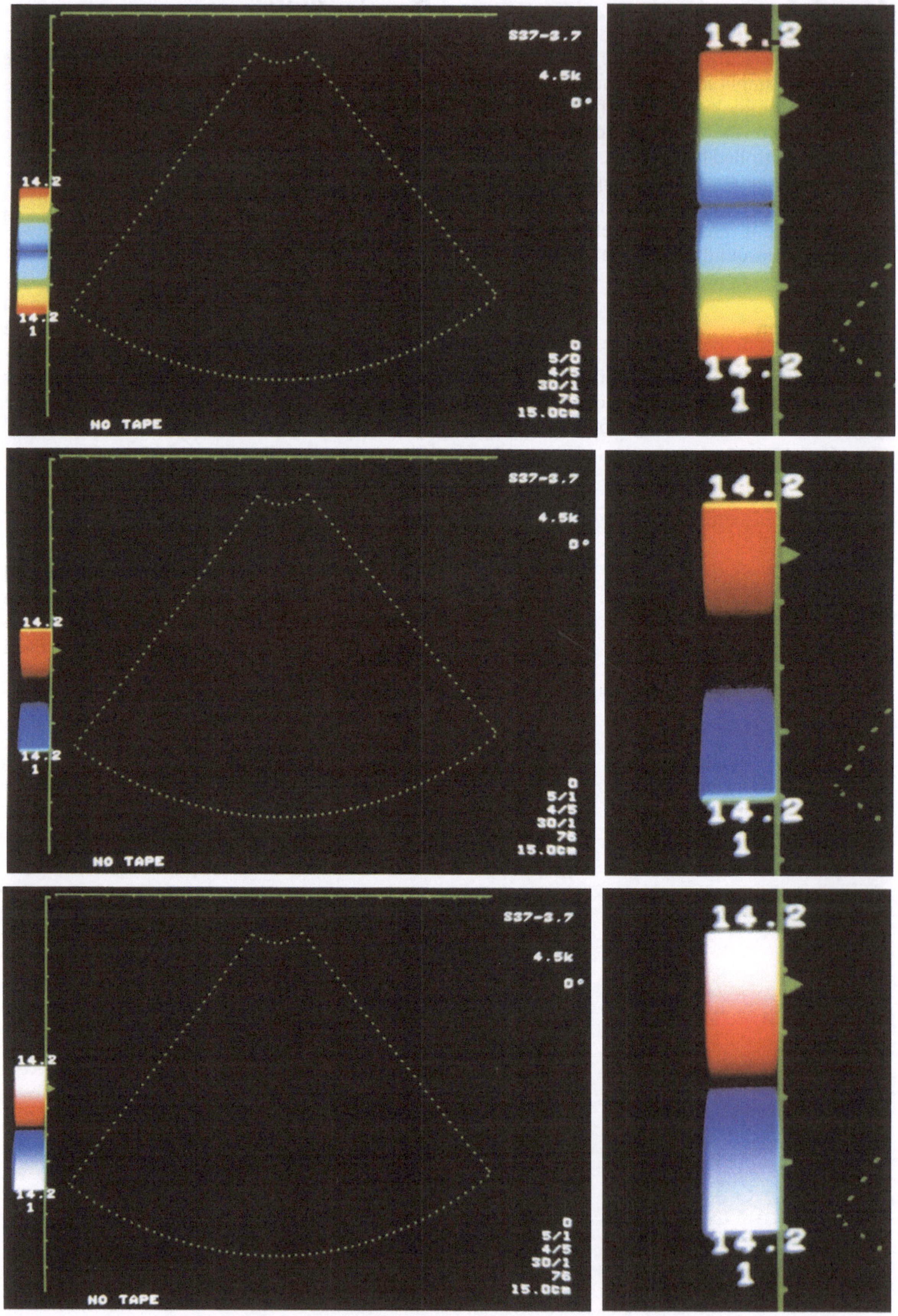

Fig. 4.2. TDE velocity maps

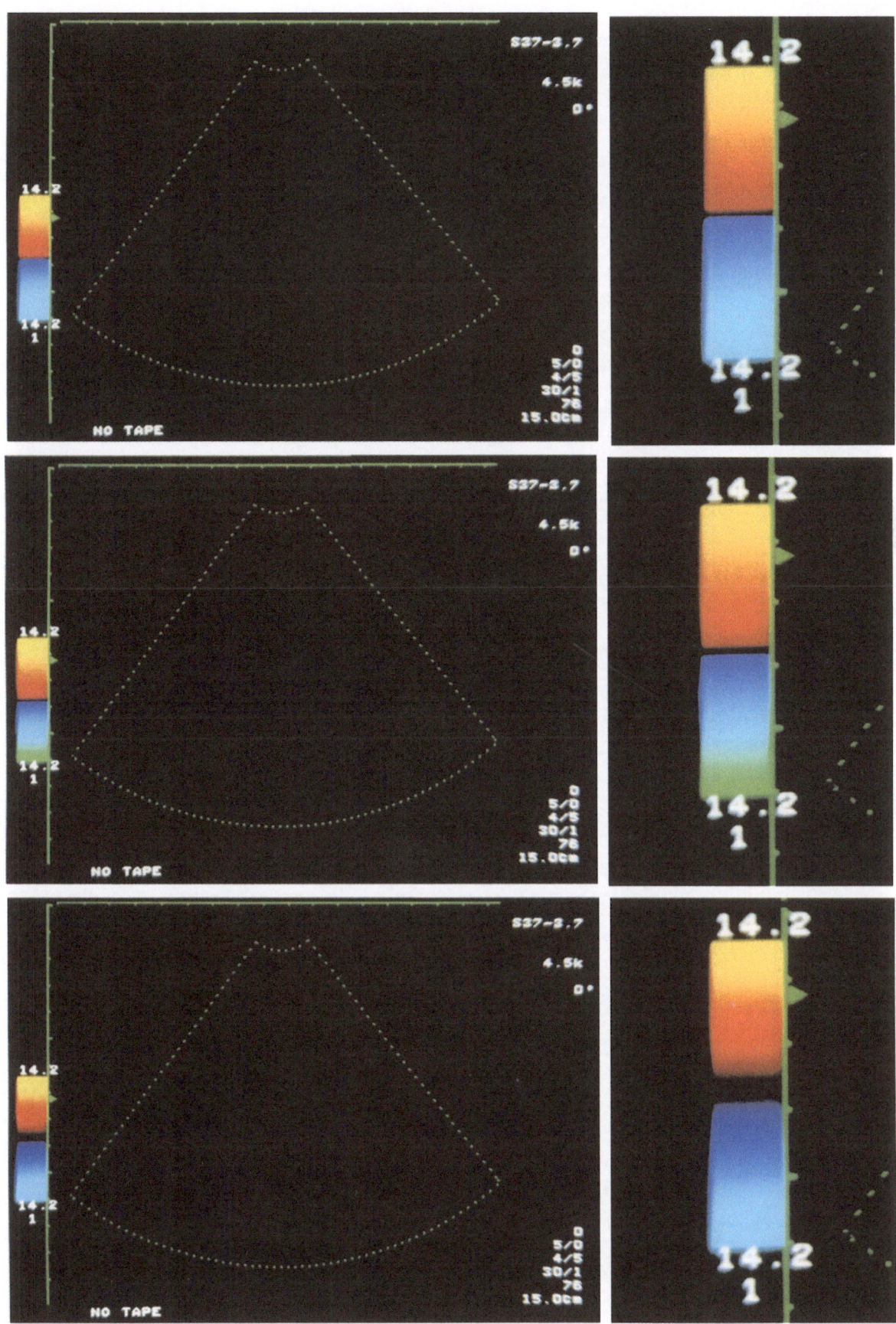

Fig. 4.2. TDE velocity maps

Chapter 5 Normal Pattern of Myocardial Velocity

J. Drozdz, R. Erbel, D. Wallbridge

Understanding of the normal pattern of myocardial wall velocities is necessary for comprehensive assessment of tissue Doppler echocardiography (TDE) [2, 3, 8, 16]. TDE examination should include imaging in multiple planes using slow-motion and frame-by-frame visualization. Due to rapid velocity changes slow-motion and frame-by-frame analysis are necessary to estimate the direction and speed of wall motion [3, 8, 16, 22]. The M-mode technique superimposed by color-coded tissue Doppler information is important in order to understand TDE. This section describes the wall velocity pattern observed in the normal heart.

TDE Examination

In two-dimensional TDE mode the same parts of the heart quickly change their color during the cardiac cycle. The reason for this is that the velocity pattern of myocardial walls are very complex. The color-coding is not simply divided into two phases of opposite velocity directions during systole and diastole. The total physiologic aspects of cardiac contraction and relaxation are reflected and superimposed by the motion of the whole heart. Not only wall motion, but also wall thickening has to be taken into account.

TDE Color-Coding

Depending on the orientation of the cardiac structures in relation to the ultrasonic beam, the velocity signals will appear either as red or blue [10, 18, 22]. The red color signifies that the cardiac tissue moves towards the transducer, and the blue color means that it moves away from the transducer. Different color-coding scales reflect different velocities: yellow reflects high velocities, red indicates low velocities toward the transducer, green and blue the opposite direction. In general, the low velocities are coded with dark colors, and the high velocities with bright colors. In every frame the actual velocity scale is presented on the left side of the image.

The intensity of color-coding changes during the cardiac cycle. The velocity signal depends on the amplitude of reflected echoes. Cyclic changes of amplitude of the reflected echoes from the same part of the cardiac wall [11] are well known from ultrasonic tissue characterization studies. In tissue Doppler examination the phenomenon seems not to play an important role. The intensity seems to be related to myocardial fibre direction, image quality and the position of the transducer [2, 12, 17].

Aliasing Effect

During TDE examination of the myocardial wall the aliasing effect cannot be seen, due to appropriate modifications of the machine. In conventional color Doppler systems the color display range is set between $\pm PRF/2$, where PRF is the ultrasound pulse repetition frequency. PRF/2 corresponds also to the measurable maximum deviation frequency [21]. The blood flow velocities above this limit are visualized with the aliasing effect.

In the tissue Doppler technique the improvement of low-velocity detection allows to enhance low velocities in the color display image [22]. The color display range is set between $\pm PRF/8$ or $\pm PRF/16$. Under normal circumstances the left ventricular wall velocity range is selected between 0 and 15 cm/s, and thus an aliasing effect is not observed. The only cardiac structures producing high-velocity tissue Doppler signals in the TDE image are the cardiac valves producing an aliasing effect.

TDE Velocity Measurement

TDE provides a velocity map of the cardiac structures and additionally the velocity values. By positioning a sample-volume, 3 by 3 pixel, on the two-dimensional TDE image, the velocity value of the region-of-interest (ROI) is displayed on the screen. The velocity values of multiple ROIs can be measured for all frames stored in the cine-loop.

Myocardial Velocity Pattern

Measurement of wall velocities in all frames covering one heart cycle by placing a ROI in the same part of the myocardium allows to construct a velocity profile. The frame number which can be used is dependent on the heart rate. The pattern of left ventricular wall velocities in a representative healthy subject is given in Fig. 5.1 (parasternal long-axis view), and in Fig. 5.2 (apical two-chamber view) for segments 1 and 9 as well as 6, 7 and 8 according to the ASE guidelines.

Wall Motion Analysis

Left ventricular shape changes have been assessed using radiopaque markers implanted into the myocardial wall in animals [7], and in man during cardiac surgery or heart transplantation [9]. The markers were visualized by fluoroscopy. Several models for regional left ventricular wall motion analysis were used. The left ventricular wall motion is assessed routinely and invasively by contrast ventriculography [1].

Noninvasive methods for left ventricular wall motion analysis include two-dimensional echocardiography with off-line epicardial and endocardial boundary delineation [5, 6, 13], acoustic quantification (AQ) for on-line wall motion analysis [14], radionuclide ventriculography, and nuclear magnetic resonance imaging using the myocardial tagging technique [19].

During systole the basal and mid segments of the left ventricle move inward toward the apex [9]. The apical segments move inward, but show hardly any movement toward the basis of the left ventricle [1]. A center of gravity of the left ventricle can be determined. The location of this center has been studied by Ingels et al. [9]. According to their findings, this center is located between the second and third part of the long axis (69% of the distance from the base to the apex) (Figs. 5.3, 5.4). This point represents the best mathematical approximation of the intersection of the left vetricular excursion lines. All ventricular segments in systole are moving toward this point with different angles and excursions. The most extensive movements are found at the base of the heart and there is hardly any movement near the apex. The work of Ingels et al. [9] is a key reference for the understanding of left ventricular TDE images.

Left Ventricular Wall Motion in TDE

Left ventricular wall velocity directions detected by TDE are consistent with the results of both invasive and noninvasive studies, but the information is visualized on-line in multiple views and planes.

In TDE the velocity pattern of the moving cardiac tissue are strongly dependent on the imaging plane. In the parasternal long axis view of the left ventricle (Figs. 5.5 and 5.6), the posterior wall moves toward the transducer during systole and is coded red, whereas the interventricular septum moves away from the transducer and is coded blue. The reason for this is that the external reference system, the transducer, is located precordially in the parasternal view.

In the apical views left ventricular basal and mid segments are moving in the same direction during systole, toward the transducer, and both are coded red. The apex in the apical view is moving away from the transducer and appears blue during systole.

Transmural Myocardial Velocity

M-mode and 2-D TDE examination demonstrates that different layers of the left ventricular wall have different velocities [15, 16, 20]. In other words, the transmural distribution of velocities is nonhomogeneous. The velocities of the subendocardial layers are higher than those of the subepicardial layers (Fig. 5.7). A transmural gradient can be calculated in systole and diastole. This is a result of differences in wall thickening during systole. The different velocities of the myocardial

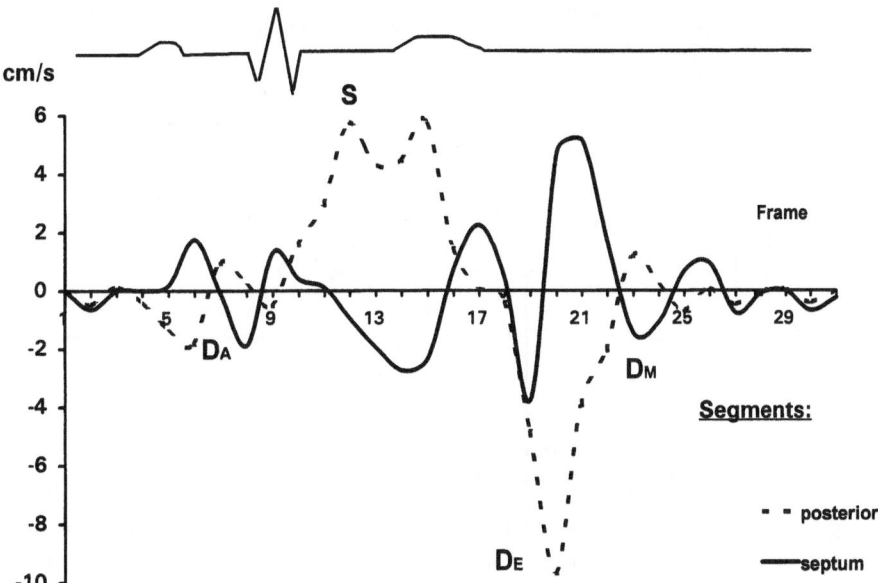

Fig. 5.1. Interventricular septum and posterior wall (segments 1, 9) velocities in subsequent frames from the parasternal view in a representative healthy subject. (S=peak systolic velocity, D_E=peak early-diastolic velocity, D_M=peak mid-diastolic velocity, D_A=peak late-diastolic velocity)

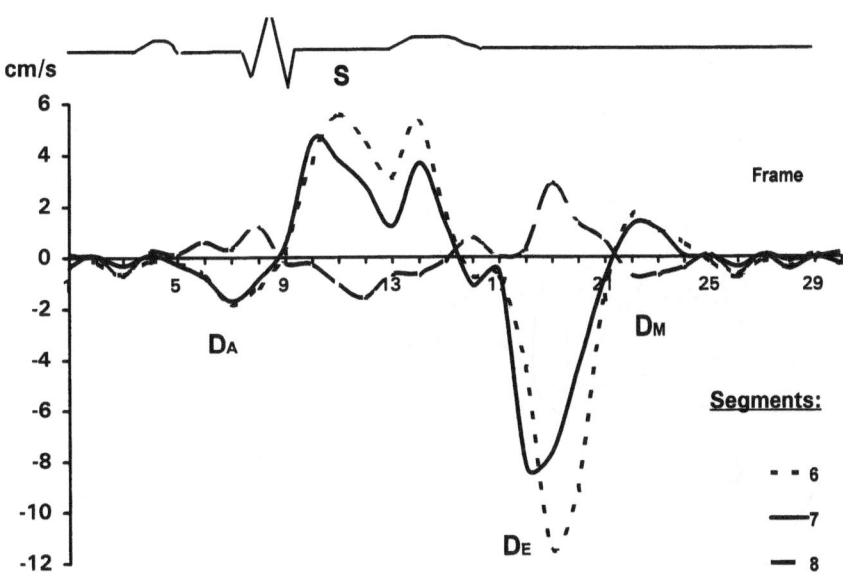

Fig. 5.2. Left ventricular posterior wall (segments 6-basal 7-mid, and 8-apical) velocities in subsequent frames from the apical two-chamber view in a representative healthy subject. (S=peak systolic velocity, D_E= peak early-diastolic velocity, D_M=peak mid-diastolic velocity, D_A=peak late-diastolic velocity)

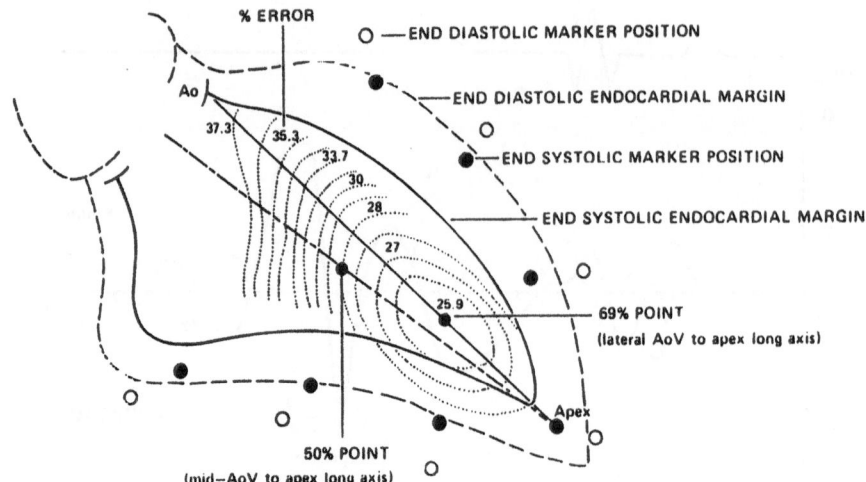

Fig. 5.3. Schematic diagram of the left ventricle in the 30° right anterior oblique projection. End-diastolic and end-systolic positions of intramyocardial markers and endocardium are shown. A point 69% of the distance along the line from the anterolateral aortic valve edge to the apex at end-systole was shown previously to be the optimum position for the polar origin of a fixed external reference system with the minimum of percent error. The choice of a fixed external reference system with polar origin at the 50% point, shown on the line from midaortic valve (AoV) to apex, would result in an increase in error of only 2.1% (see text). (From [9], with permission)

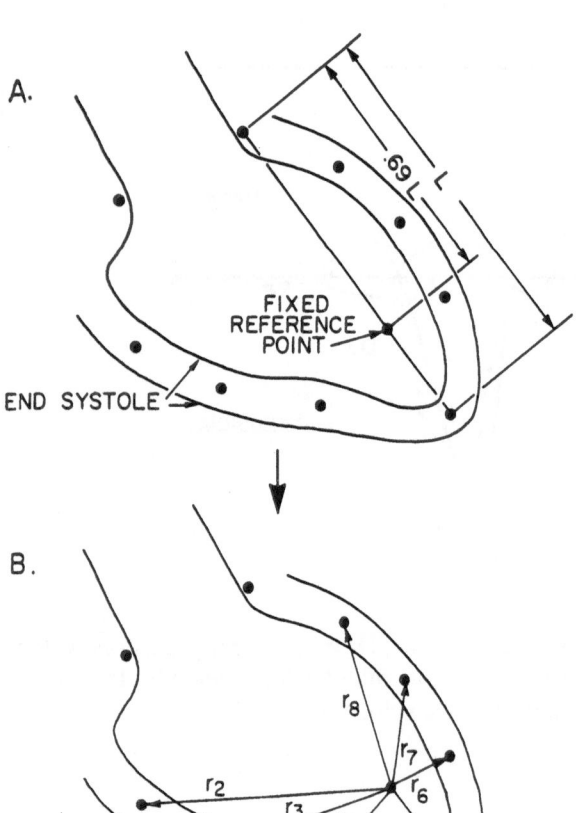

Fig. 5.4 A, B. Summary of method 5. **A** Location of polar axis at a point 69% of the distance along a line from the anterolateral aortic valve edge to the apex in the end-systolic frame. **B** Radii from this fixed reference point used to quantitate left ventricular segmental wall motion of all frames for the same beat. (From [9], with permission)

layers have previously been reported using implanted subendocardial and subepicardial markers [7]. In the parasternal view different velocity directions across the interventricular septum are seen. At the same time the left and right ventricular layers of the interventricular septum are moving in different directions in regard to the transducer (Figure 5.6).

Systole

Peak myocardial velocity and the brightest color-coding occur in the first third of the systole in healthy subjects and declines thereafter (Fig. 5.6, 5.7). TDE allows to study the onset of myocardial wall motion. The myocardial response to electrical activation in the healthy heart is not uniform. This is well known from electrophysiologic studies and can be observed in the TDE image using a high frame rate which is provided in modern TDE machines (up to 58 frames/s). The technology can be used to locate the WPW pathway and to control the effect of ablation.

A very high time-resolution is achieved with M-mode imaging (Figure 5.6). The time delay between two lines of the M-mode image depends on the pulse repetition frequency and does not exceed a few milliseconds (for example, 1.6 ms by 6 kHz pulse repetitions frequency; this corresponds to 625 M-mode lines per second). The time delay between electrical activation and mechanical response can be estimated in both the parasternal and apical M-mode TDE images.

In healthy subjects the time delay between electrical activation (Q-wave on the ECG) and mechanical response is about 50–80 ms (Fig. 5.7). This varies slightly for different structures and different transducer positions, but does not exceed 100 ms under normal circumstances. The time from the Q-wave on the ECG to peak systolic velocity visualized by the brightest color-coding is below 160 ms. The time to the end of systole depends on the heart rate. In healthy subjects, with heart rates about 60/min, it is 350–400 ms.

Diastolic Myocardial Velocities

TDE shows different phases of diastolic velocities of the left ventricular wall in healthy subjects. At early diastole an expected color reversal occurs [10, 17, 22].

During early diastole high wall velocities appear, as is shown by brighter color-coding. This corresponds to the rapid filling phase of the left ventricle. The direction of wall velocities is now opposite to that during systole. The left ventricular velocity values are in this phase the highest among all velocity values recorded in the cardiac cycle in healthy subjects: 8–14 cm/s.

After this early diastolic left ventricular expansion several phases of wall velocities are recorded. Both velocity values and directions change from phase to phase. The number of velocity phases during diastole is dependent on the imaging plane and segment studied. Surprising is the velocity pattern of the interventricular septum and posterior left ventricular wall in the parasternal view. This can be studied in both M-mode and two-dimensional TDE using a high frame-rate machine (Fig. 5.6, 5.7, 5.8).

Posterior Myocardial Wall

The posterior wall velocity is high in early diastole with corresponding bright blue/green color-coding (Fig. 5.6). The recorded velocity is above 8 cm/s. Immediately after this phase a short motion in the opposite direction takes place. The phase corresponds to the start of diastasis in mid diastole. The velocities recorded are rather low, often below 2 cm/s.

Whereas systolic and early diastolic velocities are related to well known shape changes of the left ventricle, the mid-diastolic wall velocity has not been studied. The mid-diastolic velocities occur shortly after early-diastolic ventricular expansion and their duration is rather short. The mid-diastolic velocity direction is opposite to that of the preceding phase. The velocities at mid-diastole correspond with the early-diastolic velocities. This motion is also closely related to the preceding early-diastolic phase and may be related to the elastic properties of the myocardium (Figs. 5.6, 5.7).

Subsequently, a phase occurs with slow cardiac wall backward velocities. This is indicated by dark blue coding. This phase corresponds to slow filling of the left ventricle. The velocity direction is now similar to that in the early diastole, and opposite to the mid-diastolic phase. The velocity values are below 1 cm/s when the heart rate is low.

In late-diastole the velocity increases, but still the direction corresponds to the early-diastolic phase. The velocity values are above 2 cm/s. The late-diastolic myocardial velocity occurs after the P-wave on the ECG and is related to the left ventricular filling due to atrial contraction.

Interventricular Septum

The interventricular septum velocity pattern is more complex (Figs. 5.4, 5.5, and 5.6). After the systolic backward motion a phase occurs with different velocity directions across the wall. At the end of this phase both the interventricular septum and posterior wall are moving toward the transducer. This means that in the parasternal view the heart is moving toward the transducer. This was described using conventional two-dimensional echocardiography and off-line left ventricular shape analysis [13]. This cardiac motion can be seen by nuclear magnetic resonance imaging, too. Subsequently, both the interventricular septum and posterior wall are moving away from the transducer (Figs. 5.6 and 5.7). In this phase of early diastole the left ventricular wall velocities are lower than the velocities of the whole heart. This makes it possible to visualize the whole heart motion within the chest.

During the next phase of the early diastole the interventricular septum is moving toward the transducer with the highest velocities recorded during the cardiac cycle in normal subjects (Figs. 5.1, 5.2). This wall velocity predominantly represents diastolic expansion. Finally, two opposite phases of septum velocity are observed. The mechanism of the first may be similar to the mid-diastolic phase described for the posterior left ventricular wall. In late diastole a typical velocity pattern related to the atrial contraction is observed.

The TDE pattern of apical 2-D echocardiograms of the left ventricle are given in Figs. 5.9, 5.10, and 5.11 with M-mode tracings of the interventricular septum and lateral wall in Figs. 5.12 and 5.13.

Peak Wall Velocities

Calculating in ROI the myocardial velocities in the basal, mid, and apical parts of the interventri-

cular septum and posterior wall, and plotting against time allowes the assessment of pattern peak velocities during the cardiac cycle.

Four peaks of the left ventricular wall velocity pattern were found: peak systolic velocity (S), peak early-diastolic (D_E), mid-diastolic (D_M), and late-diastolic (D_A) velocities. The values and the directions of the peak myocardial velocities are strictly dependent on the imaging plane and part of the myocardium studied. In general, peak early-diastolic velocities are higher than all remaining velocity peaks in all investigated left ventricular segments of healthy, young subjects:

S $= 4–8$ cm/s
$D_E = 8–14$ cm/s
$D_M = < 2$ cm/s
$D_A = 2–4$ cm/s

Ratios of Peak Wall Velocities

Wall velocity ratios can be calculated, which are neither dependent on the imaging plane nor the left myocardial segment studied. The ratio of peak wall velocity in early diastole to systole (D_E/S), the ratio of peak wall velocity in mid diastole to early diastole (D_M/D_E), and the ratio of peak velocity in late diastole to early diastole (D_A/D_E) can be determined. The normal ranges for peak velocity ratios for left ventricular segments in healthy, young subjects are

D_E/S $= -1.5–2.0$
$D_M/D_E = -0.03–0.1$
$D_A/D_E =   0.25–0.4$

Aortic Wall Velocities

In the parasternal view the aortic wall (Figure 5.8) is moving toward the transducer during systole and away from the transducer during diastole. This motion may correspond to heart motion in the chest. It can be expected that the movement of aortic wall and recorded velocities are related also to blood ejection during systole as well as to the left atrial contraction. Apart from the motion of the whole aorta within the chest, there are changes in the aortic diameter. The velocity of both aortic walls is not the same at each moment of the cardiac cycle.

Left Atrium Wall Velocities

Left atrial posterior wall velocities can be recorded by TDE in the parasternal and apical views (Figs. 5,5, 5,8, 5.18). In the parasternal view the left atrial wall moves toward the transducer during systole and away from the transducer during early and mid diastole. This seems to depend on the cardiac motion in the chest. The velocity values during systole and diastole are rather low. The highest velocities occur during active contraction of the left atrium in the late-diastole.

In the apical view different velocity values are recorded, depending on the contribution between heart movement and left atrial dynamics. During systole, and early and late diastole, the posterior walls of both atria move toward the transducer in the apical view. The motion depends during systole on cardiac movement, and during early and late diastole on atrial emptying.

Right Ventricular Wall Velocities

The right ventricular free wall is also visualized in TDE (Fig. 5.6). Its color-coded movement can be clearly delineated from non-moving and non-color-coding chest wall in the parasternal view. The resulting possibility to measure right ventricular myocardium exactly is presented in chapter 9.

References

1. Assmann PE, Slager CJ, Van-der-Borden SG, Tijssen JG, Oomen JA, Roeland JR (1993) Comparison of models for quantitative left ventricular wall motion analysis from two-dimensional echocardiograms during acute myocardial infarction. Am J Cardiol 71:1262–9
3. Drozdz J, Schön F, Nesser HJ, Erbel R (1994) Colour coded tissue Doppler echocardiography – a new method for quantification of cardiac wall motion (abstract). Eur J C P E 4:248
4. Erbel R, Henkel B, Ostländer C, Clas W, Brennecke R, Meyer J (1985) Normalwerte für die zweidimensionale Echokardiographie. Dtsch Med Wschr 110:123–8
5. Erbel R, Schweizer P, Pyhel N, Hadre U, Meyer J, Krebs W, Effert S (1980) Quantitative Analyse regionaler Kontraktionstörungen des linken Ventrikels im zweidimensionalen Echokardiogramm. Z Kardiol 69:562–72
6. Erbel R, Schweizer P, Meyer J, Krebs W, Yalkinoglu Ö, Effert S (1985) Sensivity of cross-sectional echocardiography in detection of impaired global and regional left ventricular function: prospective study. Int J Cardiol 7:375–89
7. Gallagher KP, Osakada G, Matsuzaki M, Miller M, Kemper WS, Ross J (1985) Nonuniformity of inner and outer systolic wall thickening in conscious dogs. Am J Physiol 249:H241–248
8. Gorcsan J, Katz WE, Mandarino WA, Pinsky MR (1994) Heterogenous left ventricular septal and posterior wall velocities: quantitative temporal assessment by myocardial color Doppler imaging (abstract). Circulation 90:I–327
9. Ingels N, Daughters G, Stinson E, Alderman E (1980) Evaluation of methods for quantitation of left ventricular segmental wall motion in man using myocardial markers as a standard. Circulation 61:966–72
10. McDicken WN, Sutherland GR, Moran CM, Gordon LN (1992) Colour Doppler velocity imaging of the myocardium. Ultrasound Med Biol 18:651–4
11. Milunski MR, Mohr GA, Perez JE (1989) Ultrasonic tissue characterisation with integrated backscatter. Circulation 80:491–503
12. Miyatake K, Yamagishi M, Tanaka N, Sasaki T, Ohe T, Yamazaki N, Mine N, Sano A, Hirama M (1993) A new method for evaluation of left ventricular wall motion by color-coded tissue Doppler echocardiography: In vitro and in vivo studies (abstract). Circulation 88:I–48
13. Pandian NG, Skorton DJ, Collins SM, Falsetti HL, Burke ER, Kerber RE (1983) Heterogeneity of left ventricular segmental wall thickening and excursion in 2-dimensional echocardiograms of normal human subjects. Am J Cardiol 51:1667–73
14. Perez JE, Klein SC, Prater DM, Fraser CE, Cardona H, Waggoner AD, Holland MR, Miller JG, Sobel BE (1992) Automated, on-line quantification of left ventricular dimensions and function by echocardiography with backscatter imaging and lateral gain compensation. Am J Cardiol 70:1200–5
15. Raisinghani A, Donaghey L, Nozaki S, Dittrich H, DeMaria A (1994) New approaches to the evaluation of LV function: assessment of transmural myocardial velocity gradients and diastolic relaxation rates by Doppler tissue imaging (abstract). Circulation 90:I–327
16. Sutherland GR, Stewart MJ, Groundstroem KW, Moran CM, Fleming A, Guell-Peris FJ, Riemersma RA, Fenn LN, Fox KA, McDicken WN (1994) Color Doppler myocardial imaging: a new technique for the assessment of myocardial function. J Am Soc Echocardiogr 7:441–58
17. Schön F, Drozdz J, Nesser HJ, Erbel R (1994) New insight into ventricular contraction by colour coded tissue Doppler echocardiography (abstract). Eur J C P E 4:248
18. Stewart MJ, Groundstroem WE, Sutherland GR, Moran CM, Fleming A, Fenn LN, McDicken WN (1993) Myocardial imaging by colour Doppler coded velocity mapping – a new method for the assessment of myocardial contractility (abstract). Eur Heart J 14 (suppl):467
19. Thomsen PQ, Stahlberg F, Henriksen O (1993) Normal left ventricular wall motion measured with two-dimensional myocardial tagging. Acta Radiol 34:450–6

20. Uematsu M, Miyatake K, Yamagishi M, Tanaka N, Nagata S, Sasaki T, Sano A, Yamazaki N, Mine Y, Hirama M (1994) Myocardial velocity gradient as a new method to quantitate regional left ventricular wall motion abnormalities (abstract). Circulation 90:I–326

21. Weyman AE (1994) Principles of color flow imaging. In: Weyman AE (Ed). Principles and practice of echocardiography. Lea & Febiger, 218-33

22. Yamazaki N, Mine Y, Sano A, Hirama M, Miyatake K, Yamagishi M, Tanaka N (1994) Analysis of ventricular wall motion using color-coded tissue Doppler imaging system. Jpn J Appl Phys 33:3141–6

Fig. 5.5. Normal heart. Two-dimensional tissue Doppler echocardiographic image. Parasternal long axis view in early diastole *(left)* and systole *(right)* using a 2.5 MHz transducer. The lowest color-coded velocity is set to be 0.42 cm/s. The highest measurable velocity is set to be 7.0 cm/s. The forward velocities are coded by red up to 2.9 cm/s, and by yellow above 2.9 cm/s. The backward velocities are coded by dark blue up to 2.9 cm/s, by light blue up to 5.4 cm/s, and by green above 5.4 cm/s. The interventricular septum and posterior wall are moving in opposite directions in both phases of the cardiac cycle. Both are moving away from the center of the left ventricle during diastole and toward the center of the left ventricle during systole. The interventricular septum is moving toward the transducer during diastole (indicated by red-yellow color-coding) and away from the transducer during systole (indicated by blue). The posterior left ventricular wall moves away from the transducer during diastole (indicated by blue) and toward the transducer during systole (indicated by yellow). Clear definition of right ventricular (RV) myocardium. The direction of movement of the right ventricular anterior wall corresponds to the direction of the movement of the interventricular septum. The anterior mitral leaflet is moving in early diastole toward the interventricular septum. The aortic wall (AO) moves blackward during diastole and forward during systole. (AO = aortic root, LA = left atrium, LV = eft ventricle, RV = right ventricle)

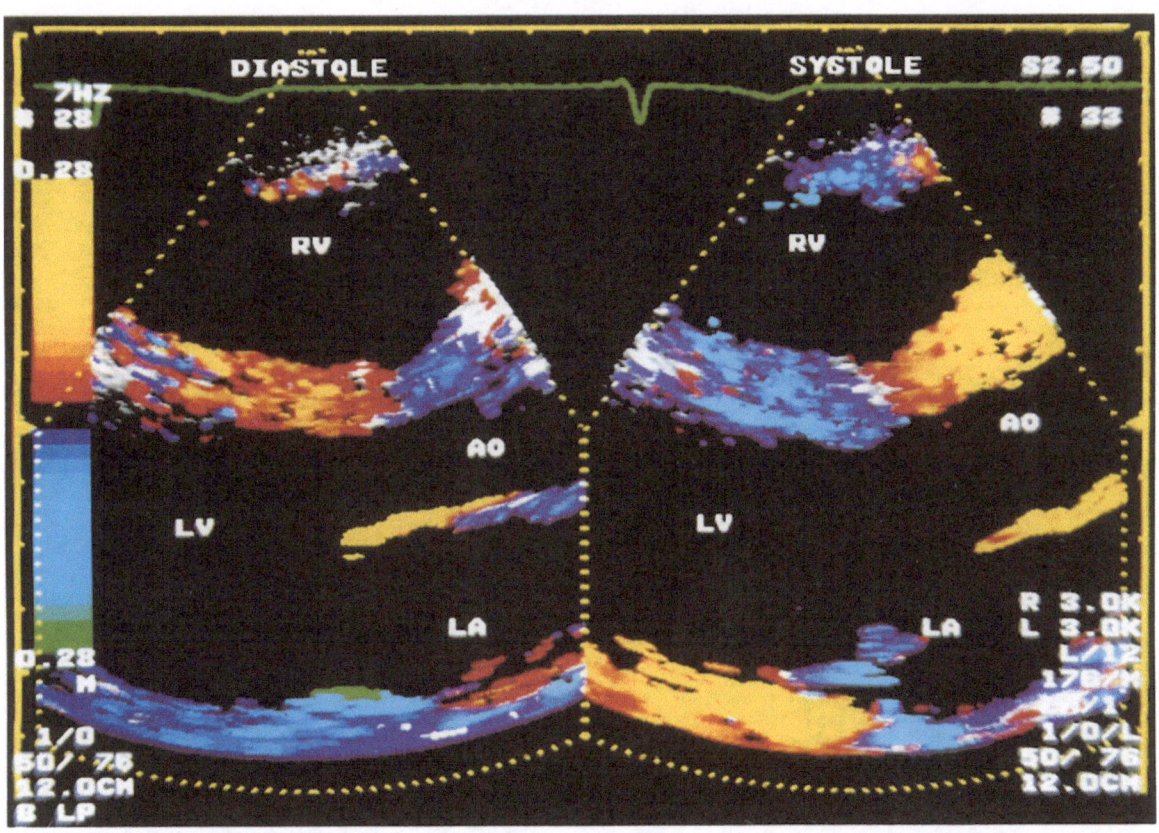

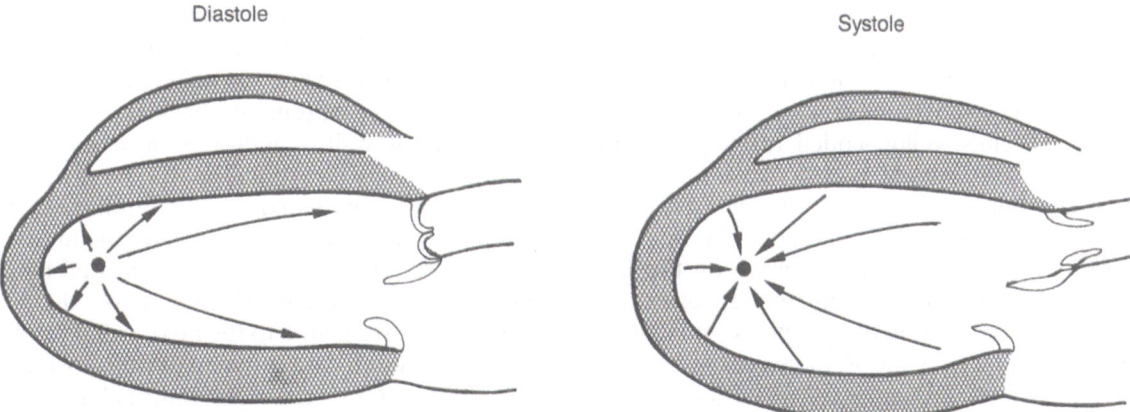

Diastole

Systole

● center of gravity of the left ventricle   → direction of left ventricular wall velocities

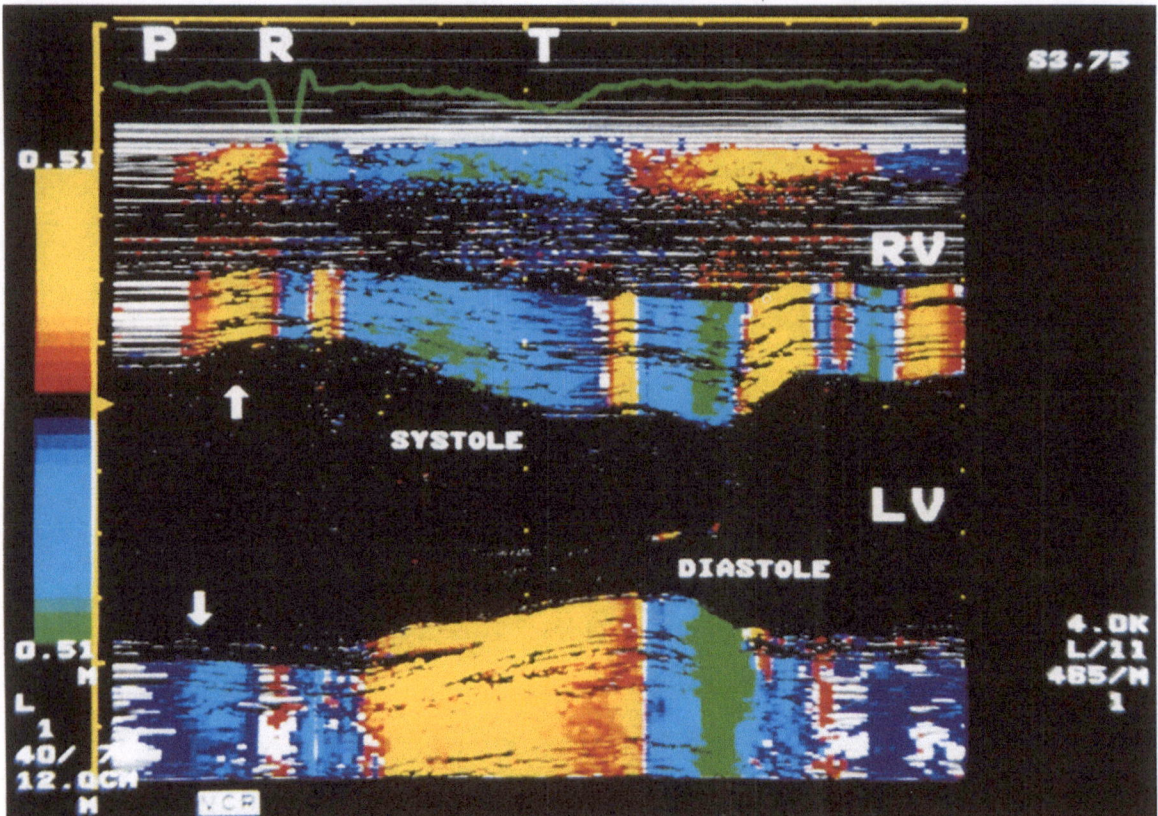

Fig. 5.6. Normal heart. M-mode tissue Doppler echocardiographic image from the parasternal long axis view using a 3.75 MHz transducer. Machine settings are: non-color-coded velocities up to 0.18 cm/s, red or dark blue-coded velocities up to 0.8 cm/s, yellow-coded forward velocities above 0.9 cm/s, bright blue-coded backward velocities from 0.8 cm/s up to 2.6 cm/s, and green-coded backward velocities above 2.6 cm/s. The posterior wall moves after P wave on the ECG away from the transducer *(arrow)*. It corresponds to the forward motion of the interventricular septum *(arrow)*. After the R-wave on the ECG the systole begins with forward posterior wall and backward interventricular septum movement. A transmural gradient due to different velocities is visible in the interventricular septum and posterior wall. The detection of red-yellow coding of the interven-tricular septum similar to the posterior wall in late systole is related to the anterior movement of the total heart. At the beginning of diastole both the interventricular septum and posterior wall are moving away from the transducer with blue-green color-coding. The velocity of the interventricular septum reverses in the next phase. It moves now in the opposite direction in regard to systole. After forward diastolic motion of the interventricular septum and backward motion of the posterior wall a mid-diastolic phase occurs with the velocity direction opposite to the preceding left ventricular expansion. Different velocities within the myocardium, particularly the interventricular septum, are visible and indicated by different colors. Different velocities across the myocardial wall are related to the myocardial thickening during systole and thinning during diastole.

Clear definition of the right ventricular anterior wall. The right ventricular anterior wall is moving away from the transducer during systole and toward the transducer during diastole. The time delay between the Q-wave on the ECG and systolic right ventricular wall motion is 38 ms in comparison with the time delay measured over the interventricular septum – 96 ms and over the posterior left ventricular wall – 99 ms. (LV = left ventricle, RV = right ventricle)

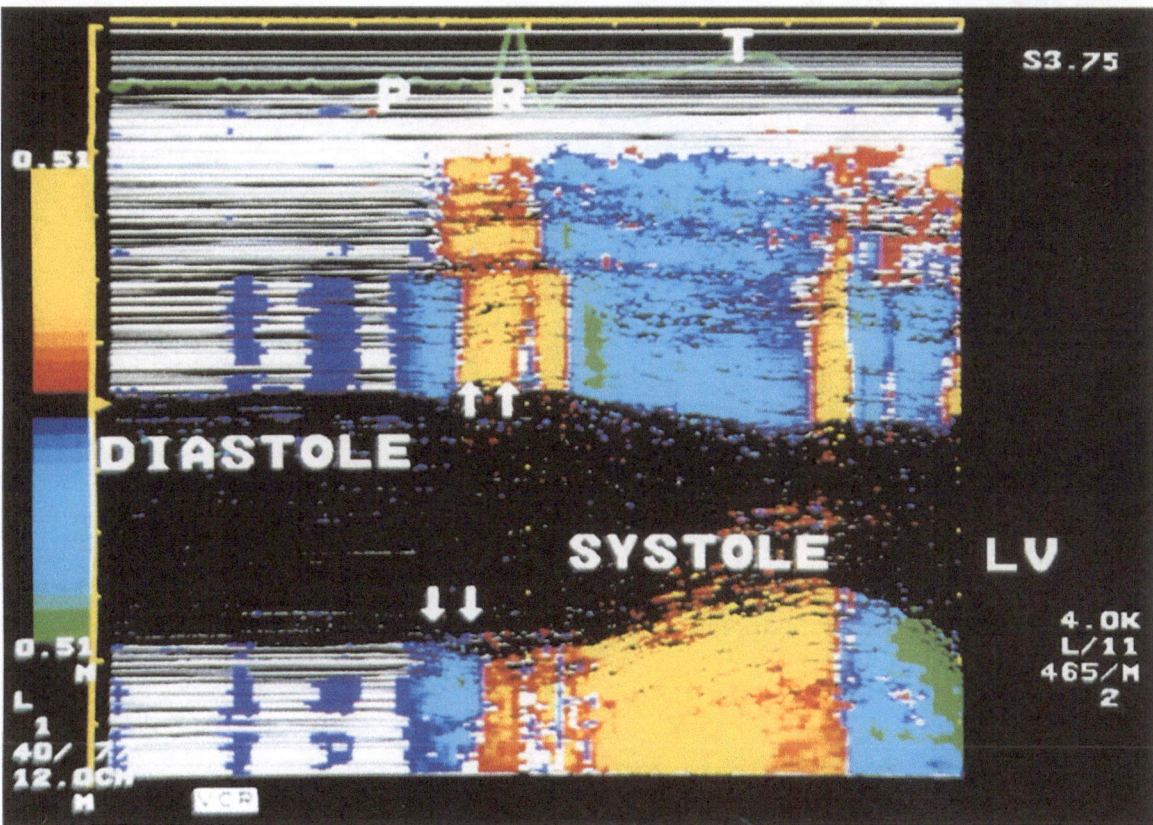

Fig. 5.7. Normal heart. M-mode TDE recording from the parasternal long axis view. Machine settings are the same as in Figure 5.6. At the end of diastole whole heart backward movement with low velocity near the non-color-coded velocity values is visualized. After P-wave on the ECG cardiac backward movement with higher velocities occurs with corresponding bright blue-coding of the interventricular septum and posterior wall. This may be related to the atrial contraction. After this short phase the left ventricular filling is recorded with the opposite velocity direction of the interventricular septum and posterior wall. The time delay between the start of the P-wave on the ECG to the onset of the interventricular septum motion is 46 ms, and to the onset of the posterior wall motion 24 ms (two arrows). The beginning of systole is also illustrated. The first part moving with systolic directed velocity is the right ventricular anterior wall. The backward movement begins 63 ms after the Q-wave on the ECG. Interventricular septum movement begins 36 ms later as visualized in the M mode image. Overestimation of the right ventricular wall thickness is due to non-perpendicular ultrasonic beam location. (LV = left ventricle)

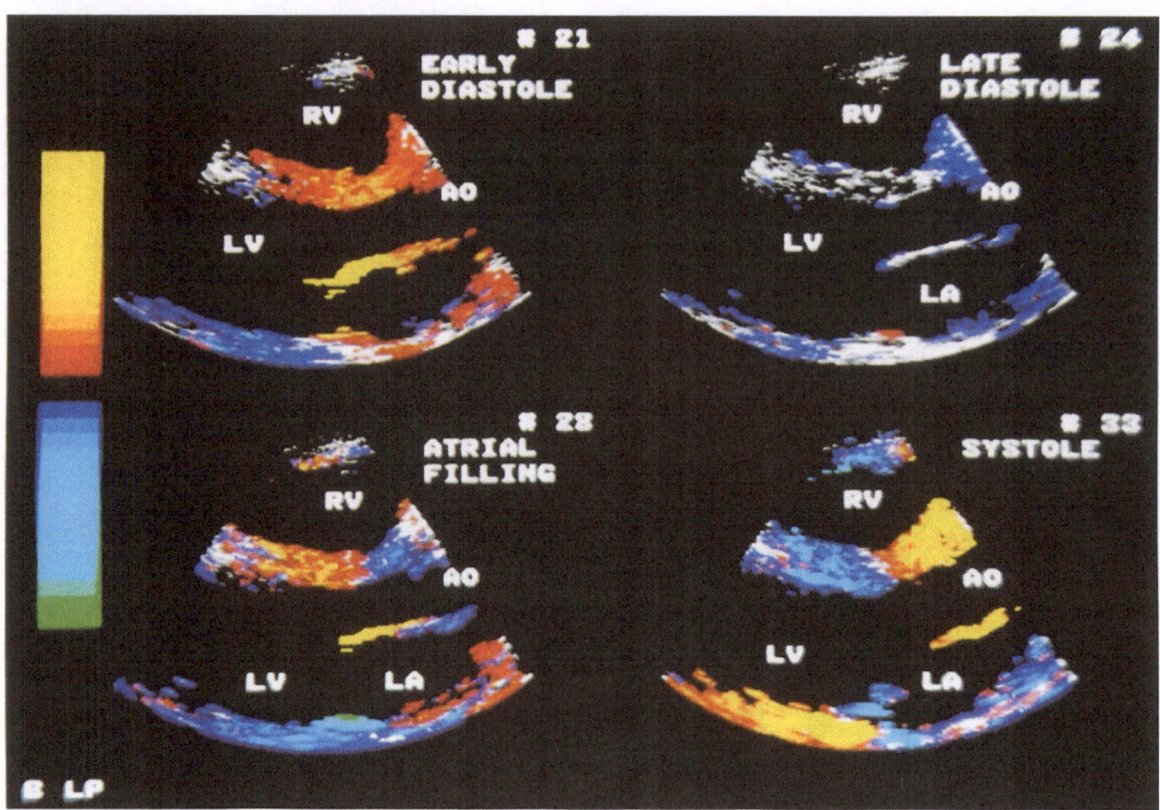

Fig. 5.8. Normal heart. Parasternal long axis view using a 2.5 MHz transducer. Machine settings are the same as in Fig 5.5. Four frames illustrating interventricular septal and posterior wall velocities during early diastole *(upper left)*, late diastole before the P-wave on the ECG *(upper right)*, after atrial contraction *(below left)*, and during systole *(below right)*. The anterior leaflet of the mitral valve is moving toward the transducer during early diastole and after atrial contraction. During the early-diastole, indicated by opened mitral valve leaflets *(upper left)*, the aortic root is still moving toward the transducer as during systole. During the next diastolic frames the aortic root moves away from the transducer as it is typical for diastolic aortic motion in this view. (AO = aortic root, LA = left atrium, LV = left ventricle, RV = right ventricle)

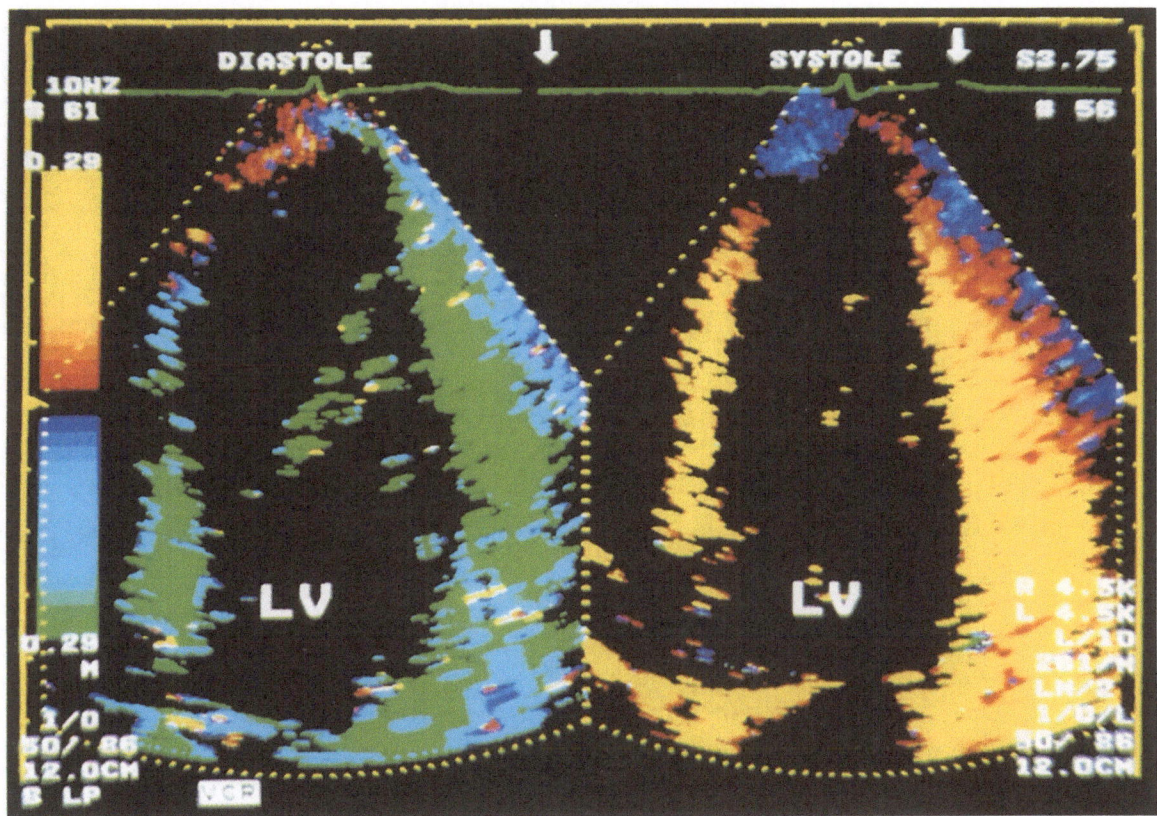

Fig. 5.9. Normal heart. Apical view in early diastole *(left)* and in systole *(right)* using a 3.75 MHz transducer. Machine settings are: non-color-coded velocities up to 0.21 cm/s, red or dark blue-coded velocities up to 0.9 cm/s, yellow-coded forward velocities above 0.9 cm/s, light blue-coded backward velocities from 0.9 cm/s up to 3.0 cm/s, and green-coded backward velocities above 3.0 cm/s. Basal and mid left ventricular segments move at different velocities during diastole away from the transducer and are coded green. The apex is moving toward the transducer and is coded red. During systole the mid and basal parts of the left ventricle move toward the transducer (red and yellow-coded depending on velocity) and the apex moves away from the transducer. (LV = left ventricle)

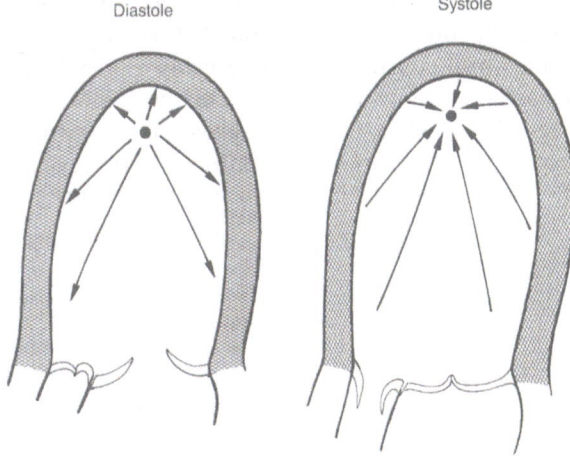

• center of gravity of the left ventricle
→ vectors of left ventricular wall velocity

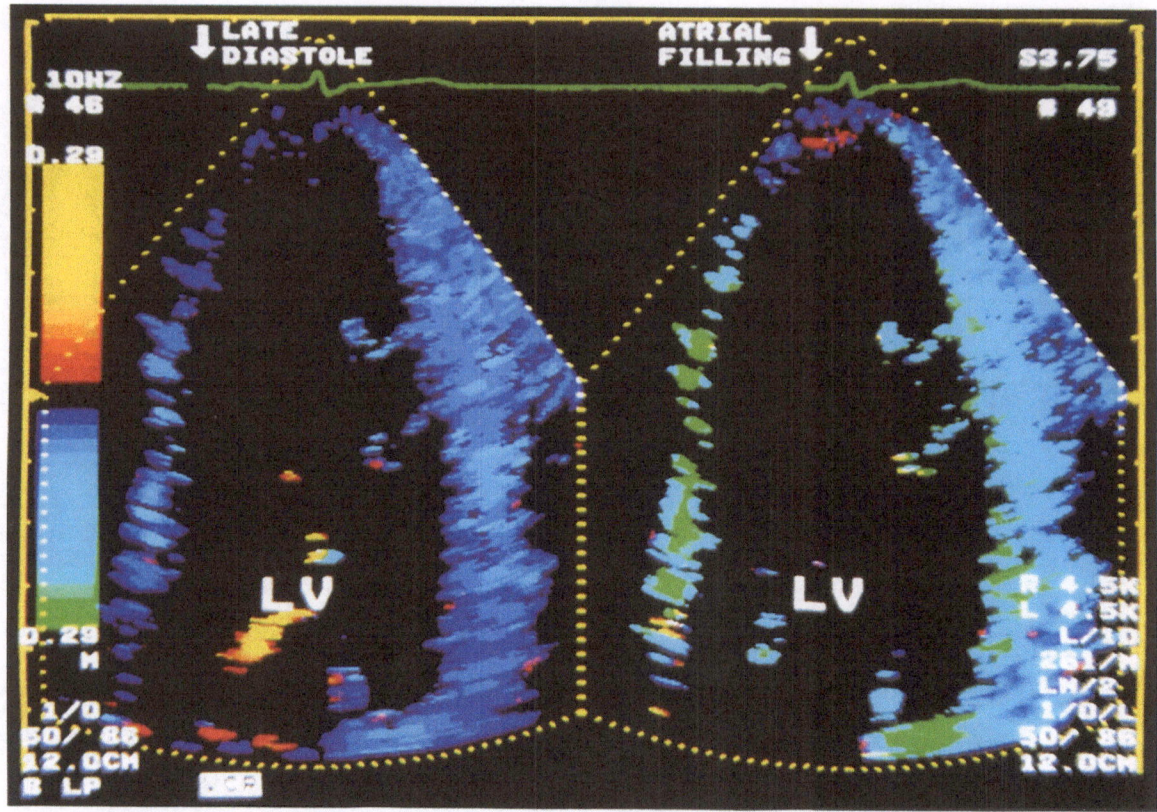

Fig. 5.10. Normal heart. Apical view of the left ventricle during late diastole before *(left)* and after atrial contraction *(right)* using a 3.75 MHz transducer. Machine settings are the same as in Fig. 5.9. Arrows indicate the phase of the cardiac cycle on the ECG. During late diastole, before the P-wave on the ECG, low backward velocities are indicated by dark blue. High myocardium backward velocities during atrial left ventricular filling are indicated by green. The only part of the left ventricle moving in the opposite direction is the apex. (LV = left ventricle). Note the synchrony of the wall velocities

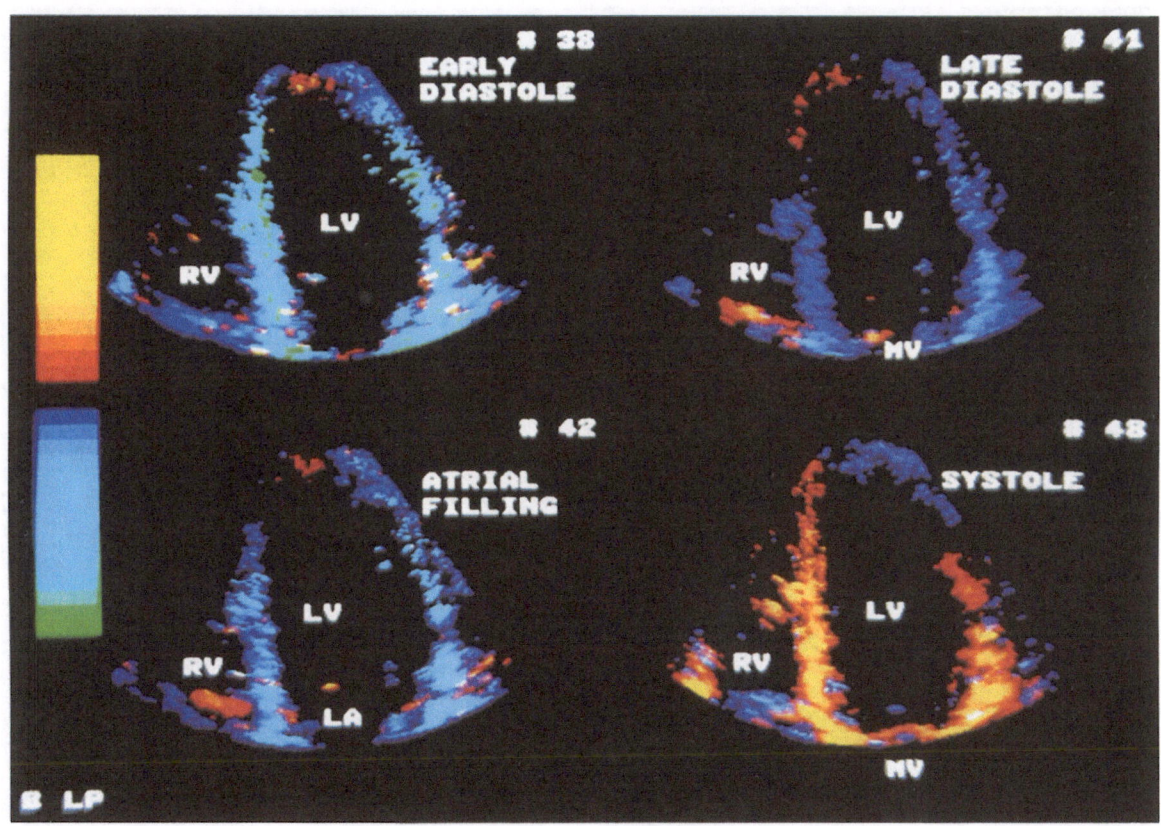

Fig. 5.11. Normal heart. Apical view using a 3.75 MHz transducer. Machine settings are: non-color-coded velocities up to 0.1 cm/s, red or dark blue-coded velocities up to 0.45 cm/s, yellow-coded forward velocities above 0.45 cm/s, bright blue-coded backward velocities from 0.45 cm/s up to 1.5 cm/s, and green-coded backward velocities above 1.5 cm/s. Four frames illustrating left ventricular wall velocities during early diastole *(upper left)*, late diastole before the P-wave on the ECG *(upper right)*, late diastole after atrial contraction *(below left)*, and during systole *(below right)*. There is synchrony of the ventricular walls throughout the cardiac cycle. Note the still opposite velocity direction of the apex in comparison to the velocity direction of the basal and mid – left ventricular segments. (LA = left atrium, LV = left ventricle, MV = mitral valve, RV = right ventricle)

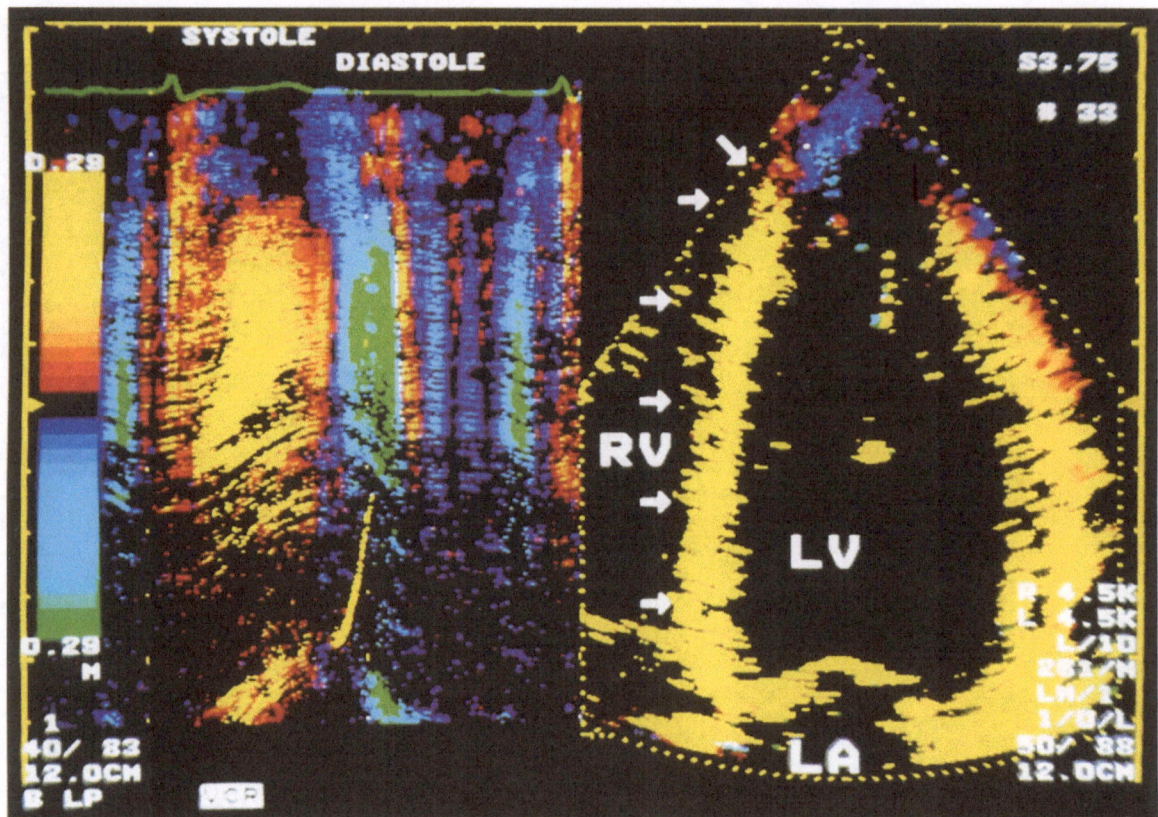

Fig. 5.12. Normal heart. M-mode recording of the interventricular septum velocities in the apical view using a 3.75 MHz transducer. Machine settings are the same as in Fig. 5.9. During systole a stable velocity direction toward the transducer is observed. The highest velocities coded by bright yellow color are located in mid-systole. After color reversal in early diastole very high backward velocities are recorded. After this early diastolic ventricular expansion a mid-diastolic phase occurs with the wall velocities in the opposite direction. The movement of the interventricular septum in late diastole can be divided into two phases. In the first phase low backward wall velocities are recorded above 0.1–0.4 cm/s. In the second phase after the P-wave on the ECG faster backward velocities are noted, indicating left ventricular filling due to atrial contraction. (LA = left atrium, LV = left ventricle, RV = right ventricle)

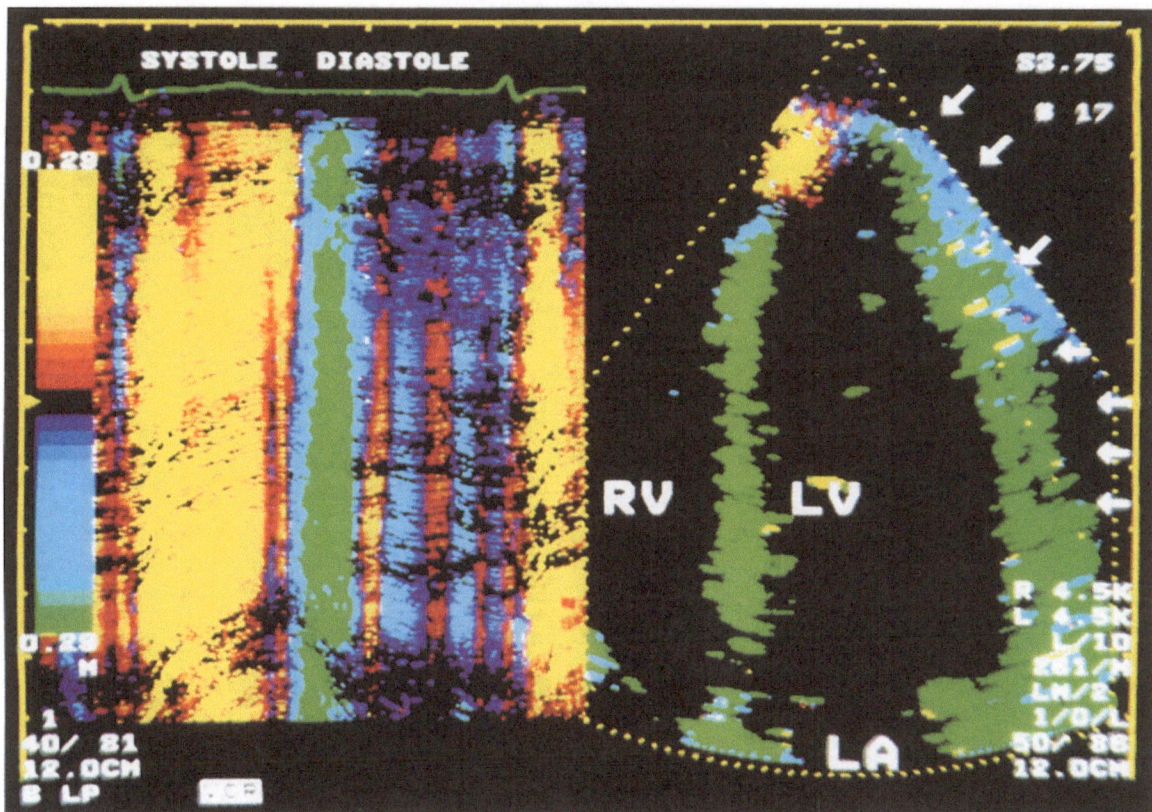

Fig. 5.13. Normal heart. M-mode recording of the lateral left ventricular wall velocities in the apical view using a 3.75 MHz transducer. Machine settings are the same as in Fig. 5.9. During systole the wall velocity is directed toward the transducer. After color reversal in early diastole very high backward velocities are recorded. After this early diastolic ventricular expansion a mid-diastolic phase occurs with the wall velocities in the opposite direction. The movement of the lateral wall in the late-diastole can be divided into two phases. In the first phase low backward and forward wall velocities are recorded above 0.1–0.4 cm/s. In the second phase after the P-wave on the ECG the faster backward velocities are noted, indicating left ventricular filling due to atrial contraction. (LA = left atrium, LV = left ventricle, RV = right ventricle)

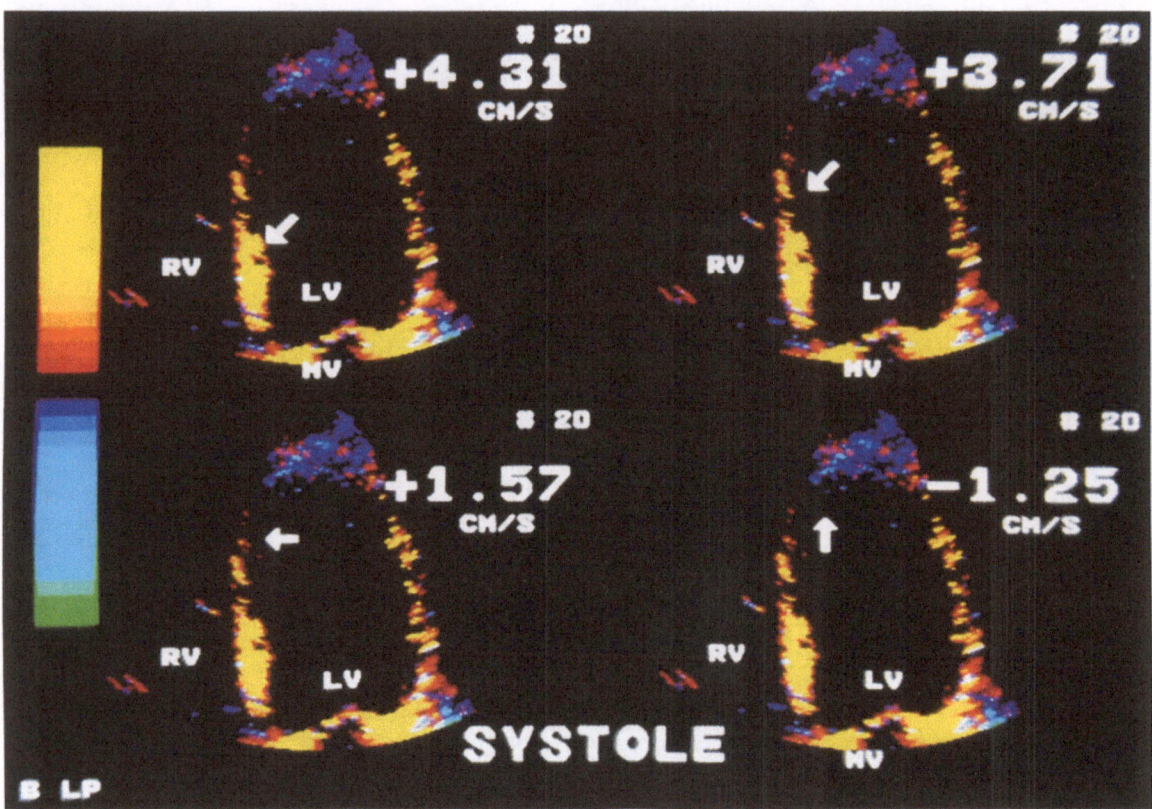

Fig. 5.14. Normal heart. Apical view of the left ventricle during mid systole using a 2.5 MHz transducer. Machine settings are: non-color-coded velocities up to 0.28 cm/s, red or dark blue-coded velocities up to 1.3 cm/s, yellow-coded forward velocities above 1.3 cm/s, bright blue-coded backward velocities from 1.3 cm/s up to 4.2 cm/s, and green-coded backward velocities above 4.2 cm/s.

All pictures represent the same mid-systolic frame. The interventricular septum velocities are measured as localized by arrows. The basal parts of the septum are moving with higher velocities than mid parts. The apex is moving at the same time away from the transducer, as indicated by negative wall velocity. Note synchrony of the interventricular septum and lateral wall velocities. (LV = left ventricle, MV = mitral valve, RV = right ventricle)

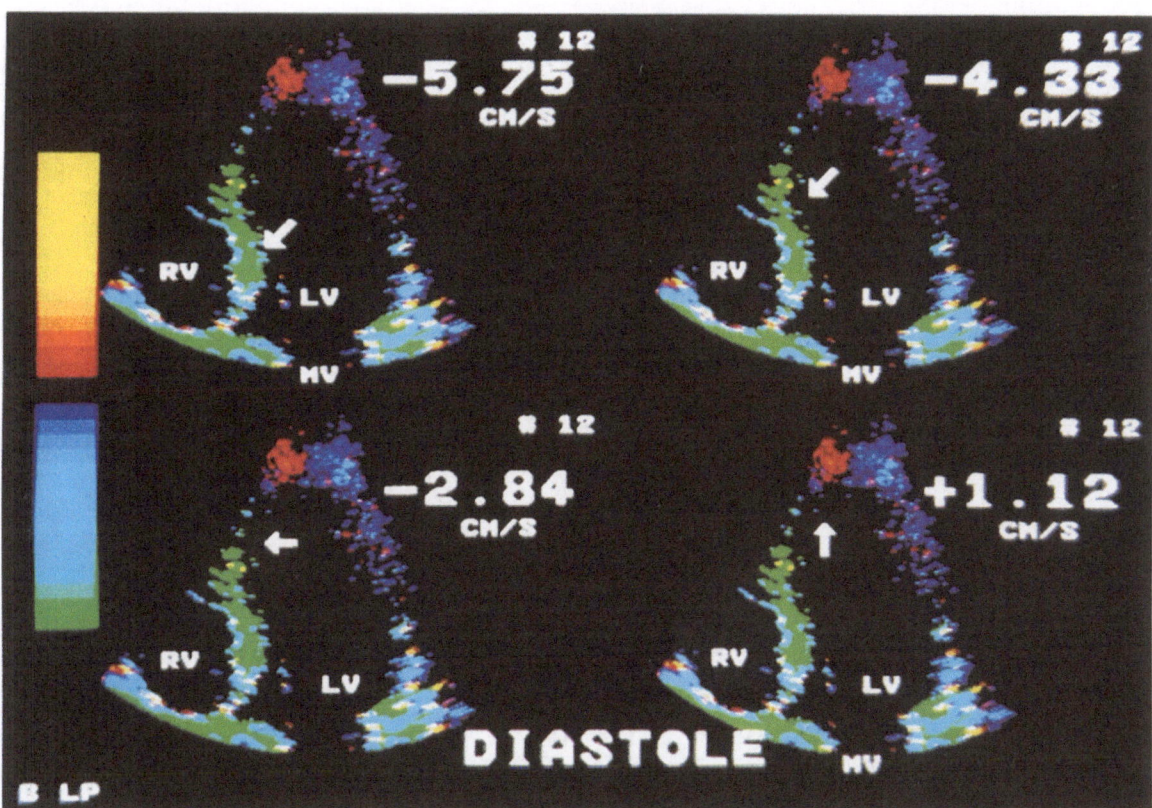

Fig. 5.15. Normal heart. Apical view of the left ventricle during early diastole using a 2.5 MHz transducer. Machine settings are the same as in Fig. 5.14. All pictures represent the same early-diastolic frame. The interventricular septum velocities are measured as indicated by arrows. The basal parts of the septum are moving with higher negative velocities than mid parts. The apex is moving at the same time toward the transducer as indicated by positive wall velocities. (LV = left ventricle, MV = mitral valve, RV = right ventricle)

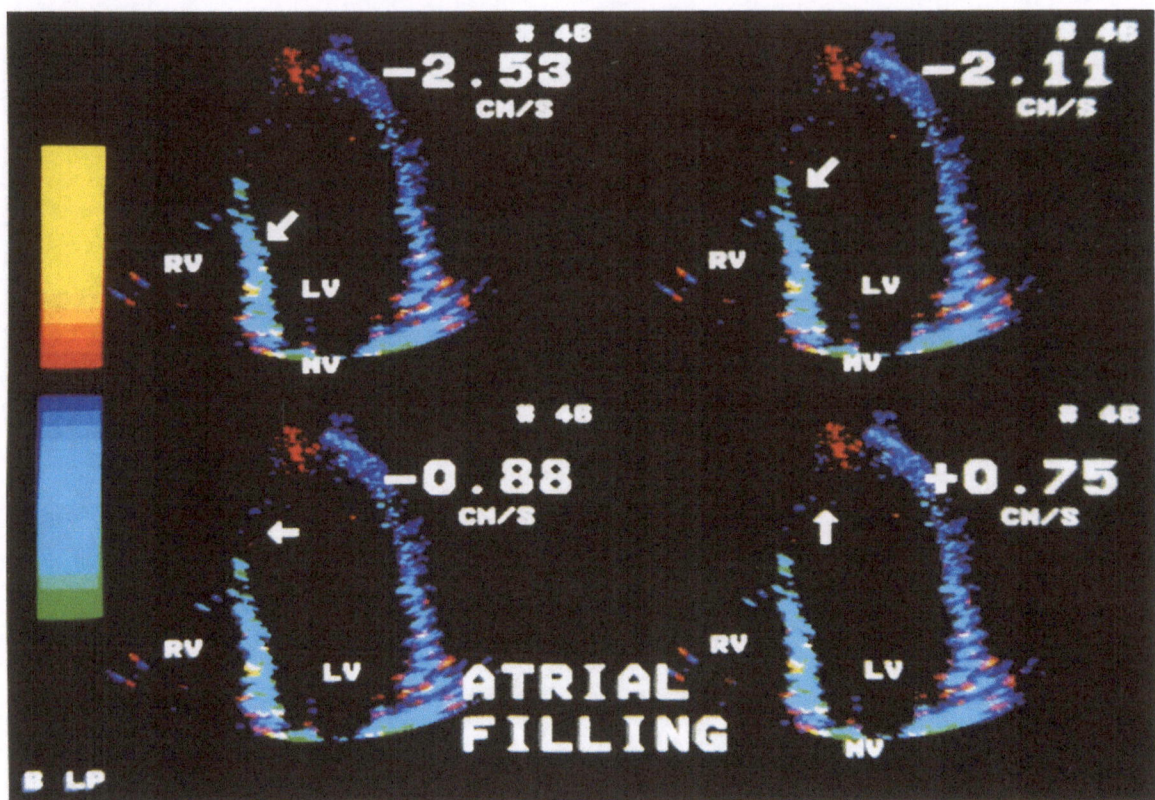

Fig. 5.16. Normal heart. Apical view of the left ventricle during late diastole using a 2.5 MHz transducer. Machine settings are the same as in Fig. 5.14. All pictures represent the same late-diastolic frame. The interventricular septum velocities are measured as indicated by arrows. The basal parts of the septum are moving with higher negative velocities than mid parts, similar to both previously described pictures. The apex is moving at the same time toward the transducer as indicated by the positive wall velocities. The velocity direction is consistent with that during early diastole, but the velocity values are lower. (LV = left ventricle, MV = mitral valve, RV = right ventricle)

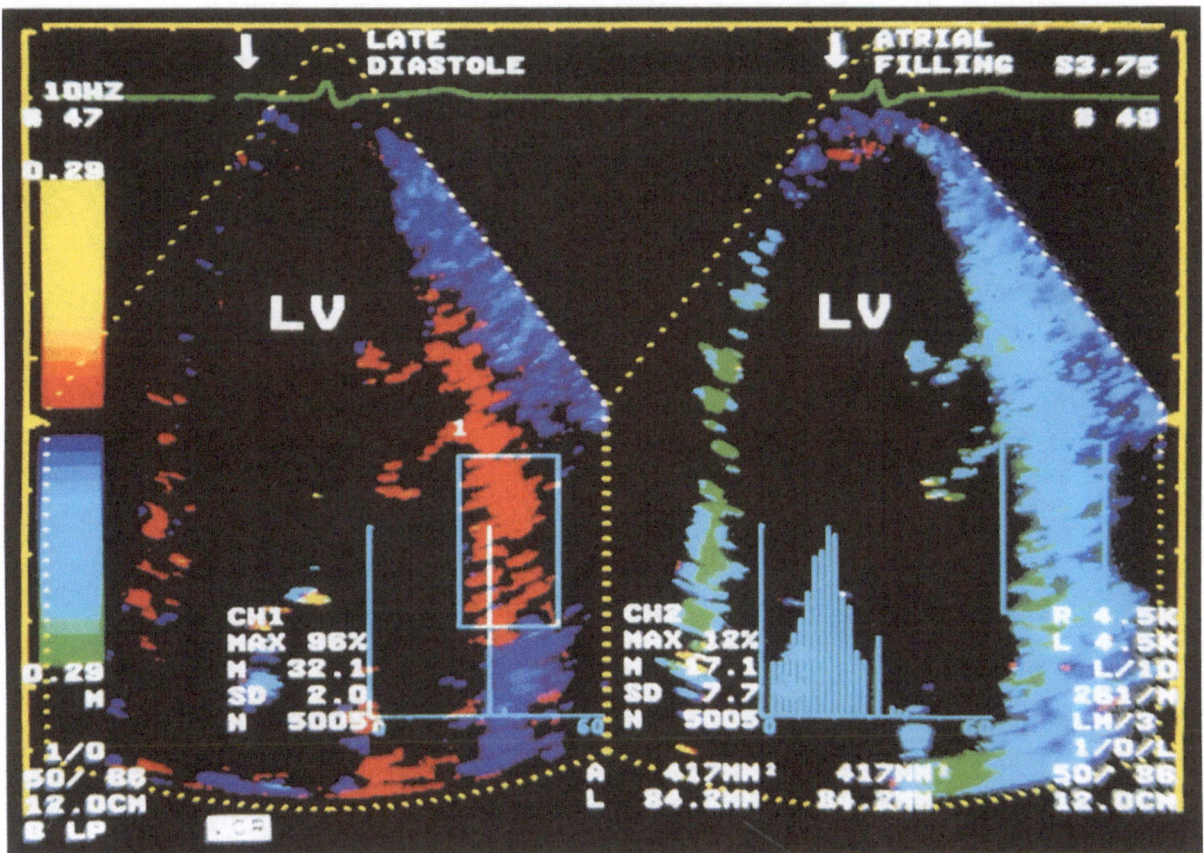

Fig. 5.17. Normal heart. Apical view of the left ventricle during late diastole before the P-wave on the ECG *(left)* and after atrial contraction *(right)* using a 3.75 MHz transducer. Machine settings are: non-color-coded velocities up to 0.1 cm/s, red or dark blue-coded velocities up to 0.45 cm/s, yellow-coded forward velocities above 0.45 cm/s, bright blue-coded backward velocities from 0.45 cm/s up to 1.5 cm/s, and green-coded backward velocities above 1.5 cm/s. The wall velocity histogram analysis is shown. In both frames the region of interest is positioned in the same part of the myocardium. The displays below each region of interest (ROI) show the velocity histogram of the myocardial wall. The values displayed on the left side of the velocity histogram are: max = percentage of the pixels, which have the maximum histogram, M = mean tissue velocity, SD = standard deviation of the tissue velocity, and N = number of pixels in the region of interest. Almost all parts of the cardiac tissue revealed the same low velocity in the late diastole. After atrial contraction the velocity dissociation occurs, indicated by increase of standard deviation of the velocity values and lower percentage of pixels with the maximum transmural velocity gradient. (LV = left ventricle)

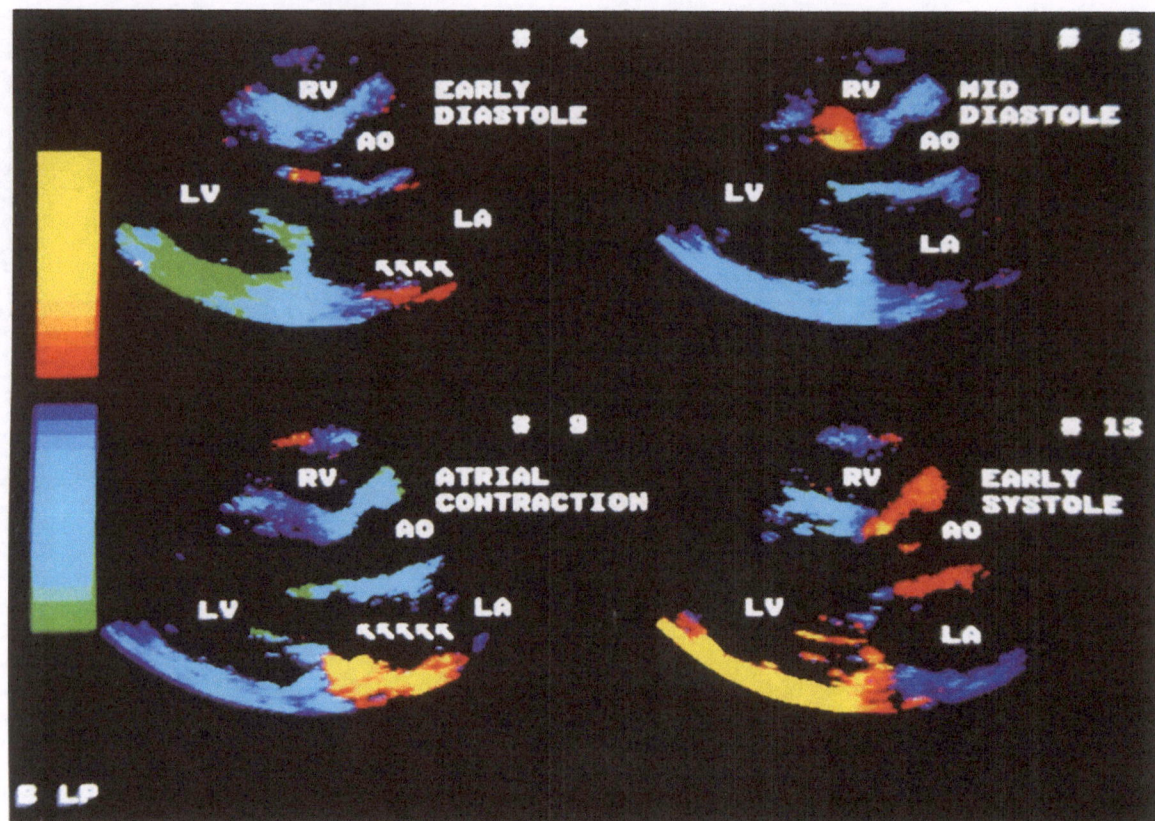

Fig. 5.18. Normal heart. Parasternal long axis view using a 3.75 MHz transducer. Machine settings are: non-color-coded velocities up to 0.28 cm/s, red or dark blue-coded velocities up to 1.3 cm/s, yellow-coded forward velocities above 1.3 cm/s, bright blue-coded backward velocities from 1.3 cm/s up to 4.2 cm/s, and green-coded backward velocities above 4.2 cm/s. Four frames illustrating wall velocities during early diastole *(upper left)*, mid-diastole *(upper right)*, after atrial contraction *(below left)*, and during early systole *(below right)*. Left atrium posterior wall is moving toward the transducer in the early diastolic image. The velocity is found to be below 1.3 cm/s. During mid-diastole the posterior left atrial wall is not color-coded (velocity below 0.28 cm/s). The highest atrial wall velocity is recorded during atrial contraction in the lower left image. In early systole filling of the left atrium is shown with forward motion of the anterior and backward motion of the posterior wall. Note closed aortic valve in the isovolumic early systolic contraction period. (AO = aortic root, LA = left atrium, LV = left ventricle, RV = right ventricle)

Chapter 6   **Movement of the Total Heart**

J. Drozdz

Left ventricular wall motion has been extensively studied using different methods, without the availability of a "gold-standard" algorithm. Several cardiovascular disorders such as coronary artery disease or cardiomyopathy affect regional left ventricular function. Different methods were proposed for regional left ventricular wall motion analysis [1, 4, 7, 9]. Some algorithms are based on systolic movement of the base of the heart toward the apex, some measure the area reduction using fixed- or floating-reference systems, and others use the centerline between the end-diastolic and end-systolic endocardial contours [1]. None of these has been proven to provide optimal results. For most of the patients, methods using a fixed center of gravity are superior to those using a floating center. In patients with enhanced cardiac motion due to the open pericardium after coronary bypass surgery, however, a method using a floating center of gravity is superior. Heterogeneity of left ventricular segmental wall excursion and heart movement within the chest during the cardiac cycle (heart translation) plays an important role [5, 6, 10, 13, 14].

This chapter describes heart translation studied by different techniques and the influences of heart translation on the wall velocity measured by tissue Doppler echocardiography (TDE). The relationship between the velocities of left ventricular wall motion during the cardiac cycle and the velocities of heart translation within the chest in healthy subjects was studied using the parasternal long-axis view.

Heart Translation Within the Chest

Left ventricular translation within the chest has been studied in humans using different modalities. According to findings from both noninvasive and invasive studies, the heart moves in a complex way within the chest [2, 3, 5, 6, 10, 11, 15, 16]. During systole the left ventricle is moving forward and

the base downward. Furthermore, the heart rotates, the degree of rotation being different for various parts of the heart and changing from early to late systole [12, 14, 15]. The rotation ranges from 3–5°.

Invasive Methods

Invasive studies have been based on the analysis of motion of implanted radiopaque markers in the myocardial wall [9, 13]. In humans this was possible during cardiac surgery or heart transplantation. The markers were visualized by fluoroscopy, which allowed determination of the regional wall motion and the translation of the heart within the chest. These studies do not reflect the normal situation as the chest had been opened and/or a new heart was implanted. The results of studies in both groups of patients are not helpful in the understanding of the normal pattern.

Noninvasive Methods

Left ventricular translation within the chest and left ventricular rotation at the papillary muscle level were also studied using echocardiography [11, 12, 14]. According to these reports the heart moves in the anterior direction during systole and shows counterclockwise rotation. Postoperative abnormal motion of the interventricular septum was found to be dependent on abnormal heart translation within the chest [5, 6].

Nuclear magnetic resonance with the technique of myocardial tagging has been introduced recently to investigate the normal left ventricular rotation [15, 16]. According to these studies the direction of the left ventricular rotation along the long axis changes from early to late systole [15]. The base and middle levels of the left ventricle rotate counterclockwise in the early systole and clockwise in the late systole, whereas the apex rotates counterclockwise. The net rotation of the left ventricle shows a clockwise trend at the base, and a counterclockwise rotation at the middle and apical segments [15]. These results reflect the typical circular- and apex-directed orientation of the myocardial fibers described from autopsies.

TDE Findings Concerning Heart Translation

Information concerning translation of the heart by TDE can be obtained by analyzing velocities of different parts of the left ventricle. The change of myocardial velocities shown for the interventricular septum is only partly dependent on left ventricular shape change during the cardiac cycle [8]. It is also influenced by the movement of the heart.

TDE Velocity Components

Quantification of wall velocity allows studying the relation between the velocity of myocardial wall, the velocity of left ventricular translation, and the velocity of left ventricular rotation.

The last component plays only a minor role, as the rotation of the interventricular septum and the posterior left ventricular wall rarely exceeds 5°. TDE velocity imaging is mainly influenced by two components: wall motion and heart translation in the antero-posterior plane. Using the parasternal view both components are superimposed for the posterior wall, but subtracted for the interventricular septum (Figs. 6.1, 6.2). As a result, the net velocity of the interventricular septum is negative during the main part of systole. The interventricular septum moves away from the transducer. The net velocity of the posterior left ventricular wall is positive (toward the transducer) and higher than the velocity of the interventricular septum.

At end-systole the movement of the heart exceeds the movement of the interventricular septum during a short phase (30–60 ms). At this end-systolic phase, the net velocity of the interventricular septum assessed by TDE is positive. The interventricular septum and the posterior left ventricular wall move toward the transducer (red-coded) (Fig. 6.3).

After the T-wave on the ECG, subsequent reversal of the color pattern occurs. During the early-diastolic phase (60–100 ms), the velocity of the interventricular septum is lower than the velocity of the whole heart. At this time the net velocity of the interventricular septum and the posterior left ventricular wall is negative and both walls move backward (Figs. 6.1, 6.2). This is presented in TDE images as an early-diastolic phase with both interventricular septum and posterior left ventricular wall coded by blue (Fig. 6.4).

Analysis of Heart Translation

Using an internal reference system localized in the center of the left ventricle, the velocities of the interventricular septum and the posterior left ventricular wall should be the same. The sum of both velocity vectors should be zero.

Using the transducer as an external reference system, opposite velocity directions and different velocity values for both structures are obtained. When both velocity values are added, the degree of heart movement is obtained (Fig. 6.2).

In general, the velocity direction of the heart obtained according to this model is in anterior direction during systole and in posterior direction during diastole (Fig. 6.2). This is consistent with findings from other imaging modalities. Additionally, the velocity pattern of the heart within the chest can be provided by TDE.

The velocity pattern of heart movement in normal subjects is flat during systole, and during the main part of diastole, with a peak during early diastole. The pattern of the interventricular septum and the posterior left ventricular wall velocities in a representative healthy subject (Fig. 6.7), and resulting pattern of heart translation are presented in Figs. 6.2 and 6.3, respectively.

Studying the velocity pattern of the heart may be of interest concerning pericardial diseases, diseases of the chest, and after open-heart surgery. However, there are some limitations. The right ventricular shape changes may influence the left ventricular translation assessed by TDE. Furthermore, left ventricular wall motion abnormalities will make the application of the model difficult.

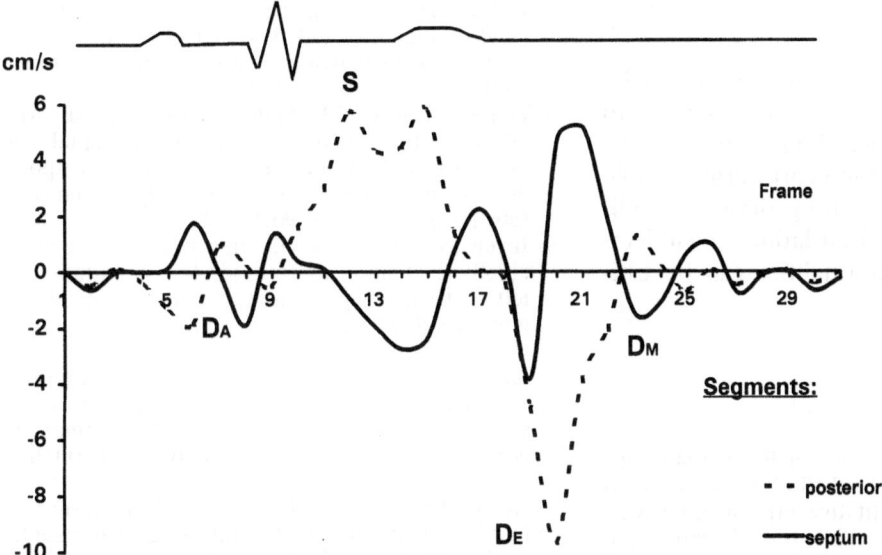

Fig. 6.1. Velocities of the interventricular septum and the posterior left ventricular wall in subsequent frames from the parasternal view in a representative healthy subject. (S=peak systolic velocity, D_E=peak early-diastolic velocity, D_M= peak mid-diastolic velocity, D_A=peak late-diastolic velocity)

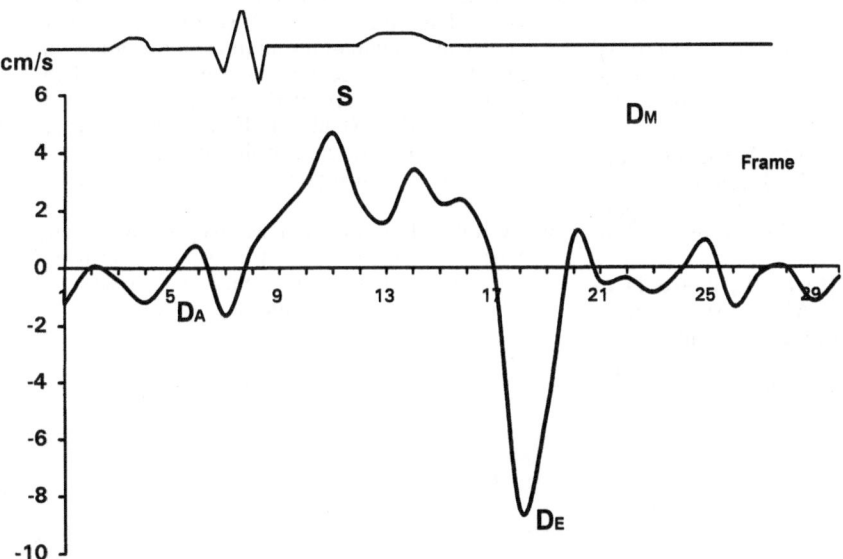

Fig. 6.2 Total heart movement: The result of subtraction of the velocities of the interventricular septum and the posterior left ventricular wall in subsequent frames from the parasternal view in a representative healthy subject. (S=peak systolic velocity, D_E=peak early-diastolic velocity, D_M= peak mid-diastolic velocity, D_A=peak late-diastolic velocity)

Conclusion

Total heart movement within the chest can be detected by TDE, and has to be taken into account when TDE is analyzed. TDE confirms the anterior displacement of the heart during systole and posterior translation during diastole. Additionally, the velocity of translation in subjects without wall motion abnormalities can be estimated.

References

1. Assmann PE, Slager CJ, Van-der-Borden SG, Tijssen JG, Oomen JA, Roeland JRTC (1993) Comparison of models for quantitative left ventricular wall motion analysis from two-dimensional echocardiograms during acute myocardial infarction. Am J Cardiol 71:1262–9
2. Cao T, Shapiro SM, Bersohn MM, Liu SC, Ginzton LE (1993) Influence of cardiac motion on Doppler measurements using in vitro and in vivo models. J Am Coll Cardiol 22:271–6
3. Cape EG, Kim YH, Heinrich RS, Grimes RY, Muralidharan E, Broder JD, Schwammenthal E, Yoganathan AP, Levine RA (1993) Cardiac motion can alter proximal isovelocity surface area calculations of regurgitant flow. J Am Coll Cardiol 22:1730–7
4. Chaitman, BR, Bristow JD, Rahimtoola SH (1973) Left ventricular wall motion assessed by using a fixed external reference system. Circulation 48: 1043–54
5. Feneley M, Kearney L, Farnsworth A, Shanahan M, Chang V (1987) Mechanism of the development and resolution of paradoxical interventricular septal motion after uncomplicated cardiac surgery. Am Heart J 114:106–14
6. Force T, Bloomfield P, O'Boyle JE, Pietro DA, Dunlap RW, Khuri SF, Parisi AF (1983) Quantitative two-dimensional echocardiographic analysis of motion and thickening of the interventricular septum after cardiac surgery. Circulation 68:1013–20
7. Gelberg HJ, Brundage BH, Glantz S, Parmley WW (1979) Quantitative left ventricular wall motion analysis: a comparison of area, chord and radial methods. Circulation 59:991–1000
8. Gorcsan J, Katz WE, Mandarino WA, Pinsky MR (1994) Heterogeneous left ventricular septal and posterior wall velocities: quantitative temporal assessment by myocardial color Doppler imaging (abstract). Circulation 90:I–327
9. Ingels N, Daughters G, Stinson E, Alderman E (1980) Evaluation of methods for quantitation of left ventricular segmental wall motion in man using myocardial markers as a standard. Circulation 61:966–72
10. Kerber RE, Marcus ML, Wison R, Ehrhardt J, Abboud FM (1976) Effects of acute coronary occlusion on the motion and perfusion of the normal and ischemic interventricular septum. Cirulation 54:928–35
11. Kessler KM, Pefkaros K, Sequeira R, Myerburg RJ (1982) Quantitation and significance of horizontal cardiac motion in M-mode and two dimensional echocardiography. Am J Cardiol 50:520–34.
12. Mirro MJ, Rogers EW, Weyman AE, Feigenbaum H (1979) Angular displacement of the papillary muscles during the cardiac cycle. Circulation 60:327–33
13. Nguyen TN, Glantz SA (1993) Floating axis does not reduce motion artifacts in a model of left ventricular wall motion in dogs. Am J Physiol 264: H631–8
14. Pandian NG, Skorton DJ, Collins SM, Falsetti HL, Burke ER, Kerber RE (1983) Heterogeneity of left ventricular segmental wall thickening and excursion in 2-dimensional echocardiograms of normal human subjects. Am J Cardiol 51:1667–73
15. Thomsen PQ, Stahlberg F, Henriksen O (1993) Normal left ventricular wall motion measured with two-dimensional myocardial tagging. Acta Radiol 34:450–6
16. Zerhouni EA, Parish DM, Rogers WJ, Yang A, Shapiro E (1988) Human heart. Tagging with MR imaging – a method for noninvasive assessment of myocardial motion. Radiology 169:59–63

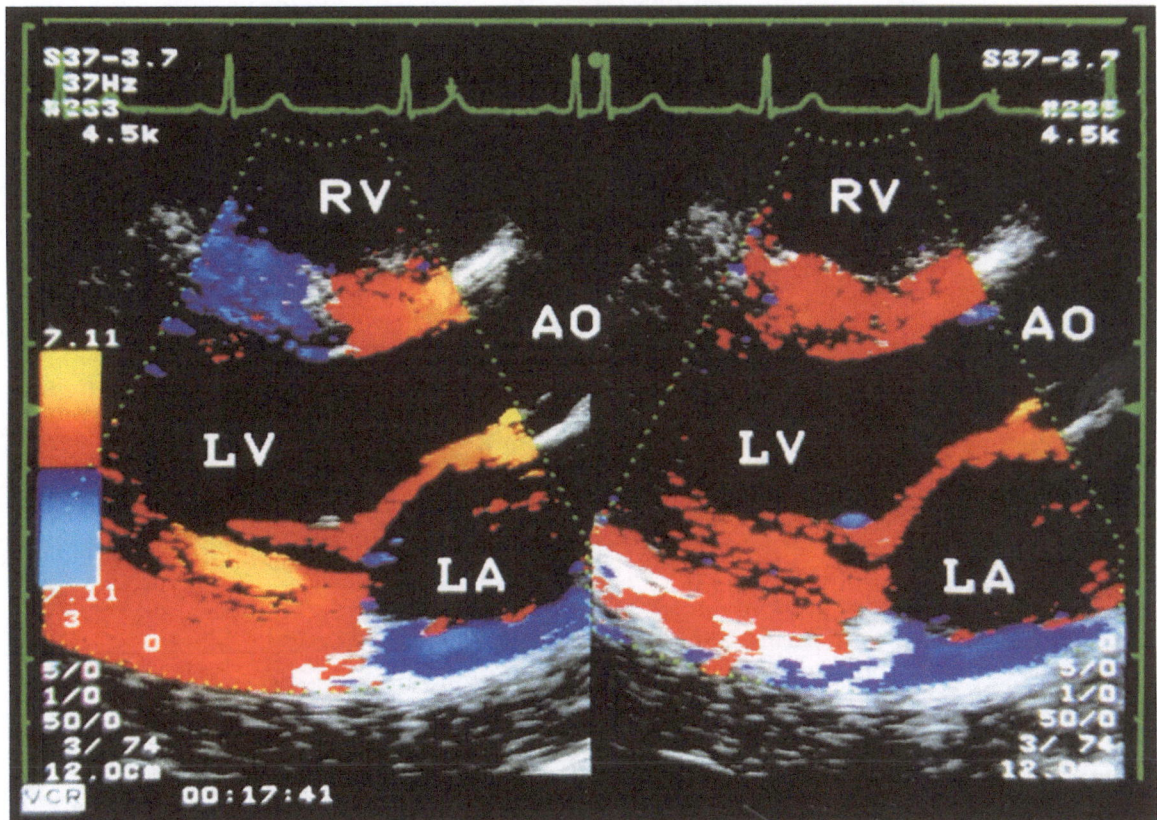

Fig. 6.3. Normal heart. Two-dimensional tissue Doppler echocardiographic image. Parasternal long axis view in mid systole *(left)* and late systole *(right)* using a 3.75 MHz transducer. Opposite directions of the interventricular septum and the posterior wall velocity in the mid-systolic frame. At late systole both the interventricular septum and the posterior left ventricular wall move in the same direction: toward the transducer, and both are coded by red. The whole heart moves toward the transducer in the parasternal view at this time. Note thickening of the posterior wall in the mid-systolic frame with enhanced velocity of the endocardial compared to epicardial layers. Endocardial layers are coded and yellow epicardial layers are red. Transmural velocity gradient (AO = aortic root, LA = left atrium, LV = left ventricle, RV = right ventricle)

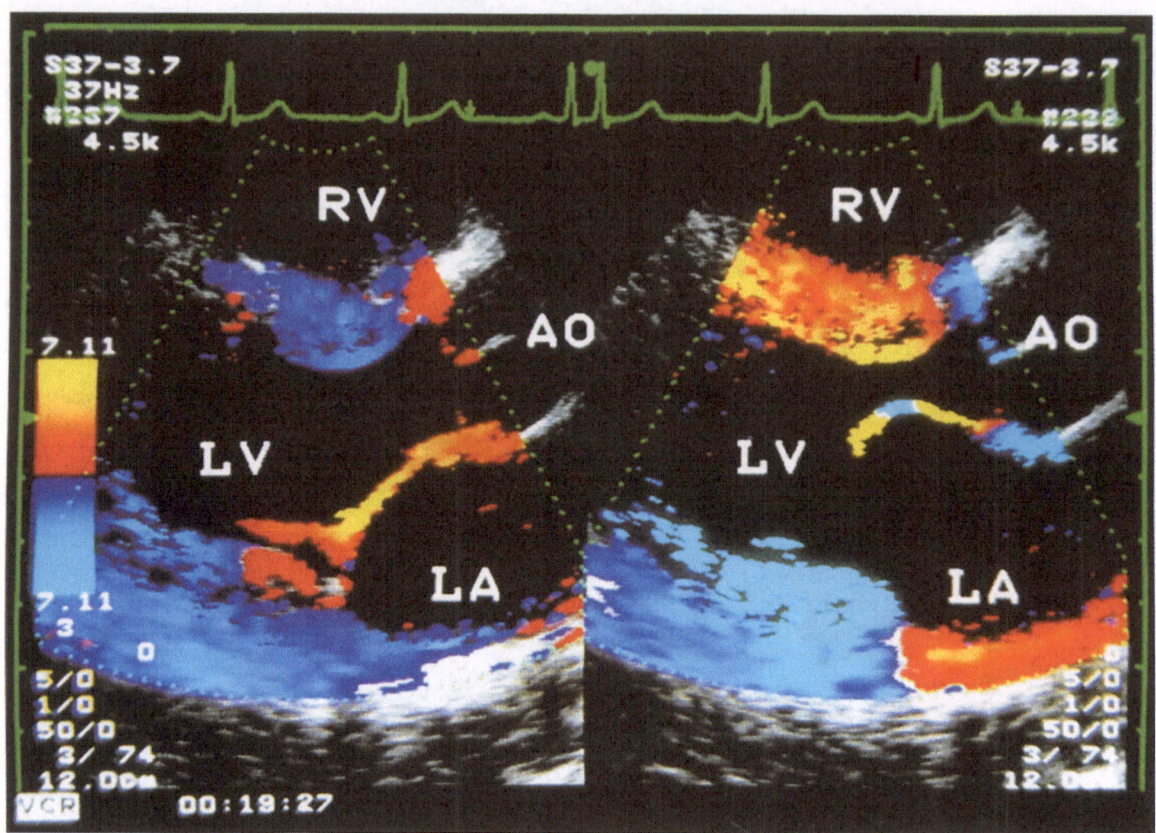

Fig. 6.4. Normal heart. Two-dimensional tissue Doppler echocardiographic image of the same subject as in Figure 6.3. Parasternal long axis view during isovolumic relaxation *(left)* and during rapid left ventricular filling *(right)* using a 3.75 MHz transducer. During isovolumic relaxation both the interventricular septum and the posterior left ventricular wall move in the same direction: away from the transducer. Note closed mitral and aortic valves. After opening of the mitral valve the rapid left ventricular filling starts. Both the interventricular septum and the posterior left ventricular wall move in opposite directions. (AO = aortic root, LA = left atrium, LV = left ventricle, RV = right ventricle)

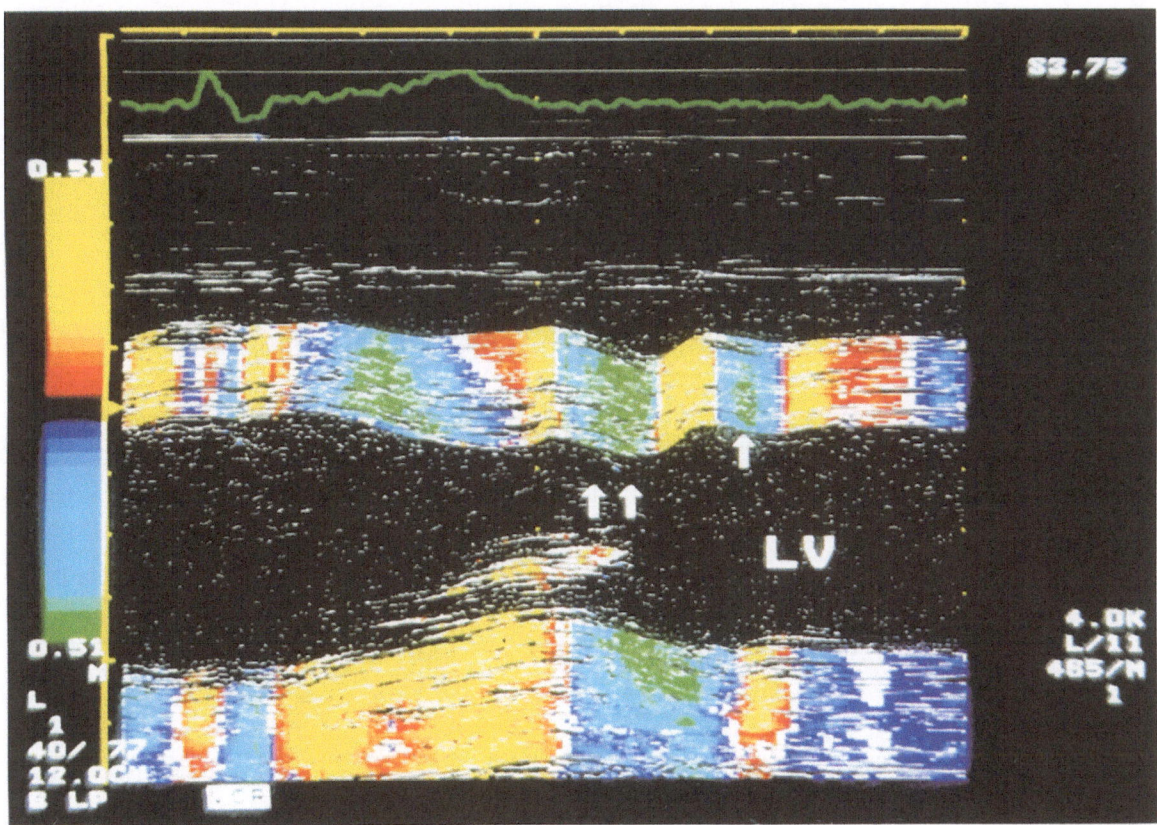

Fig. 6.5. Normal heart. M-mode tissue Doppler echocardiographic image of the interventricular septum and posterior left ventricular wall in the parasternal long axis view. Different velocities within the myocardium, particularly the interventricular septum, are indicated by different colors, green for high velocity values, and blue for low ones, representing the transmural velocity gradient. Backward movement of the interventricular septum preceding early diastolic rapid filling (*2 arrows*), and mid diastole (*1 arrow*). The color-coded display of the interventricular septum similar to the posterior wall in late systole and early diastole is clearly illustrated. This is related to movement of the heart within the chest in the antero-posterior direction. (LV = left ventricle)

Chapter 7 Assessment of Right Ventricular Wall Thickness by Tissue Doppler Echocardiography

H. J. Nesser

Introduction

Echocardiographic measurement of left ventricular wall thickness and its feasibility have been established with a good correlation to ventriculography [3] and surgical inspection [2], whereas the number of reports related to the thickness of the right ventricular wall is limited and the results remain controversial.

Sahn et al. [7] discussed poor recordings by a standard approach with the 2.25 MHz transducer, the most frequently used technique in adult echocardiography. Matsukubo et al. [5] could visualize echos from the right ventricular wall adequately in 90% of patients studied using the subxiphoid technique. On the other hand, this was not reproducible by Tsuda et al. [8], who had only a 50% success rate. They recommended an anterior approach with a 5.0 MHz transducer with the patient in a sitting position, which may limit image quality in clinical routine.

Other authors particularly refer to the fact that right ventricular mass measurement is less accurate because of unavoidable inclusion of epicardial fat [4].

Certainly, Doppler echocardiography allows an estimation of pulmonary artery pressure with good results in comparison to invasive studies [1, 9], but it offers only little or no information concerning the duration of pulmonary hypertension. Therefore, there is a need for a noninvasive technique providing an assessment of right ventricular wall morphology and function as accurate as possible, and a clear delimitation to the paracardial non moving tissue and the right ventricular cavity. Since tissue Doppler echocardiography offers a new imaging potential, we used this technique to compare the results with conventional echocardiography measuring right ventricular wall thickness in adults.

Subjects and Methods

Forty-one consecutive patients (mean age 52 ± 8 years) with various heart diseases were first examined by conventional echocardiography from parasternal technique in a left lateral position (TTE p), and subsequently by the subxiphoidal technique (TTE s). Imaging of the right ventricular free wall was performed simultaneously by two-dimensional echocardiography and the M-mode technique. Right ventricular (RV) wall thickness was measured at enddiastole and endsystole.

Color Coded Tissue Doppler Echocardiography (TDE)

Examinations were performed using a hard- and software modified ultrasound device (Toshiba Corp. Tokyo, Japan) with a phased array 3.75 or 2.5 MHz sector scanner. Pulse repetition frequency was 4.5–6 KHz, and frame rate 26–38/s, later on up to 58/s in the tissue Doppler mode.

To get optimal RV-wall images, four velocity scales at 2 cm/s, 4 cm/s, 8 cm/s, and 33 cm/s were used. The last 63 frames from the memory could be analyzed. M-mode and 2DE recordings were superimposed by the color-coded technique. RV-wall thickness was measured at enddiastole and endsystole using ECG recordings simultaneously for determining time correlation; thus, systolic increase of RV-wall was estimated.

Conventional Transesophageal Echocardiography (TEE)

was used as the reference method (Toshiba, biplane, 5 MHz probe).

Results

Feasibility

Whereas right ventricular wall could be imaged perfectly in only 63% of the patients from the transthoracic approach, and in 49% from the subcostal view by conventional echocardiography, useful measurements were possible in 100% of the patients by parasternal Tissue Doppler Echocardiography.

Especially in patients with endocardial and epicardial borders difficult to define by standard echocardiography, TDE showed a clear delineation of right ventricular tissue to the right ventricular cavity and paracardial structures (Figs. 7.1 a, b; 7.5 a, b; 7.6 a, b; 7.7 a).

Wall Measurements

Wall thickness estimated by TEE ranged from 2.2 to 11.7 mm in diastole, and from 2.4 to 12.2 mm in systole (Figs. 7.1 b, 7.2, 7.3 b).

The best correlation was obtained between TEE and TDE in diastole ($r = 0.92$/SEE ± 0.6 mm) as well as in systole ($r = 0.94$/SEE ± 0.7 mm). Correlation coefficients were $r = 0.85$/SEE ± 1.1 mm when TEE was compared with TTEp, and $r = 0.87$/SEE ± 1.1 mm with TTEs in systole; $r = 0.87$/SEE ± 1.1 mm and $r = 0.86$/SEE ± 0.9 mm in diastole, respectively.

Systolic increase of right ventricular wall thickness corresponded best between TDE and TEE ($r = 0.72$), and was worst comparing TTE s with TEE ($r = 0.27$).

Summary

Although six various views for RV-wall thickness measurements by two-dimensional echocardiography have been described by McKenna et al. [6], this method is still of limited value in clinical routine examinations. Tissue Doppler Echocardiography as a new quick, on-line and non-invasive technique seems to be accurate and feasible to estimate right ventricular wall thickness and to separate RV-cavity and paracardial stuctures from RV-wall tissue using the transthoracical parasternal approach (Figs. 7.5 a, b; 7.6 a, b; 7.7 a).

In our series TDE was superior to conventional echocardiography when using TEE as a reference method.

Since the correct delineation of RV endocardial border plays an important role in the assessment of RV-volume and -function, TDE has an additional potential to investigate right ventricular disease (Fig. 7.8).

References

1. Berger M, Haimowitz A, Van Toch A, Berdoff RL, Goldberg E (1985) Quantitative assessment of pulmonary hypertension in patients with tricuspid regurgitation. J Am Coll Cardiol 6:359–65
2. Feigenbaum H, Popp RL, Chip JN, Haine CL (1968) Left ventricular wall thickness measured by ultrasound. Arch Intern Med 121:391–5
3. Feigenbaum H, Popp RL, Wolfe SB et al. (1972) Ultrasound measurements of the left ventricle. A correlative study with angiography. Arch Intern Med 129:461–7
4. Kopelman HA et al. (1985) Right ventricular myocardial infarction in patients with chronic lung disease; possible role of right ventricular hypertrophy. J Am Coll Cardiol 5:1302–07
5. Matsukubo H, Matsuura T, Endo N et al. (1980) Echocardiographic measurement of right ventricular wall thickness in adults by anterior approach. Br Heart J 44:55–61
6. McKenna WJ, Kleinebenne A, Nihoyannopoulos P, Foal R (1988) Echocardiographic measurement of right ventricular wall thickness in hypertrophic cardiomyopathy; Relation to clinical and prognostic features. J Am Coll Cardiol 11:351–8
7. Sahn DJ, Demaria A, Kisslo J, Weyman A (1978) Recommendations regarding quantitation in M-mode echocardiographiy: results of a survey of echocardiographic measurements. Circulation 58:1072–83
8. Tsuda T, Sawayama T, Kawai N et al. (1980) Echocardiographic measurement of right ventricular wall thickness in adults by anterior approach. Br Heart J 44:55–61
9. Yock PG, Popp RL (1984) Noninvasive estimation of right ventricular systolic pressure by Doppler ultrasound in patients with tricuspid regurgitation. Circulation 70:657–62

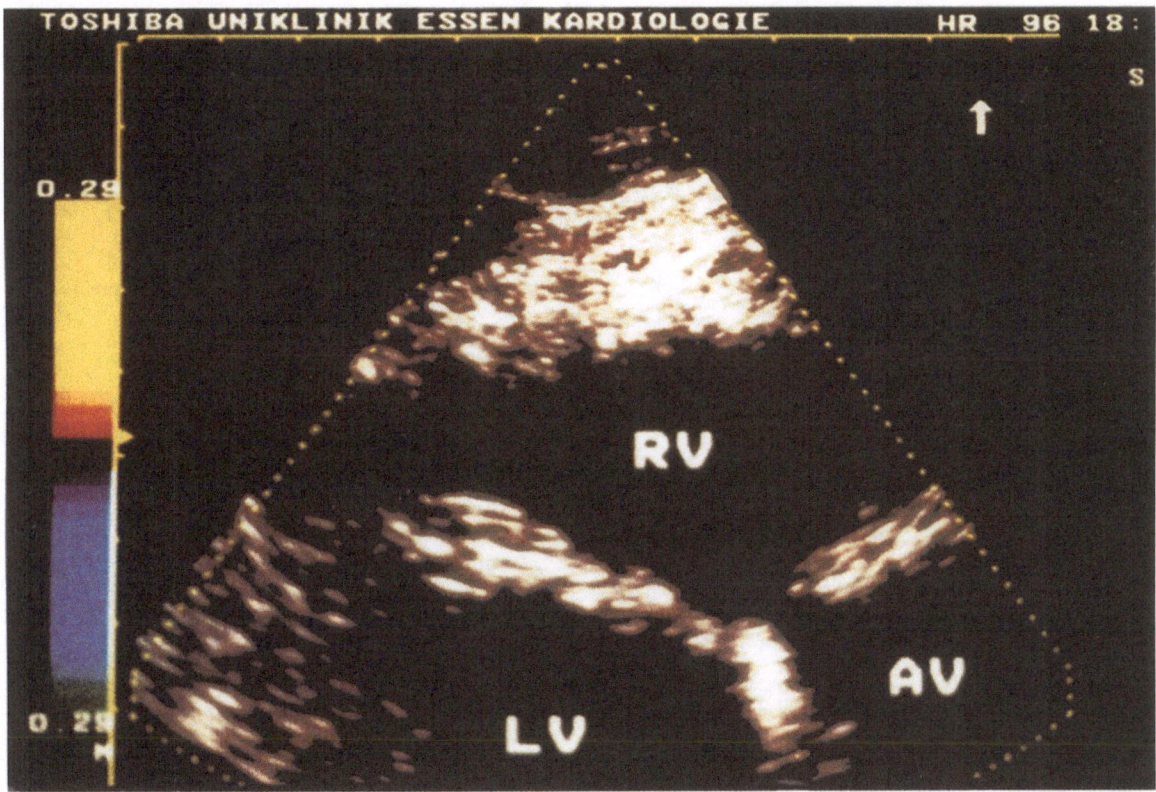

Fig. 7.1a. Conventional two-dimensional echocardiogram (magnified detail), parasternal long-axis view of the left side of the heart with proximal right ventricular outflow tract. Note that the right ventricular endocardium cannot be defined very clearly. Right ventricular pericardium cannot be separated from paracardial structures. (RV = right ventricle, AV = aortic valve, LV = left ventricle)

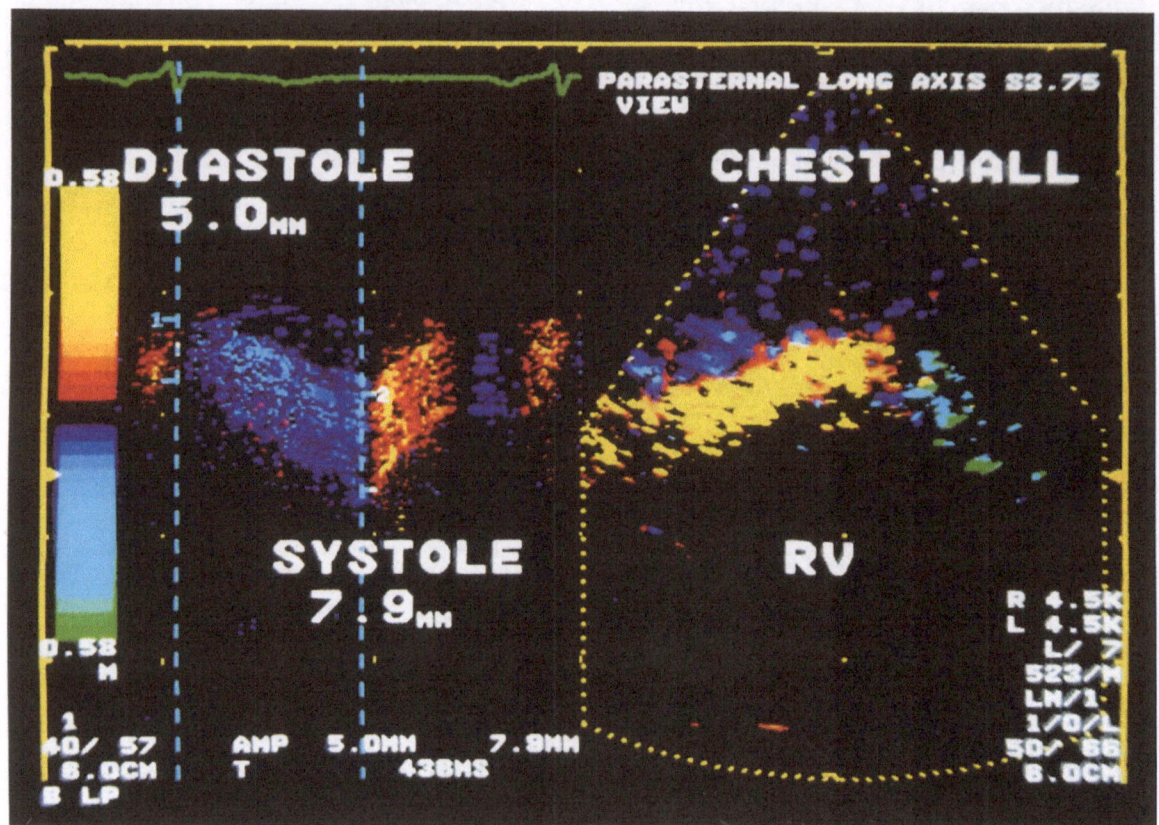

Fig. 7.1 b. TDE (magnified detail), parasternal long-axis view of the left side of the heart with proximal right ventricular outflow tract. *Right:* Two-dimensional imaging of the right ventricular endocardium, myocardium and pericardium during systole *(yellow color)*. The borders to the right ventricular cavity and paracardial structures are much better identifyable than in Fig. 1a. RV = right ventricle. *Left:* Simultaneous Tissue Doppler M-mode of right ventricular wall movement. Measurement of right ventricular wall thickness during endsystole *(blue color)* and end-diastole *(red color)* based on the clear edge detection. Thus, systolic increase and possible right ventricular hypertrophy can be estimated easier than with conventional echocardiography. Wall thickness during diastole: 5.6 mm, wall thickness during systole: 7.9 mm

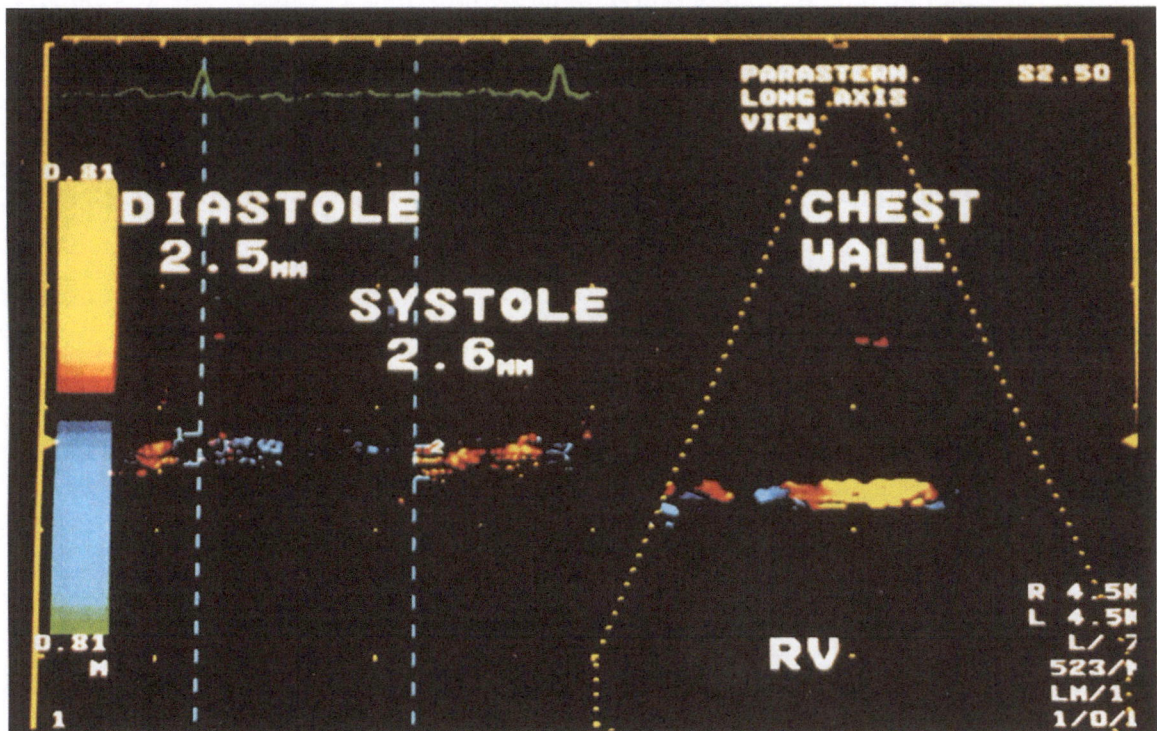

Fig. 7.2. Right ventricular myocardial infarction: TDE (magnified detail), parasternal long-axis view of the proximal right ventricular outflow tract. *Right:* Two-dimensional imaging of the right ventricular wall during diastole *(yellow color)*. Borders of the right ventricular cavity and paracardial structures are well defined. *Left:* Simultaneous Tissue Doppler M-mode of right ventricular wall. Note myocardial thinning and the lack of systolic increase of wall thickness due to myocardial infarction. (RV = right ventricle). Wall thickness during diastole 2.5 mm, wall thickness during systole: 2.6 mm

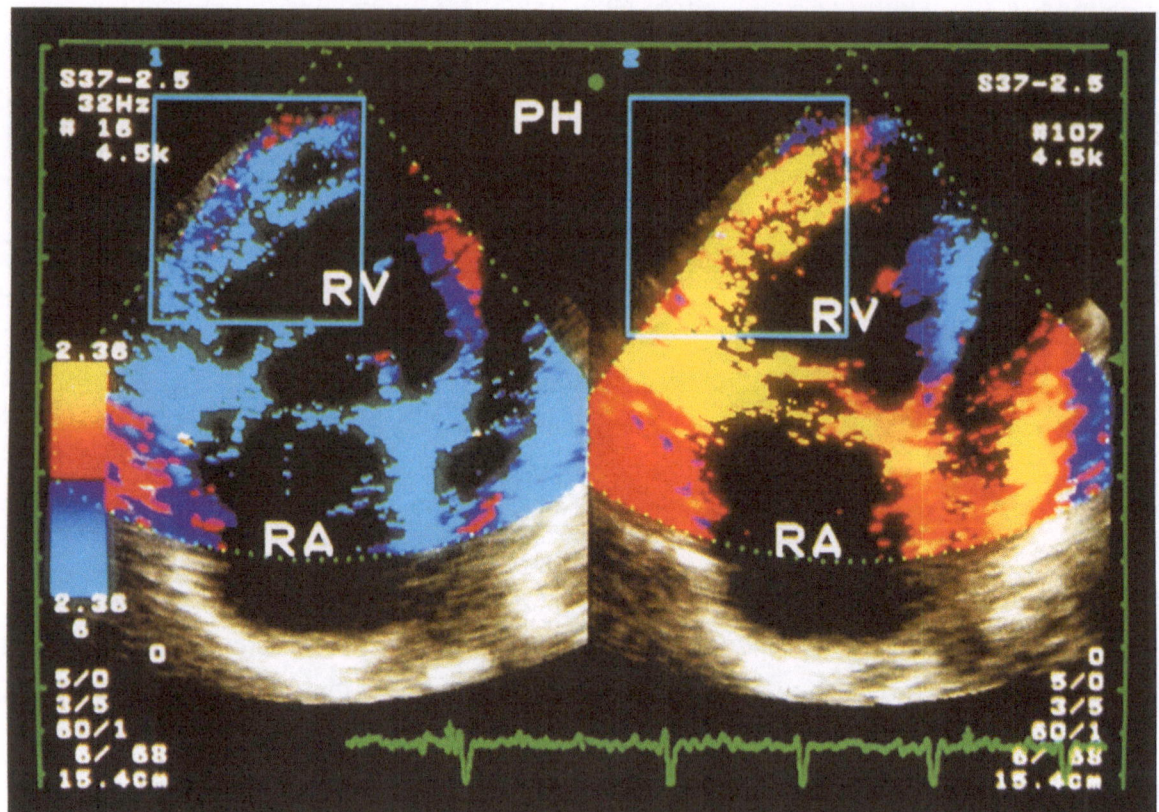

Fig. 7.3a. Chronic pulmonary hypertension (patient: female, 35 years). TDE, apical four-chamber view of the right ventricular lateral wall. Predominant right heart due to chronic pressure overload (cor pulmonale III). *Left:* Right ventricular wall during systole *(blue color, rectangle)*. Note paradoxical septal movement *(red color)* at the same time due to chronic right ventricular pressure overload. Asynchrony. *Right:* Right ventricular lateral wall during diastole *(yellow color, rectangle)*. Note paradoxical septal movement *(blue color)* at the same time. Significant right ventricular hypertrophy is visible. (RV = right ventricle, RA = right atrium, PH = pulmonary hypertension)

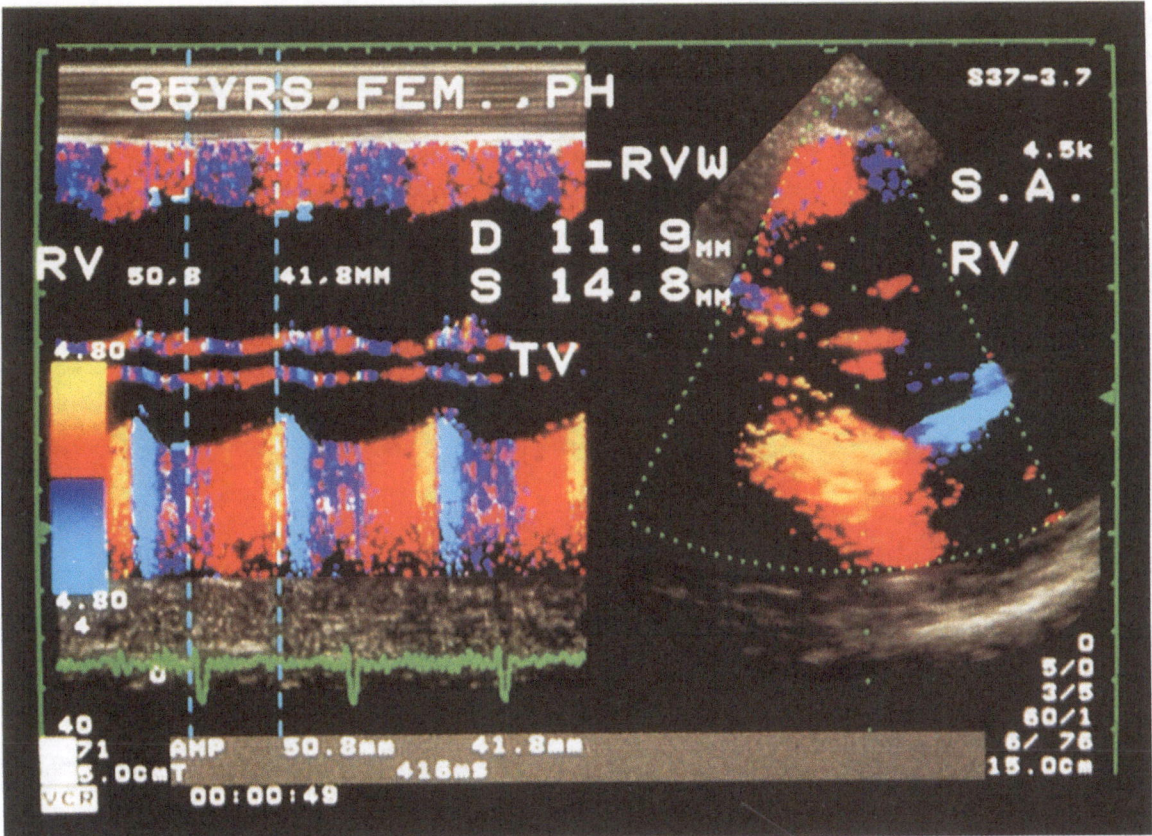

Fig. 7.3 b. Chronic pulmonary hypertension (patient female, 35 years). TDE, parasternal short axis view of the right ventricle. *Right:* Two-dimensional imaging of the hypertrophied right ventricle during systole. *Left:* Simultaneous Tissue Doppler M-mode of right ventricular wall movement. Measurement of right ventricular wall thickness during enddiastole *(red color)* and end-systole *(blue color, RVW)*. Note reduced systolic increase of right ventricular wall thickness and significant hypertrophy. Clear delineation of right ventricular borders. (RV = right ventricle, RVW = right ventricular wall, TV = tricuispid valve). Wall thickness during diastole: 11.9 mm, wall thickness during systole: 14.8 mm

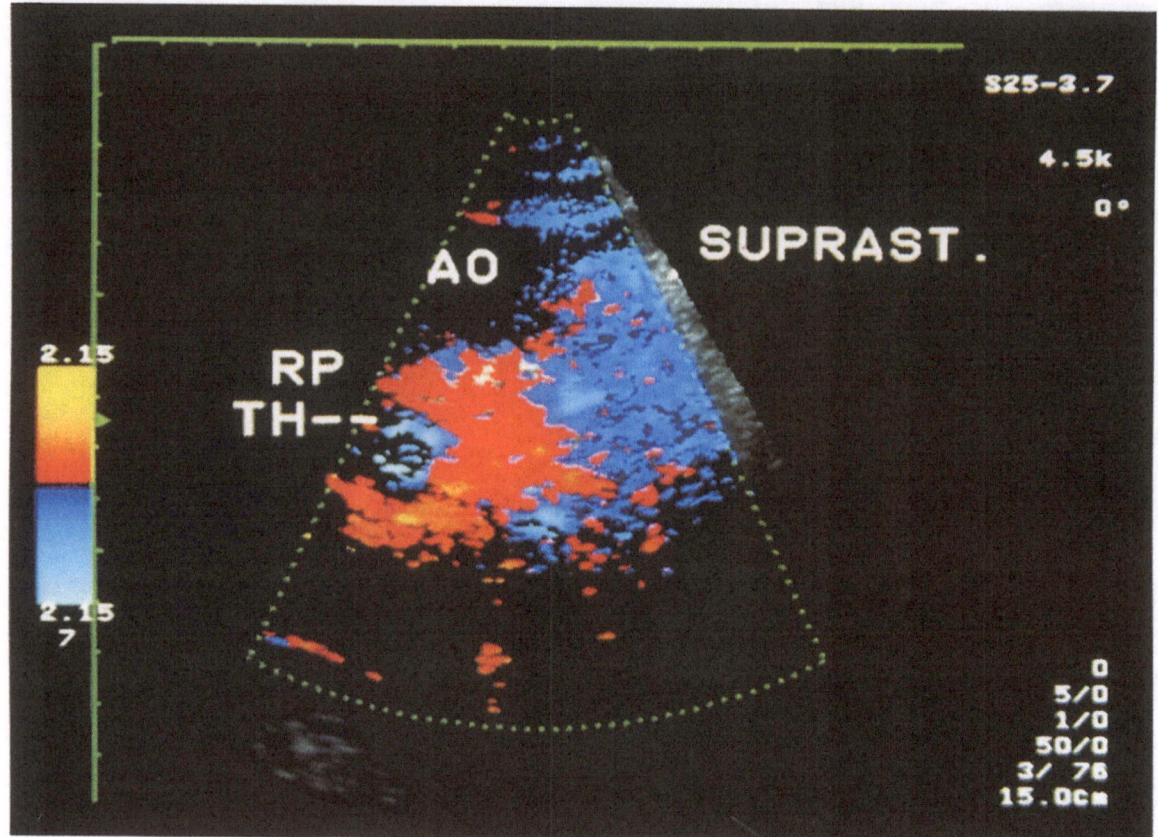

Fig. 7.4.a. Acute pulmonary embolism (patient: female, 57 years, acute pulmonary embolism postoperatively). TDE, suprasternal view, short axis of right pulmonary artery. During systole the right pulmonary artery is represented in red colors (movement anteriorly towards transducer). Structures within the vessel moving in opposite direction, represented in blue color, allow the identification of an intravascular thrombus which disappeared after thrombolysis

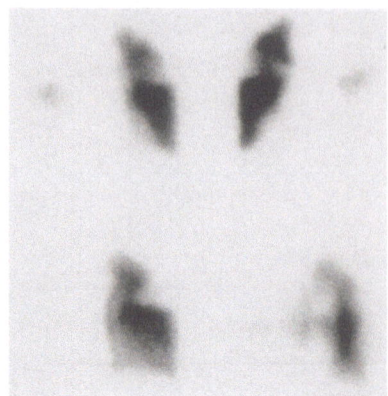

Fig. 7.4b. Lung perfusion scintigraphy, 60 m BqTc 99m MAA. *Above left:* ventral view, *above right:* dorsal view. *Below left:* right posterior oblique view (RPO), *below right:* left posterior oblique view (LPO). Amost complete perfusion defect of the right lung. Subsegmental perfusion defects of the anterior upper lobe and superior lower lobe of the left lung. (Reproduced with permission of B. Markt, M.D., Head of the Institute of Nuclear Medicine)

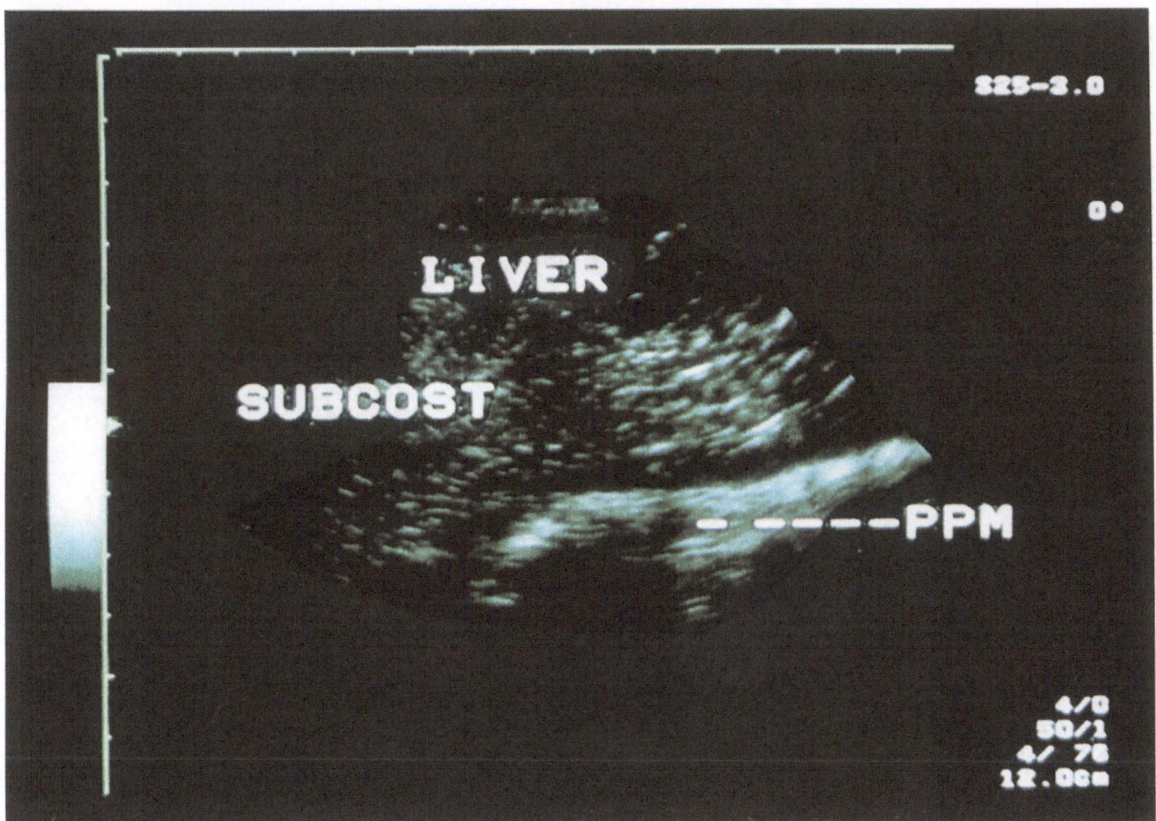

Fig. 7.5 a. Conventional two-dimensional echocardiogram (magnified detail), subcostal long-axis view of the heart showing the right ventricular diaphragmatic wall. (PPM = papillary muscle)

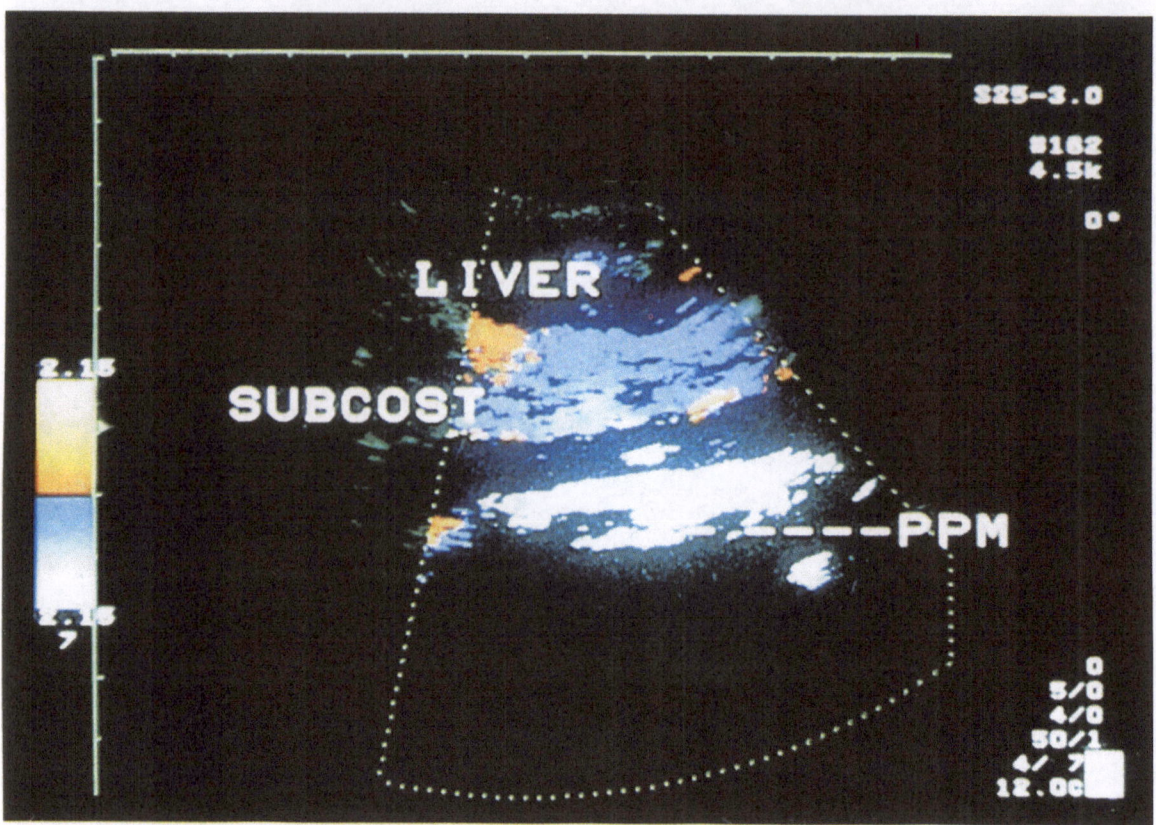

Fig. 7.5 b. TDE (magnified detail) during systole, subcostal long-axis view, right ventricular diaphragmatic wall. In comparison to Fig. 7.5 a, better imaging of the right ventricular wall is possible. Additionally, separation from the liver due to paracardial fat (without color because of lack of velocities) is imaged very well. As the structures are moving away from the transducer, blue colors are displayed. Right ventricular wall is moving much faster during systole (bright blue) than the liver during respiration (dark blue). (PPM = papillary muscle)

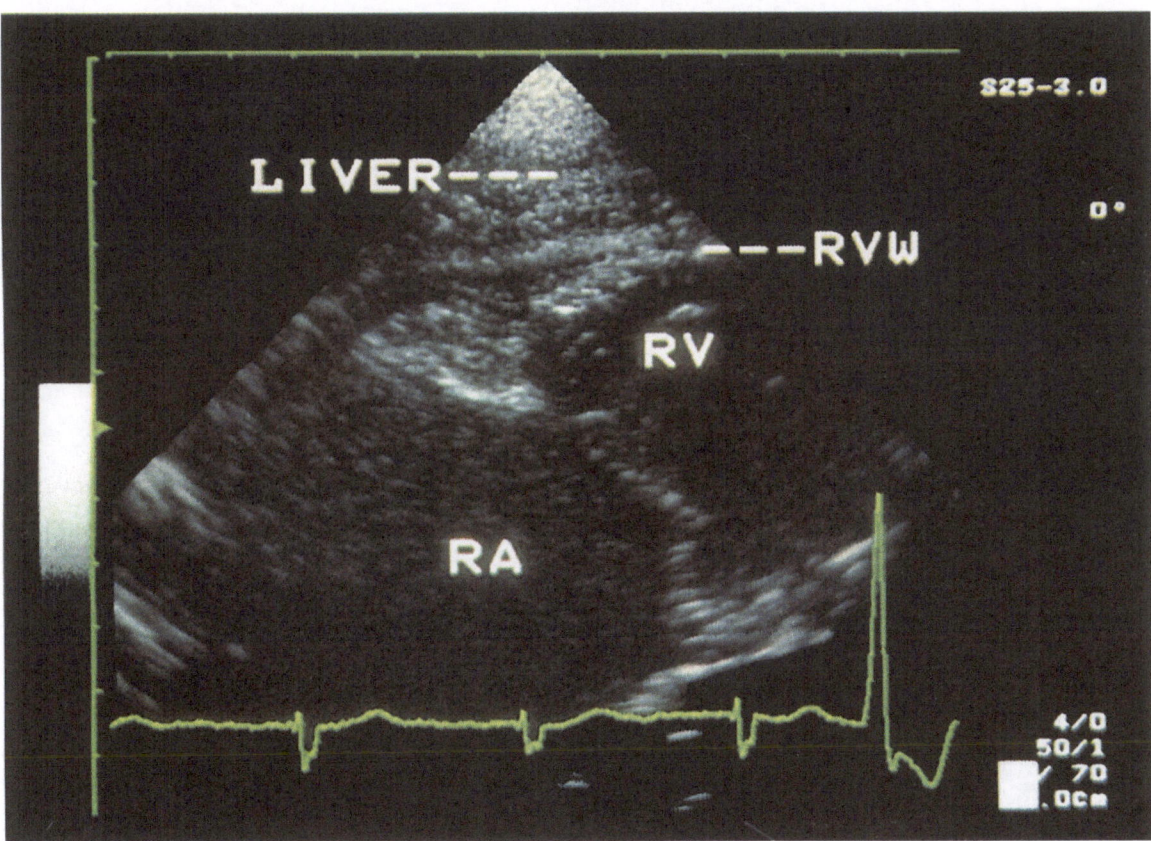

Fig. 7.6a. Structure identification by TDE. Conventional two-dimensional echocardiogram (magnified detail), subcostal long-axis view of the heart, right ventricular diaphragmatic wall. Unclear tissue at the atrioventricular area. (RVW = right ventricular wall, RV = right ventricle. RA = right atrium.)

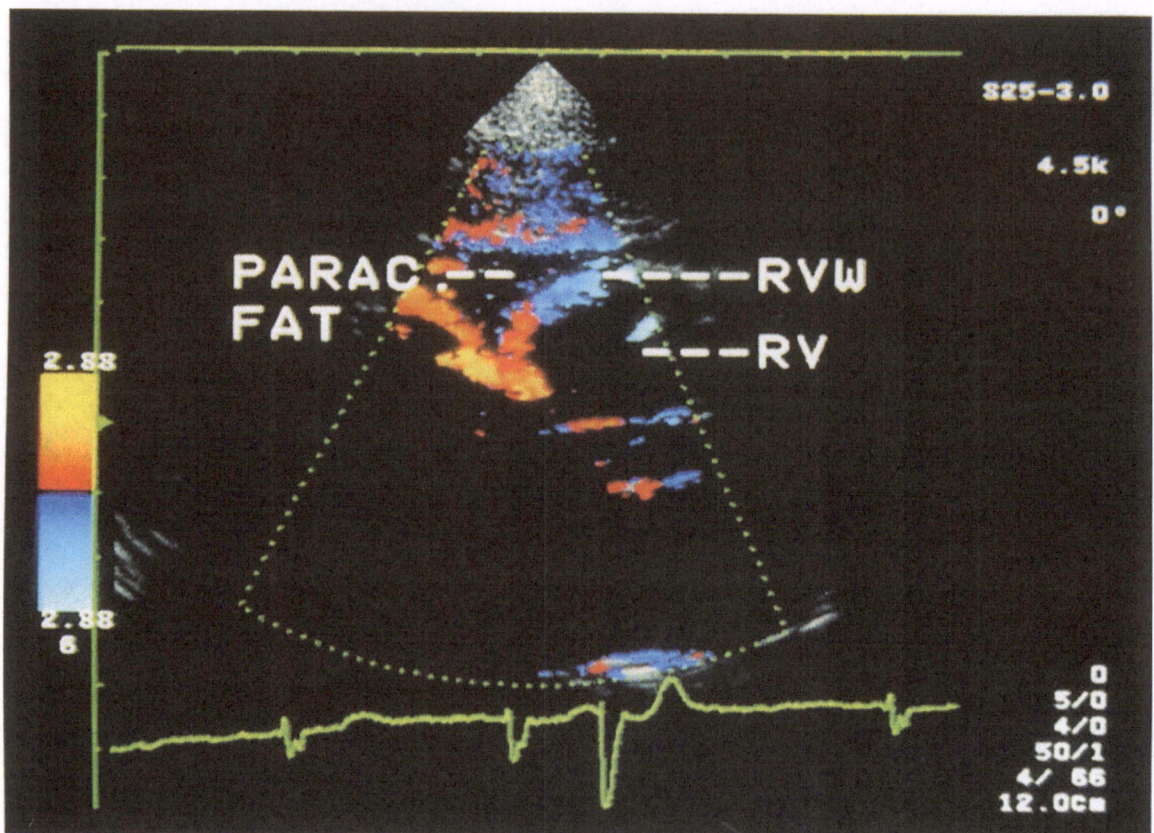

Fig. 7.6b. Structure identification by TDE. TDE (magnified detail), subcostal long-axis view, right ventricular diaphragmatic wall. In comparison to Fig. 6a, the liver, right ventricular and right atrial wall are clearly defined and separated from a tri- angular structure, which can be assessed as para- cardial fat. Due to lack of relevant velocities no colors are displayed within the structure. (RVW = right ventricular wall, RV = right ventricle)

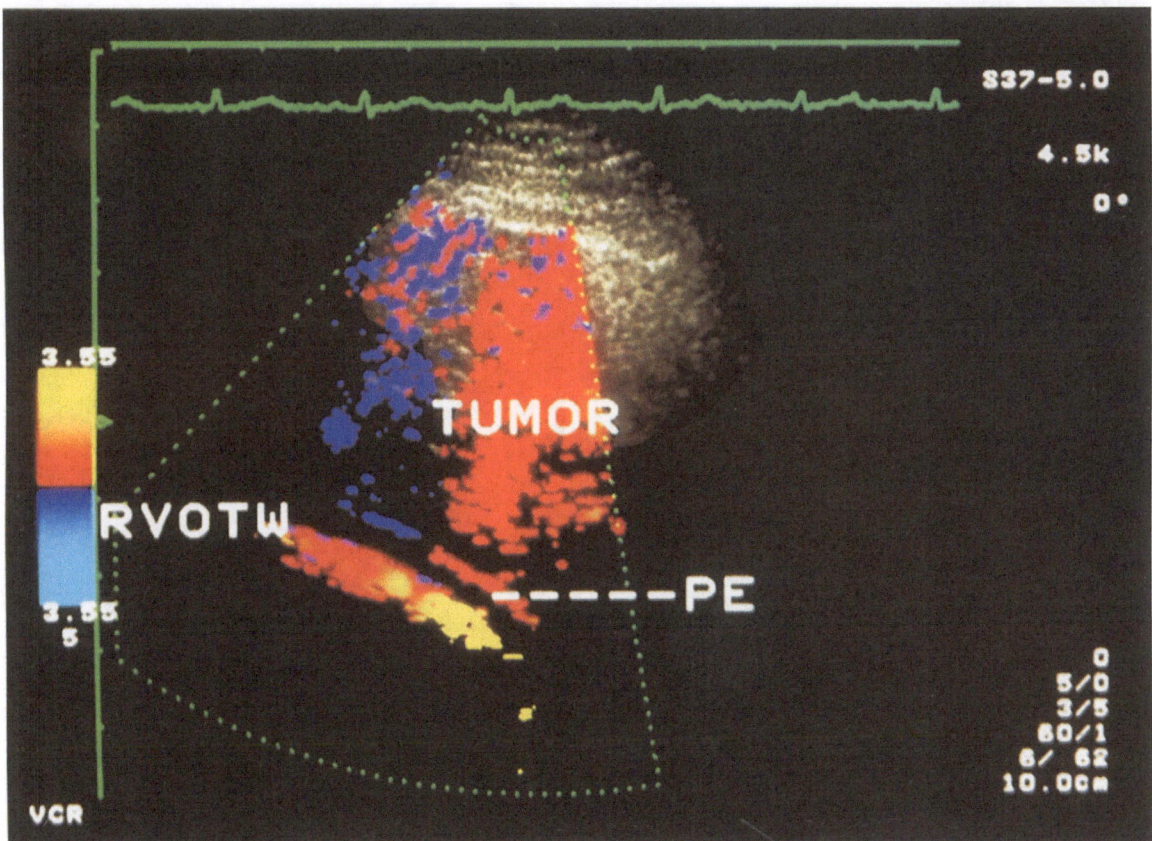

Fig. 7.7 a. Non-Hodgkin lymphoma (T-lymphoblastic). TDE (magnified detail), parasternal right ventricular outflow tract view of the right ventricular outflow tract. Structure identification.

Clear differentiation of the right ventricular outflow tract wall from pericardial effusion and a large malignant tumor mass (lymphoma). (RVOTW = right ventricular outflow tract wall, PE = pericardial effusion)

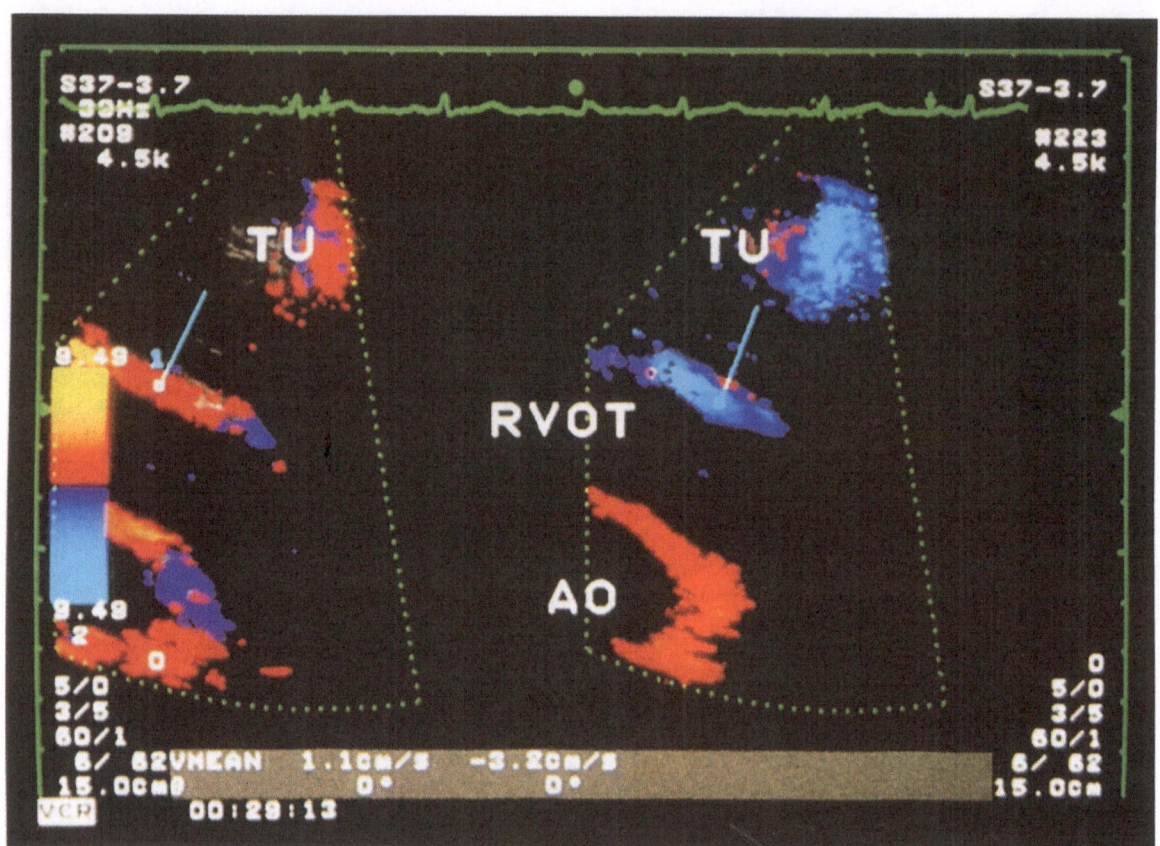

Fig. 7.7 b. Non-Hodgkin lymphoma (T-lymphoblastic). TDE (magnified detail), parasternal short-axis view of the aortic root. *Left:* right ventricular wall movement during systole *(red color)*. Due to myocardial involvement into the pericardial process a very low v_{mean} of 1.1 cm/s (1) is shown. *Right:* Right ventricular movement during diastole *(blue color)*. Diastolic v_{mean}: 3.2 cm/s. TU = tumor. (RVOT = right ventricular outflow tract, AO = aorta)

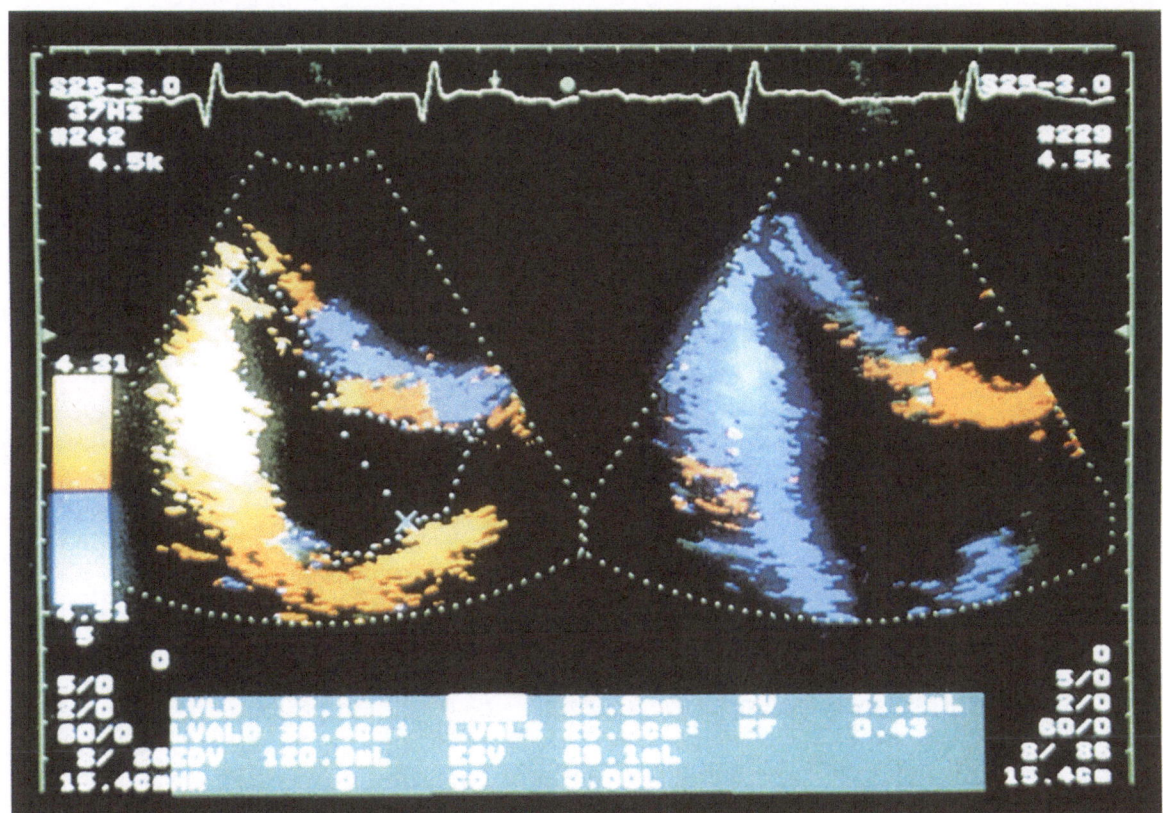

Fig. 7.8. TDE, modified apical view of the right ventricle. *Left:* Freeze frame of the right ventricle in endsystole. *Right:* Freeze frame of the right ventricle in enddiastole. In comparison to two-dimensional echocardiography tissue Doppler echocardiography allows a better definition of the right ventricular endocardial contour. Thus, better results in estimating right ventricular function, e.g., ejection fraction and RV volumes, can be expected.

Fig. 7.2. T1ω-modified ...

Chapter 8   Ischemic Heart Disease

J. Drozdz, R. Erbel

Cardiovascular ultrasound is the most convenient and most suitable technique of all cardiac imaging modalities. Worthwhile is the noninvasive registration of left ventricular shape changes in real time. Sensitivity and specificity in detecting left ventricular wall asynchrony has been reported [1, 4, 5, 7]. But there are still limitations and a need for ongoing development for quantification of global and regional left ventricular function [4, 5, 7, 8, 11, 18].

Analysis of global left ventricular function has meanwhile been standardized [21]. For quantification of left ventricular wall motion three main methods have been proposed: hemichordal, radial and trapezoid methods (Figs. 5.3, 6.1/6.2), and all can use floating-axis or fixed-axis referencing systems [1, 11, 16]. However, many disadvantages of each method still exist and manual tracing of the endocardial borders is necessary [10, 11, 18]. No standardization has been reached.

Newly introduced to the clinical routine are automatic border detection systems which make on-line analysis of left ventricular shape changes possible [19]. However, there is still a need for new methods for on-line noninvasive quantification of left ventricular function, particularly those which will be independent of geometric assumptions.

The newest echocardiographic method for on-line determination of myocardial wall velocity is tissue Doppler echocardiography (TDE) [2, 3, 9, 14, 15, 20, 22–25]. The normal pattern of myocardial wall velocity estimated by TDE is described in chapter 5. The velocities of ischemic left ventricular myocardium differ from those in the healthy subject [2, 3, 15, 22, 24]. This chapter summarizes the experiences in TDE evaluation of patients with ischemic heart disease.

New Diagnostic Approach by TDE

Wall Motion vs. Wall Velocity

TDE provides new information that has not been previously available: myocardial wall velocity [3, 17, 24, 27]. It is of interest to distinguish wall motion and wall velocity. Wall motion reflects the amplitude of the wall movement. Conventional two-dimensional (2-D) echocardiography provides the possibility to study wall motion [4, 5, 7, 8, 17, 18] and has been used for detecting disturbed regional function at rest as well as during exercise, or during pharmacological stimulation. In order to detect left ventricular asynchrony, cine ventriculograms were digitized and plotted against time in a three-dimensional mode. The on-line evaluation is not possible. Analysis of time relations of myocardial wall motion is based mainly on M-mode echocardiographic studies [6, 12, 13].

Velocities of every part of the heart at every moment of the cardiac cycle can be visualized and quantified by TDE. Moreover, recognizing different phases of myocardial velocity, estimation of peak wall velocity, and velocity dissociation across the wall are possible [2, 3, 15, 20, 24].

Very promising parameters are systolic and diastolic time intervals measured by TDE M-mode and the ECG.

TDE Assessment of Left Ventricular Function

Assessment of myocardial wall velocity can be based on visual observation of color-coding of the myocardial wall. However, the visual assessment of wall velocity in real-time is not useful, as the velocities change rapidly. Frame-by-frame and slow-motion analysis are necessary (Figures 8.1–8.4). The ultrasonic beam should be directed to regions of interest from different transducer positions starting with standard parasternal and apical views.

Myocardial velocities can also be semi-quantitatively assessed by the analysis of the color-coding of the same part of the myocardium at different times in the TDE M-mode image with very high temporal and axial resolution (Figures 8.9–8.12).

The examination includes M-mode investigation from standard parasternal view, but also from apical views. However, the ultrasonic beam does not scan the same part of the wall during the entire cardiac cycle, because of the cardiac movement (Figures 8.9–8.12).

Adjustment of machine settings gives the possibility to increase the visualization of every range of wall velocity by assigning different colors to different velocities among the range of interest. Even the velocity scale, which differentiated only velocity values independent of velocity direction, can be used. This allows semiquantitative, visual comparison between systole and diastole.

The examination of patients with poor image quality is possible using color-coded TDE. In general, TDE improves image quality and both endocardial and epicardial borders can be more easily differentiated. The differentiation of myocardial structures from artifacts becomes possible. Helpful is switching off the conventional black and white image, and using only the Doppler signals, which help to analyze myocardial wall velocities.

The examination technique in patients with poor image quality may be primarily based on the TDE M-mode recording.

A semi-quantitative analysis of the regional myocardial function can be performed by comparison of the images obtained in patients with those obtained in healthy subjects. Frame-by-frame TDE image sequence and TDE M-mode analysis is important in order to detect the abnormal myocardial velocity pattern.

Dyskinesis

In the two-dimensional TDE image left ventricular dyskinesis can be visualized as a part of myocardial wall moving during systole away from the center of gravity of the left ventricle. The center of gravity was previously localized along the axis from the antero-lateral aortic valve edge to the apex at a point equal to 69% of the distance [11].

The center of gravity can be localized by TDE as the point of color reversal between apical and the remaining segments of the left ventricle. The dyskinetic segments in systole show an outward movement when the other parts are moving inward.

M-mode TDE renders information about when and how long the systolic dyskinetic motion persists (Figure 8.13). The time of peak velocity of dyskinetic motion can be estimated. The time estimation of diastolic motion of the dyskinetic region is provided. Only interpretation of the color reversal is necessary, whereas, conventionally, sophisticated analysis with frame-by-frame outlining endocardial border segments had to be done.

Akinesis

The akinetic left ventricular wall does not move during the cardiac cycle in regard to the center of gravity. However, akinetic regions of the left ventricle may show a passive movement due to cardiac motion, which is most pronounced in the posterior wall. Thus, these segments may still be color-coded by TDE. The akinesis can be confirmed by TDE using the model of subtraction of velocities from left ventricular wall velocity.

Hypokinesis/Asynchrony

A more substantial problem of myocardial hypokinesis is assessment by TDE. The hypokinetic myocardial wall is moving toward the center of gravity of the left ventricle, but its excursion is below the normal range. An analysis of wall thickening instead of wall motion is independent of geometric assumption. For TDE, again the analysis of the velocity pattern is very helpful (Figure 8.14). As a result of perfusion abnormality asynchrony of the ventricular wall develops as an early sign Fig. 8.1. By TDE a disturbed pattern of velocity is clearly seen because the homogeneous inward or outward movement is absent. This sign has a high sensitivity and specificity (Figure 8.1). It seems to be that analysis of the regional diastolic TDE pattern is even more helpful than the systolic pattern. This reflects the fact that diastolic dysfunction occurs before systolic changes are observed.

Peak Systolic and Early-Diastolic Wall Velocities in Hypokinesis

Most often the mean and peak systolic velocities are lower than those of the same part of the myocardium in healthy subjects [3, 15]. More affected are early diastolic velocities. In coronary artery disease the peak early-diastolic velocity to peak systolic myocardial velocity ratio is markedly reduced (Figures 8.10, 8,13, 8.16).

In patients with ischemic artery disease, the peak late diastolic velocity seems to be higher than the peak early diastolic velocity, as M-mode TDE image suggests. This may be due to an increased atrial pressure during ventricular filling as indicated by Doppler analysis of the mitral inflow with increased A-wave and reduced E-wave velocity (Figure 8.15). But TDE offers analysis of regional diastolic dysfunction, whereas conventional Doppler only reflects changes of the global function.

Transmural Velocity Pattern

In addition to the reduction of left ventricular wall velocities and temporal sequences, it can be observed that the endocardial layers of the left ventricle lose their higher velocities compared to the epicardial layers [24]. The endocardial to epicardial velocity ratio is reduced (myocardial velocity gradient reduction), and the velocities across the myocardial wall become more homogeneous. The endocardial layers are first involved when coronary flow decreases or increased oxygen consumption occurs with inadequate coronary blood flow.

The calculation of the myocardial velocity gradient across the myocardial wall may be a new useful parameter for analyzing myocardial function in coronary artery disease, and cardiomyopathy [24].

Contrast echocardiography is available as an alternative method to study regional transmural flow disturbances. But this method has been, up to now, invasive, as the contrast material has to be injected into the coronary artery. Agents, which can be injected intravenously and opacify left ventricular myocardium will be more helpful, but are not yet available. Therefore, the detection and measurement of the transmural velocity gradient is important for clinical cardiology.

Time Sequence Analysis

The onset of systolic velocity occurs after the Q-wave in the ECG in healthy subjects (preejection period, PEP $= 66 \pm 15$ ms). Subtraction of the isovolumic contraction time (ICT) from the PEP time represent the electrical activation. ICT represents the time from mitral valve closure to aortic valve opening. Previously, this could be determined using dual M-mode recordings or dual Doppler flow velocity recordings of the mitral inflow and the aortic outflow. But the results reflect only the global hemodynamics. TDE allows the assessment of the time sequences in selected regions of the left or right ventricular myocardium.

Regional PEP is prolonged in patients with angiographically documented severe hypokinesis (>80 ms). The time delay can be used as a parameter of regional systolic myocardial function. A further potentially useful parameter of the systolic function seems to be the time between Q-wave on the ECG to peak systolic velocity (in healthy subjects: 129 ± 23 ms). It was also prolonged in patients with significant coronary artery disease and documented hypokinesis (>150 ms) (Figures 8.17, 8.18).

New analysis of regional myocardial function in diastole revealed prolongation of such time intervals as regional isovolumic relaxation time and the time between color reversal and peak early diastolic velocity. This time can be prolonged in some patients with coronary artery disease (>130 ms, normal values 94 ± 36 ms).

Conclusion

TDE offers several new parameters for assessing systolic and diastolic regional left ventricular function. Coronary artery disease shows in TDE asynchrony of the left ventricle. This may be a new sign to demonstrate myocardial viability. Significant coronary luminal narrowing leads to disturbed color pattern of the walls in systole as well as in diastole.

In coronary artery disease the increase of myocardial velocities in the subendocardial layers compared to the epicardial layers disappears.

Parameters based on TDE systolic and diastolic time intervals allow a quantitative assessment of regional myocardial function. Not only global but also regional time intervals can be determined. New parameters of regional myocardial function are found.

References

1. Assmann PE, Slager CJ, Van-der-Borden SG, Tijssen JG, Oomen JA, Roeland JR (1993) Comparison of models for quantificative left ventricular wall motion analysis from two-dimensional echocardiograms during acute myocardial infarction. Am J Cardiol 71:1262–9

2. Bach DS, Armstrong WF, Donovan CL, Hummel JD, Bolling SF, Muller DW (1994) Quantitative assessment of regional systolic and diastolic myocardial velocities during transient ischemia and reperfusion. Circulation 90:I-327

3. Drozdz J, Schön F, Nesser HJ, Erbel R (1994) Colour-coded tissue Doppler echocardiography – a new method for quantification of cardiac wall motion (abstract). Eur J C P E 4:248

4. Erbel R, Brennecke R, Görge G, Mohr-Kahaly S, Wittlich N, Zotz R, Meyer J (1989) Accuracy and limitations of two-dimensional echocardiography in quantitative evaluation of left ventricular function. Z Kardiol 78:131–42

5. Erbel R, Schweizer P, Meyer J, Krebs W, Yalkinoglu Ö, Effert S (1985) Sensivity of cross-sectional echocardiography in detection of impaired global and regional left ventricular function: prospective study. Int J Cardiol 7:375–389

6. Erbel R, Schweizer P (1980) The diagnostic value of echocardiography in coronary artery disease – I. M-mode echocardiography. Z Kardiol 69:391–7

7. Erbel R, Schweizer P, Meyer J, Krebs W, Effert S (1980) Regional myocardial function in coronary artery disease at rest and during atrial pacing. Eur J Cardiol 11:183–99

8. Erbel R, Schweizer P, Pyhel N, Hadre U, Meyer J, Krebs W, Effert S (1980) Quantitative Analyse regionaler Kontraktionstörungen des linken Ventrikels im zweidimensionalen Echokardiogramm. Z Kardiol 69:562–72

9. Gorcsan J, Katz WE, Mandarino WA, Pinsky MR (1994) Heterogenous left ventricular septal and posterior wall velocities: quantitative temporal assessment by myocardial color Doppler imaging (abstract). Circulation 90:I-327

10. Görge G, Erbel R, Brennecke R, Rupprecht HJ, Todt M, Meyer J (1992) High-resolution two-dimensional echocardiography improves the quantification of left ventricular function. J Am Soc Echocardiogr 5:125–34

11. Ingels N, Daughters G, Stinson E, Alderman E (1980) Evaluation of methods for quantitation of left ventricular segmental wall motion in man using myocardial markers as a standard. Circulation 61:966–72

12. Kounis NG, Zavras GM, Papadaki PJ, Soufras GD, Kitrou MP (1989) Effects of nitroglycerin on myocardial excursions and velocities in the early hours of acute myocardial infarction. Angiology 40:783–90

13. Kounis NG, Zavras GM, Soufras GD, Kitrou M (1989) Systolic and diastolic septal and posterior wall echocardiographic measurements in normal subjects. Angiology 40:521–6

14. McDicken WN, Sutherland GR, Moran CM, Gordon LN (1992) Colour Doppler velocity imaging of the myocardium. Ultrasound Med Biol 18:651–4

15. Miyatake K, Yamagishi M, Tanaka N, Sasaki T, Ohe T, Yamazaki N, Mine Y, Sano A, Hirama M (1993) A new method for evaluation of left ventricular wall motion by color-coded tissue Doppler echocardiography: in vitro and in vivo studies (abstract). Circulation 88:I-48

16. Nguyen TN, Glantz SA (1993) Floating axis does not reduce motion artifacts in a model of left ventricular wall motion in dogs. Am J Physiol 264:H631–8

17. Pandian NG, Kerber RE (1982) Two-dimensional echocardiography in experimental coronary stenosis. I. Sensitivity and specificity in detecting transient myocardial dyskinesis: comparison with sonomicrometers. Circulation 66:597–602

18. Pandian NG, Skorton DJ, Collins SM, Falsetti HL, Burke ER, Kerber RE (1983) Heterogeneity of left ventricular segmental wall thickening and excursion in 2-dimensional echocardiograms of normal human subjects. Am J Cardiol 51:1667–73

19. Perez JE, Waggoner AD, Barzilai B, Melton HE, Miller JG, Sobel BE (1992) On-line assessment of ventricular function by automatic boundary detection and ultrasonic backscatter imaging. J Am Coll Cardiol 19:313–20

20. Raisinghani A, Donaghey L, Nozaki S, Dittrich H, DeMaria A (1994) New approaches to the evaluation of LV function: assessment of transmural myocardial velocity gradients and diastolic relaxation rates by Doppler tissue imaging (abstract). Circulation 90:I-327

21. Schiller NB, Shah PM, Crawford M, DeMaria A, Devereux R, Feigenbaum H, Gutgessell H, Reichek N, Sahn D, Schnittger I, Silverman NH, Tajik AJ (1989) Recomendation for quantification of the left ventricle by two-dimensional echocardiography. J Am Soc Echocardiogr 2:358–64

22. Stewart MJ, Groundstroem KW, Sutherland GR, Moran CM, Fleming A, Fenn LN, McDicken WN (1993) Myocardial imaging by colour Doppler coded velocity mapping – a new method for the assessment of myocardial contractility (abstract). Eur Heart J 14:467

23. Sutherland GR, Stewart MJ, Groundstroem KW, Moran CM, Fleming A, Gueil-Peris FJ, Riemersma RA, Fenn LN, Fox KA, McDicken WN (1994) Color Doppler myocardial imaging: a new technique for the assessment of myocardial function. J Am Soc Echocardiogr 7:441–58

24. Uematsu M, Miyatake K, Yamagishi M, Tanaka N, Nagata S, Sasaki T, Sano A, Yamazaki N, Mine Y, Hirama M (1994) Myocardial velocity gradient as a new method to quantitate regional left ventricular wall motion abnormalities (abstract). Circulation 90:I-326

25. Yamazaki N, Mine Y, Sano A, Hirama M, Miyatake K, Yamagishi M, Tanaka N (1994) Analysis of ventricular wall motion using color-coded tissue Doppler imaging system. Jpn J Appl Phys 33:3141–6

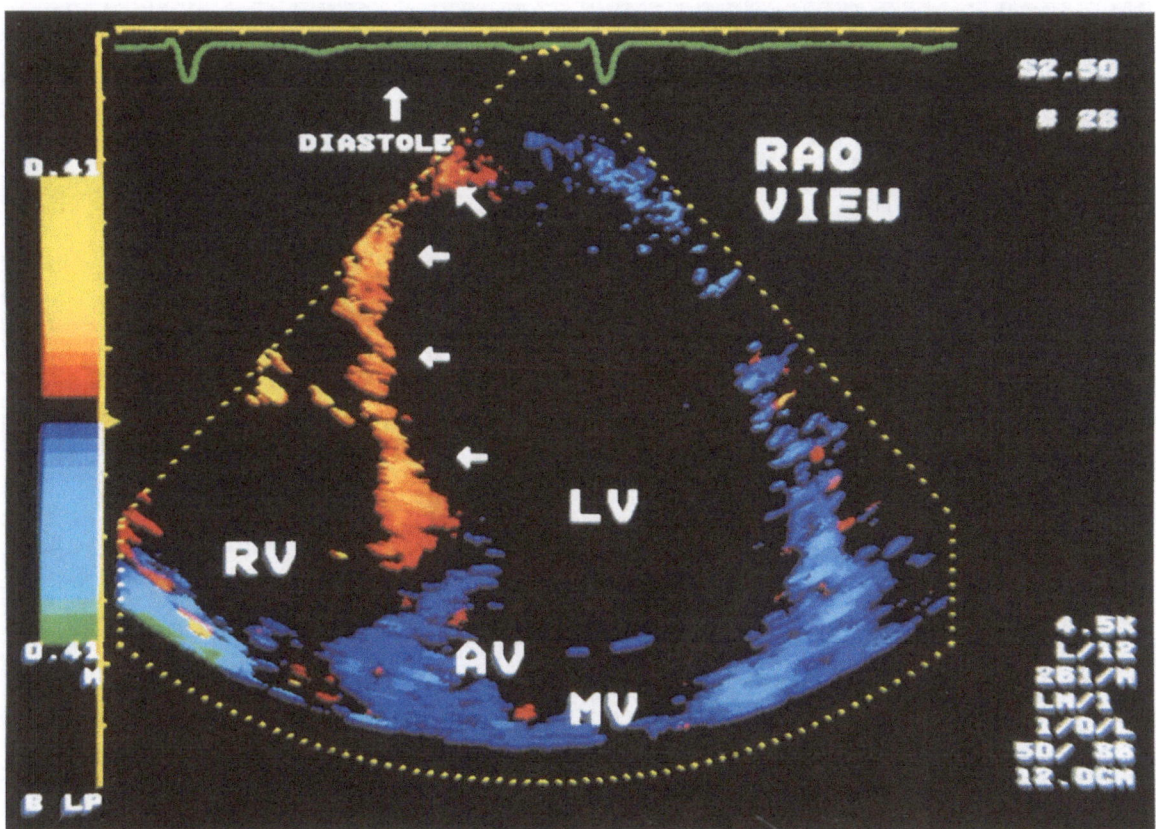

Fig. 8.1. Coronary artery disease. Asynchrony of the left ventricle. Apical long axis view using a 2.5 MHz transducer. Early diastolic frame. Machine settings are: non-color-coded velocities up to 0.30 cm/s, red- or dark blue-coded velocities up to 1.3 cm/s, yellow-coded forward velocities over 1.3 cm/s, bright blue-coded backward velocities from 1.3 cm/s up to 4.2 cm/s, and green-coded backward velocities over 4.2 cm/s. During early diastole the lateral wall of the left ventricle, mitral annulus and aortic root are moving away from the transducer. In contrast, the interventricular septum moves toward the transducer. The velocity of the asynchrony of the interventricular septum is about 1.3 cm/s in regard to the ultrasonic beam. After angle correction the velocity of the interventricular septum is about 1.9 cm/s. (AV = aortic valve, LV = left ventricle, MV = mitral valve, RV = right ventricle)

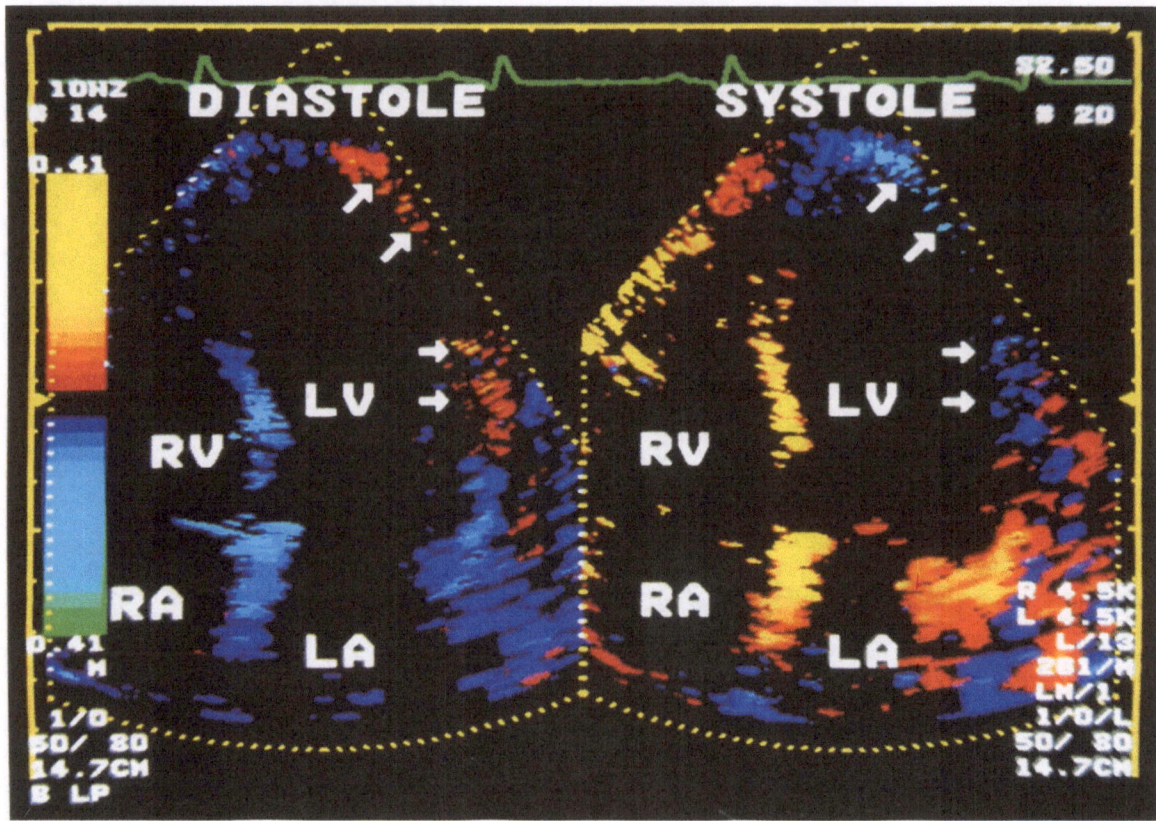

Fig. 8.2. Coronary artery disease. Asynchrony of the lateral left ventricular wall *(arrows)*. Apical four-chamber view using a 2.5 MHz transducer. Early diastolic *(left)* and mid-systolic frame *(right)*. Machine settings are: non-color-coded velocities up to 0.15 cm/s, red- or dark blue-coded velocities up to 0.7 cm/s, yellow- or bright blue-coded velocities over 0.7 cm/s. During early dias-tole interventricular septum and mitral annulus are moving away from the transducer. In contrast, the lateral wall of the left ventricle moves toward the transducer. During mid-systole the velocity directions reverse. Still opposite direction of the lateral wall velocity. (LA = left atrium, LV = left ventricle, RA = right atrium, RV = right ventricle)

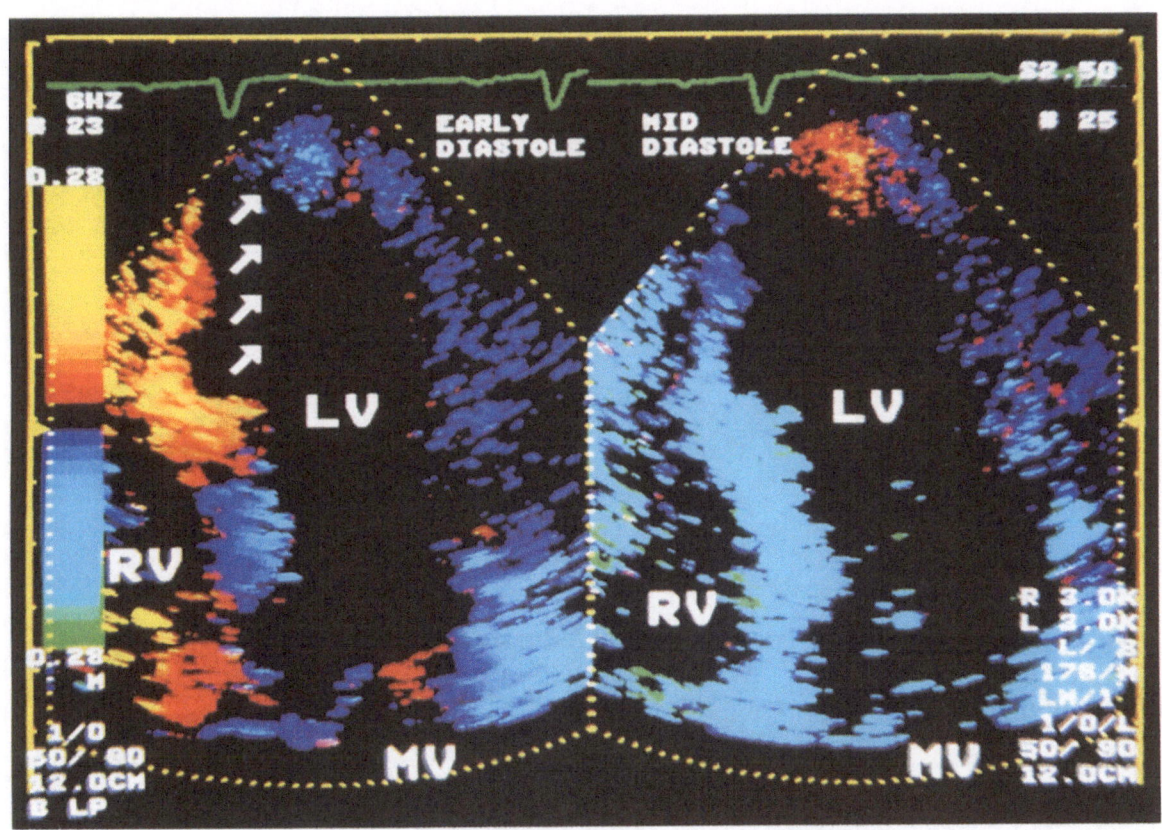

Fig. 8.3. Coronary artery disease. Asynchrony of the interventricular septum *(arrows)*. Apical long axis view using a 2.5 MHz transducer. Early diastolic *(left)* and mid-diastolic frame *(right)*. Machine settings are: non-color-coded velocities up to 0.21 cm/s, red- or dark blue-coded velocities up to 0.86 cm/s, yellow- or bright blue-coded velocities over 0.86 cm/s. During early diastole the lateral wall of the left ventricle moves away from the transducer as characteristic normal pattern for this phase. In contrast, the mid- and apical segments of the interventricular septum are moving toward the transducer. During mid-diastole the velocity direction of the interventricular septum corresponds to that of the lateral wall. The apex is moving in its typical diastolic direction, but not before mid-diastole. (LV = left ventricle, MV = mitral valve, RV = right ventricle)

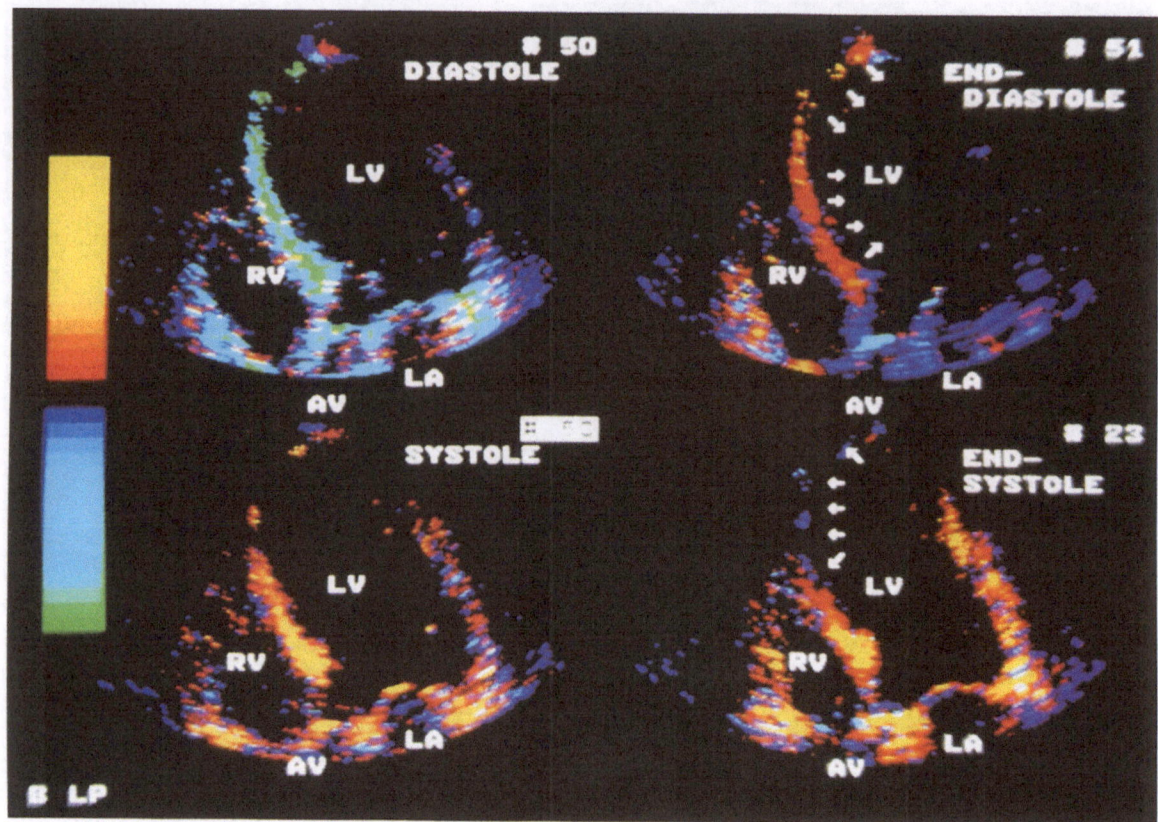

Fig. 8.4. Coronary artery disease. Asynchrony of the interventricular septum *(arrows)*. Apical long-axis view using a 2.5 MHz transducer. Four frames illustrating left ventricular wall velocity directions during early-diastole *(upper left)*, late-diastole before P-wave on the ECG *(upper right)*, early-systole *(below left)* and late-systole *(below right)*. Machine settings are: non-color-coded velocities up to 0.21 cm/s, red- or dark blue-coded velocities up to 0.86 cm/s, yellow- or bright blue-coded velocities over 0.86 cm/s, green-coded backward velocities over 2.8 cm/s. During early diastole the interventricular septum and lateral wall of the left ventricle move away from the transducer as is characteristic for this phase. During late dias-tole the interventricular septum is moving toward the transducer with the velocities above 0.8 cm/s. Similar velocity patterns are observed during systole. During early systole the velocity direction of the interventricular septum is typical for this phase: toward the transducer. In late systole the velocity direction reverses, indicated by blue cod-ing. Arrows indicate the asynchronic movement of the interventricular septum during late-diastole and late-systole. The aortic root is moving away from the transducer during diastole and toward the transducer during systole as a typical aortic root velocity pattern in this view. (AV = aortic valve, LA = left atrium, LV = left ventricle, RV = right ventricle)

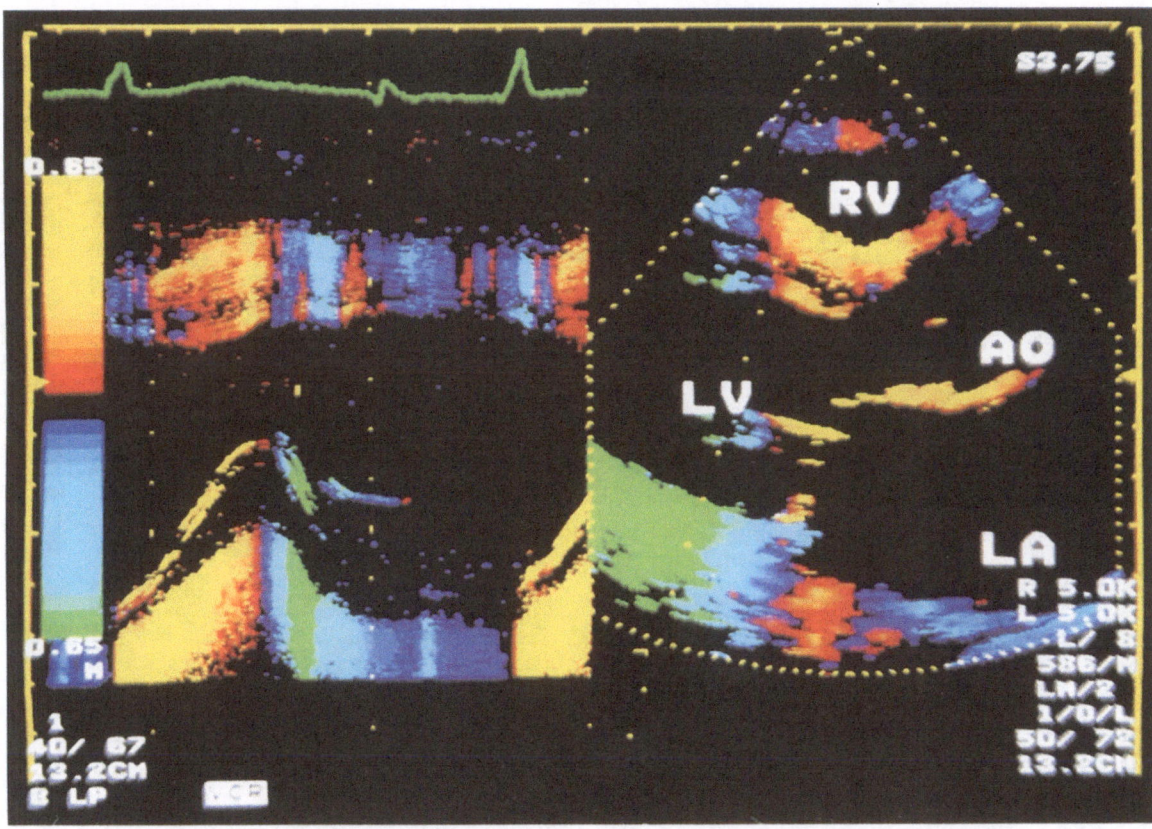

Fig. 8.5. Coronary artery disease. Paradoxical motion of the interventricular septum in a patient with coronary artery disease after coronary artery bypass surgery. Parasternal long-axis view using a 3.75 MHz transducer with tissue Doppler M-mode recording. Machine settings are: non-color-coded velocities up to 0.25 cm/s, red- or dark blue-coded velocities up to 1.0 cm/s, yellow- or bright blue-coded velocities over 1.0 cm/s, green-coded backward velocities over 3.3 cm/s. During systole both the posterior wall and the interventricular septum move toward the transducer. Transmural myocardial gradient by TDE with adequate septum thickening during systole. Abnormal color-coding of the interventricular septum depends on contribution of both velocities: toward the center of the left ventricle and the velocity of whole left ventricular movement. During diastole the velocities of the posterior wall and interventricular septum turn upward. Note long PQ time (280 ms). After the P-wave on the ECG the backward velocities of the posterior left ventricular wall increase. The velocities of the interventricular septum reverse after atrial contraction, as indicated by red-coding. However, the time delay between the P-wave on the ECG and septum forward motion is prolonged and very low velocities are recorded (0.3 cm/s). (AO = aortic root, LA = left atrium, LV = left ventricle, RV = right ventricle)

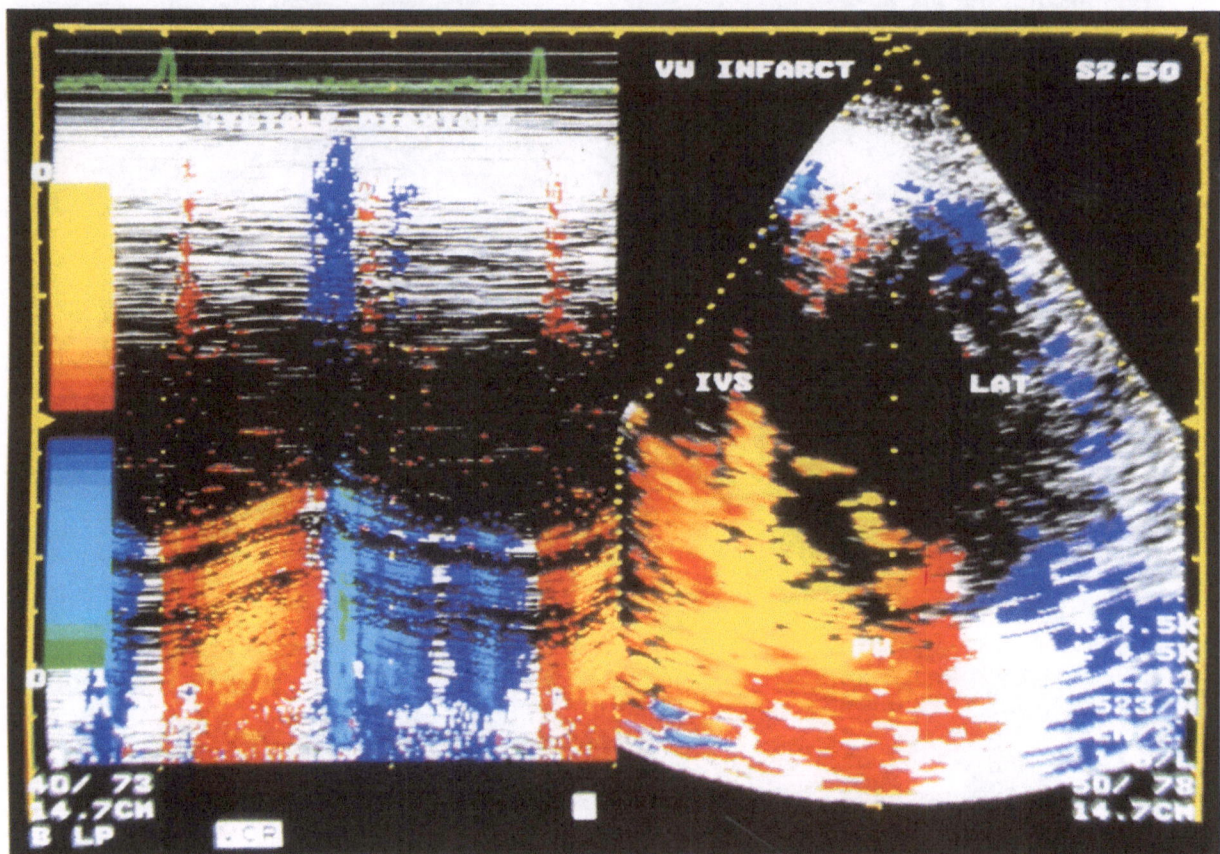

Fig. 8.6. Coronary artery disease. Akinesis of the antero-lateral left ventricular wall in a patient after anterior myocardial infarction. Parasternal short-axis view at the midpapillary level using a 2.5 MHz transducer with tissue Doppler M-mode recording. Machine settings are: non-color-coded velocities up to 0.30 cm/s, red- or dark blue-coded velocities up to 1.25 cm/s, yellow- or bright blue-coded velocities over 1.25 cm/s, green-coded backward velocities over 4.1 cm/s. Systolic frame in a two-dimensional image. Left ventricular anterior wall and lateral wall are not color-coded, indicating wall velocities below 0.30 cm/s. The M-mode recording reveals normal systolic and diastolic velocity direction of the left ventricular posterior wall with a transmural gradient. The interventricular septum moves with velocities below 0.30 cm/s. The dark blue-coded phase at the early diastole corresponds to the heart motion. (IVS = interventricular septum, LAT = left ventricular lateral wall, PW = left ventricular posterior wall)

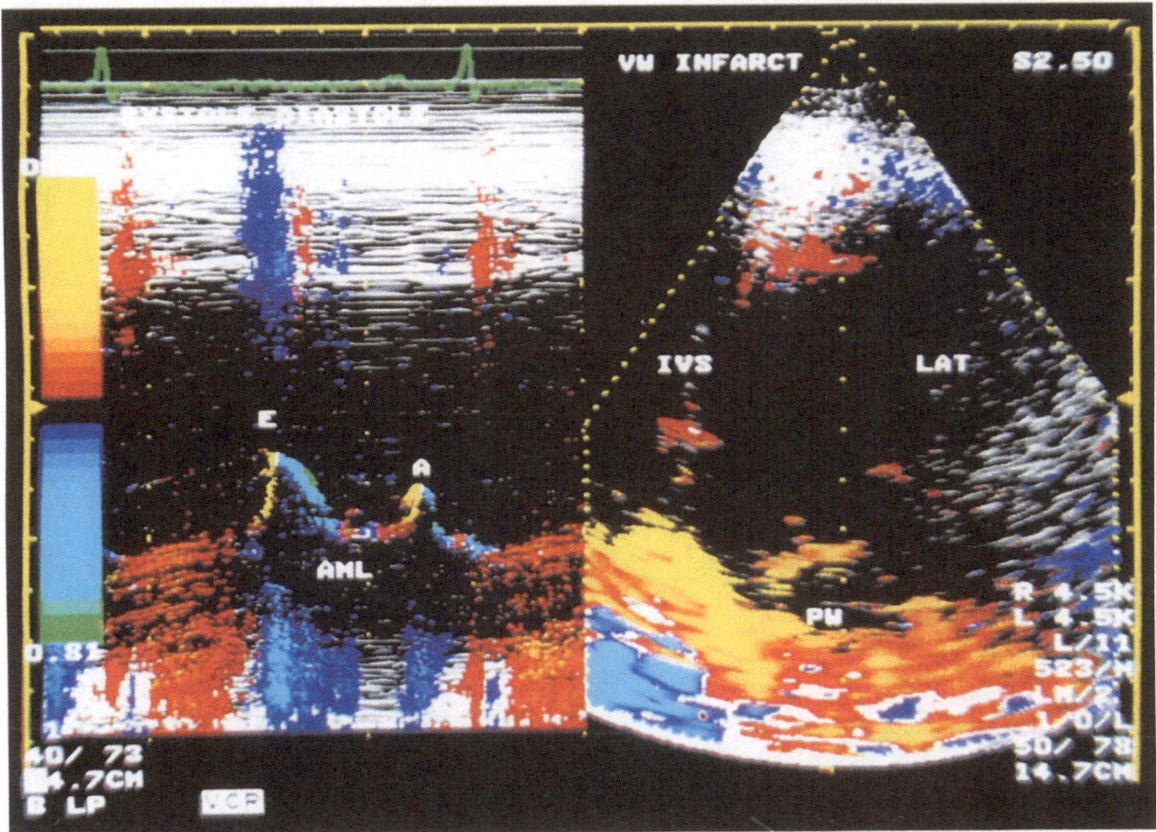

Fig. 8.7. Coronary artery disease. Akinesis of the antero-lateral left ventricular wall in a patient after anterior myocardial infarction. Parasternal short-axis view at the mitral leaflets level using a 2.5 MHz transducer with TDE M-mode recording. Machine settings are the same as in Fig. 8.6. Systolic frame in a two-dimensional image. Left ventricular anterior wall and lateral wall are not color-coded, indicating wall velocities below 0.30 cm/s. The M-mode recording reveals pathologic systolic and diastolic velocities of the left ventricular posterior wall, because the transmural velocity gradient is absent. The dark blue-coded phase at the early diastole corresponds to the heart motion. (A = atrial movement of the anterior mitral leaflet, AML = anterior mitral leaflet, E = early diastolic movement of the anterior mitral leaflet, IVS = interventricular septum, LAT = left ventricular lateral wall, PW = left ventricular posterior wall)

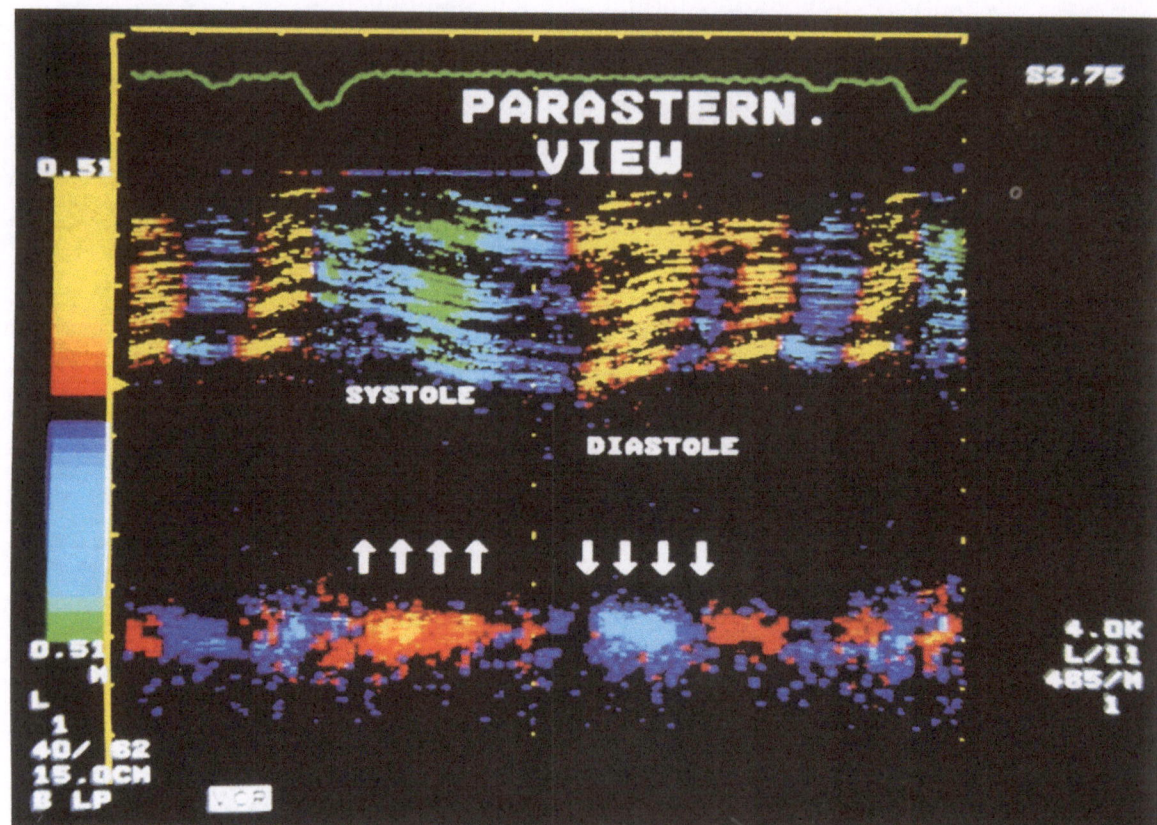

Fig. 8.8. Coronary artery disease. Severe hypokinesis of the posterior left ventricular wall in a patient after inferior myocardial infarction. TDE M-mode recording from parasternal long axis view using a 3.75 MHz transducer. Machine settings are: non-color-coded velocities up to 0.20 cm/s, red- or dark blue-coded velocities up to 0.8 cm/s, yellow- or bright blue-coded velocities over 0.8 cm/s, green-coded backward velocities over 2.6 cm/s. The interventricular septum is moving away from the transducer during systole and toward the transducer during diastole. The posterior wall moves in physiological directions during the cardiac cycle but the velocities are diminished and the onset of systolic forward motion is delayed. Typical image of severe hypokinesis of left ventricular wall. The time difference between the systolic motion of the interventricular septum and the posterior wall may be a new parameter of the regional left ventricular systolic function

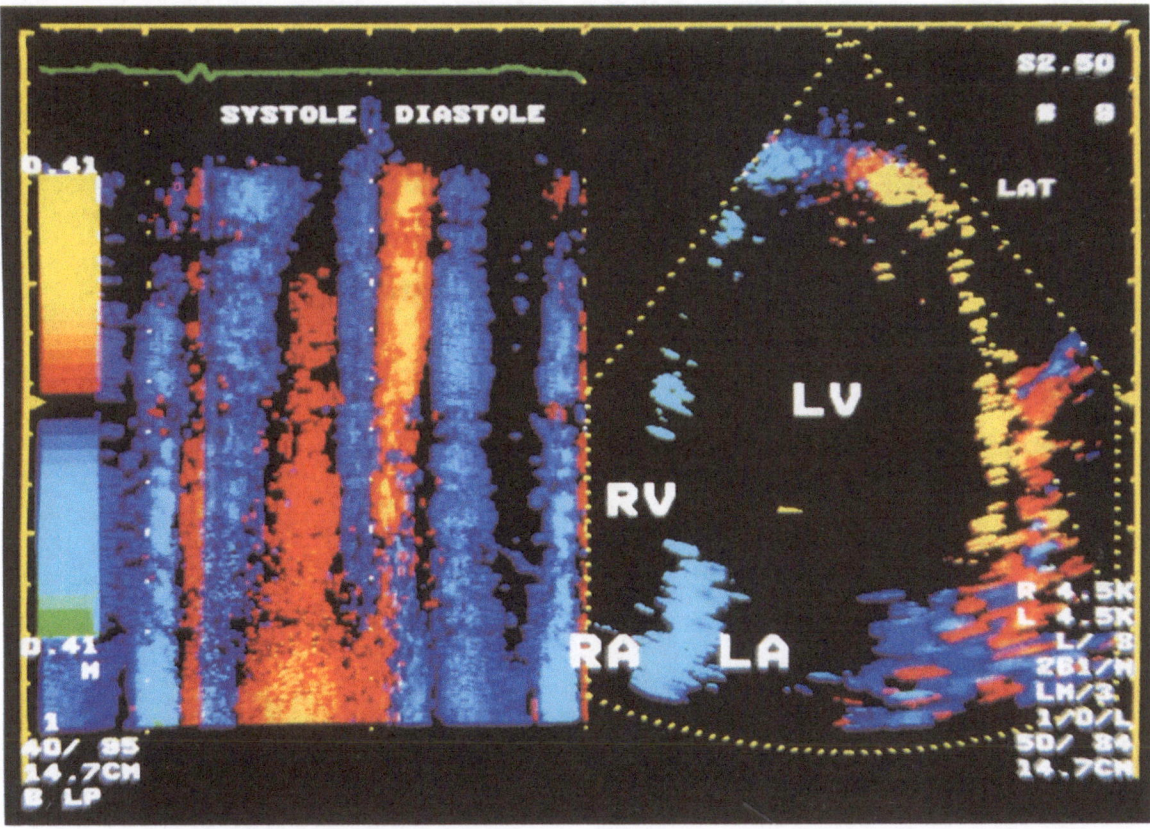

Fig. 8.9. Coronary artery disease. Asynchronous left ventricular lateral wall motion in a patient after anterior lateral myocardial infarction. Apical four-chamber view using a 2.5 MHz transducer with tissue Doppler M-mode recording. Machine settings are: non-color-coded velocities up to 0.30 cm/s, red- or dark blue-coded velocities up to 1.25 cm/s, yellow- or bright blue-coded velocities over 1.25 cm/s, green-coded backward velocities over 4.1 cm/s. Early-systolic frame in two dimensional image. The left ventricular lateral wall moves in the opposite direction from interventricular septum and mitral annulus. The M-mode recording shows the mechanism of the lateral wall motion abnormality. After the QRS complex on the ECG the backward motion of the lateral wall starts (asynchrony). In the mid- and late-systole the lateral wall moves toward the transducer, but the velocities are lower than in normal subjects (about 1 cm/s). In early diastole the velocities reverse briefly, but in mid-diastole a second forward motion is visible. The highest velocities during the cardiac cycle occur at the atrial filling phase. The conventional two-dimensional echocardiographic examination reveal a dyskinetic lateral wall of the left ventricle. (LA = left atrium, LV = left ventricle, RA = right atrium, RV = right ventricle)

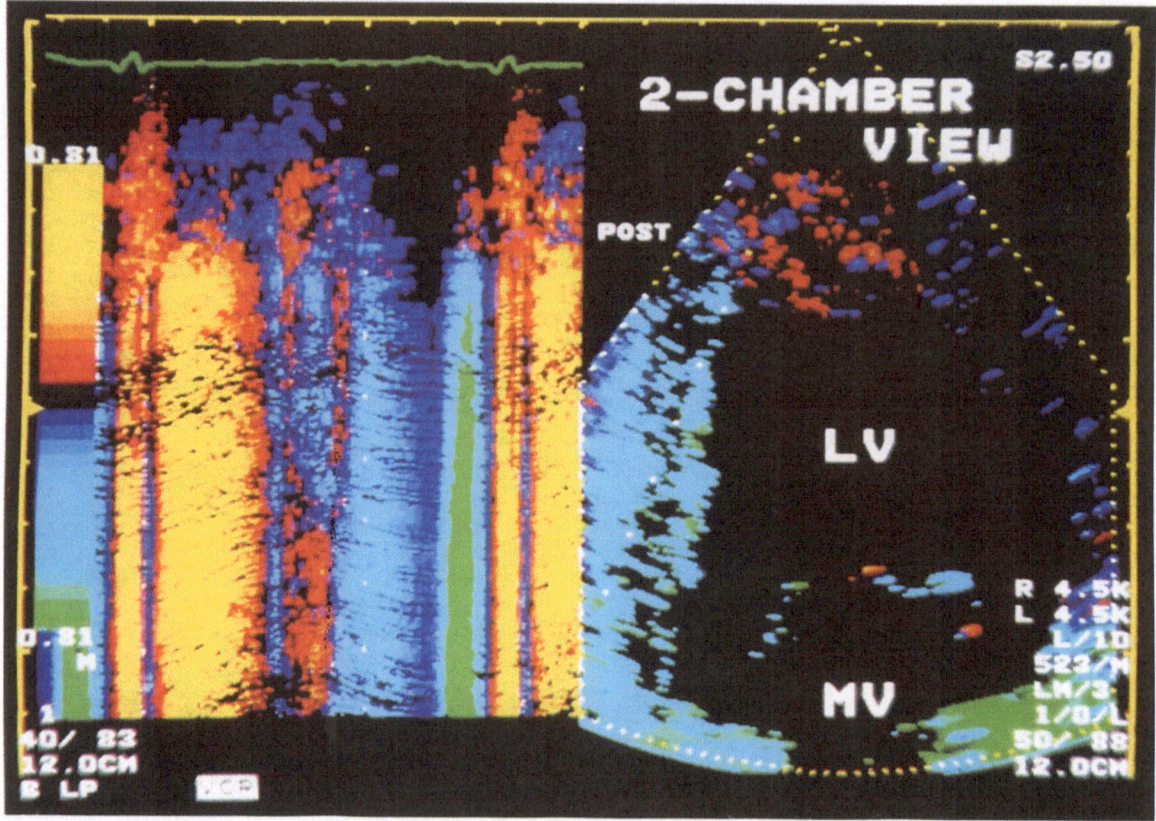

Fig. 8.10. Coronary artery disease. Left ventricular posterior wall velocities in the same patient with coronary artery disease as in Fig. 8.9. Apical two-chamber view using a 2.5 MHz transducer with TDE M-mode recording. Machine settings are: non-color-coded velocities up to 0.30 cm/s, red- or dark blue-coded velocities up to 1.25 cm/s, yellow- or bright blue-coded velocities over 1.25 cm/s, green-coded backward velocities over 4.1 cm/s. Diastolic TDE 2D-frame. The left ventricular posterior wall is moving toward the transducer during systole and away from the transducer during diastole, as found in normal subjects. However, the TDE M-mode recording shows an abnormality of posterior wall velocities. During early diastole the velocities found over the posterior wall are 2.25 cm/s, and lower than peak systolic velocities (4.6 cm/s). The highest velocities during the cardiac cycle occur at the atrial filling phase. The measured velocities are 6.13 cm/s. (LV = left ventricle, MV = mitral valve, POST = left ventricular posterior wall)

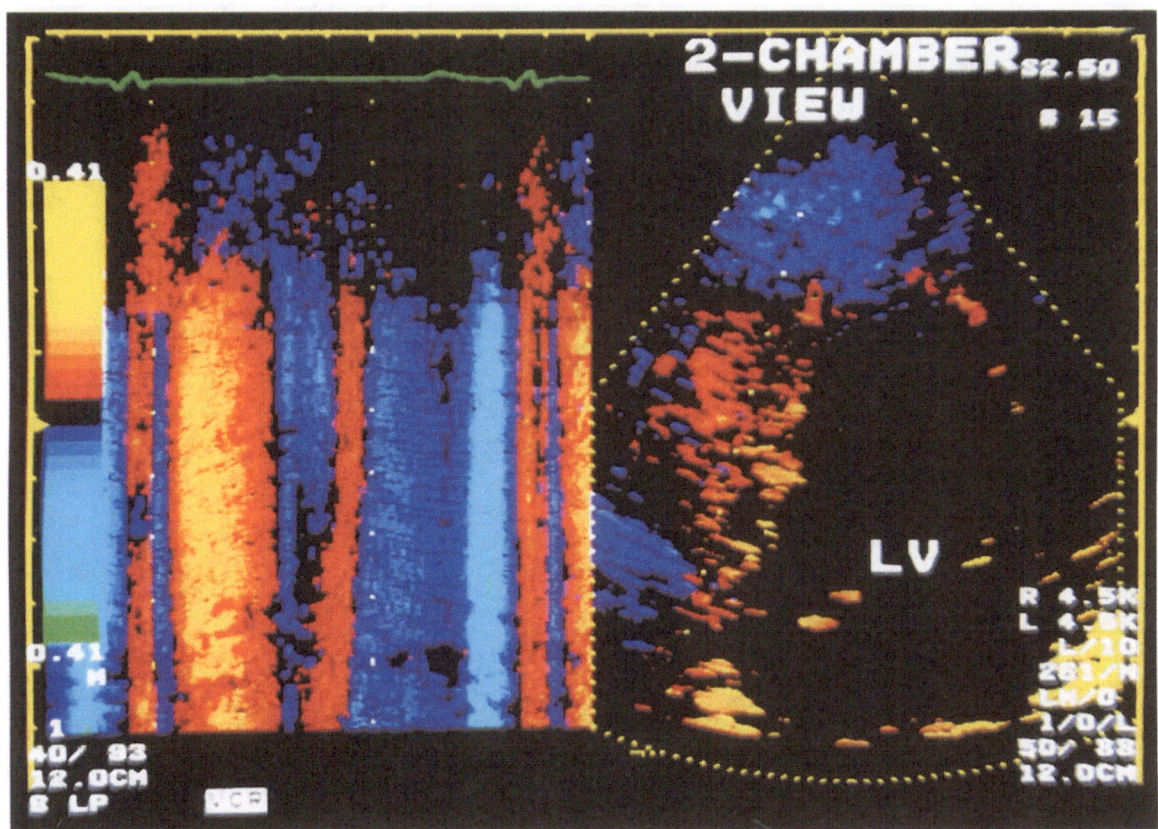

Fig. 8.11. Coronary artery disease. Left ventricular posterior wall velocities in the same patient with coronary artery disease, as in Fig. 8.10. Machine settings are now changed: non-color-coded velocities up to 0.60 cm/s, red- or dark blue-coded velocities up to 2.5 cm/s, yellow- or light blue-coded velocities over 2.5 cm/s, green-coded backward velocities over 8.1 cm/s. At the machine settings the peak backward velocity during late-diastole is clearly seen. (LV = left ventricle)

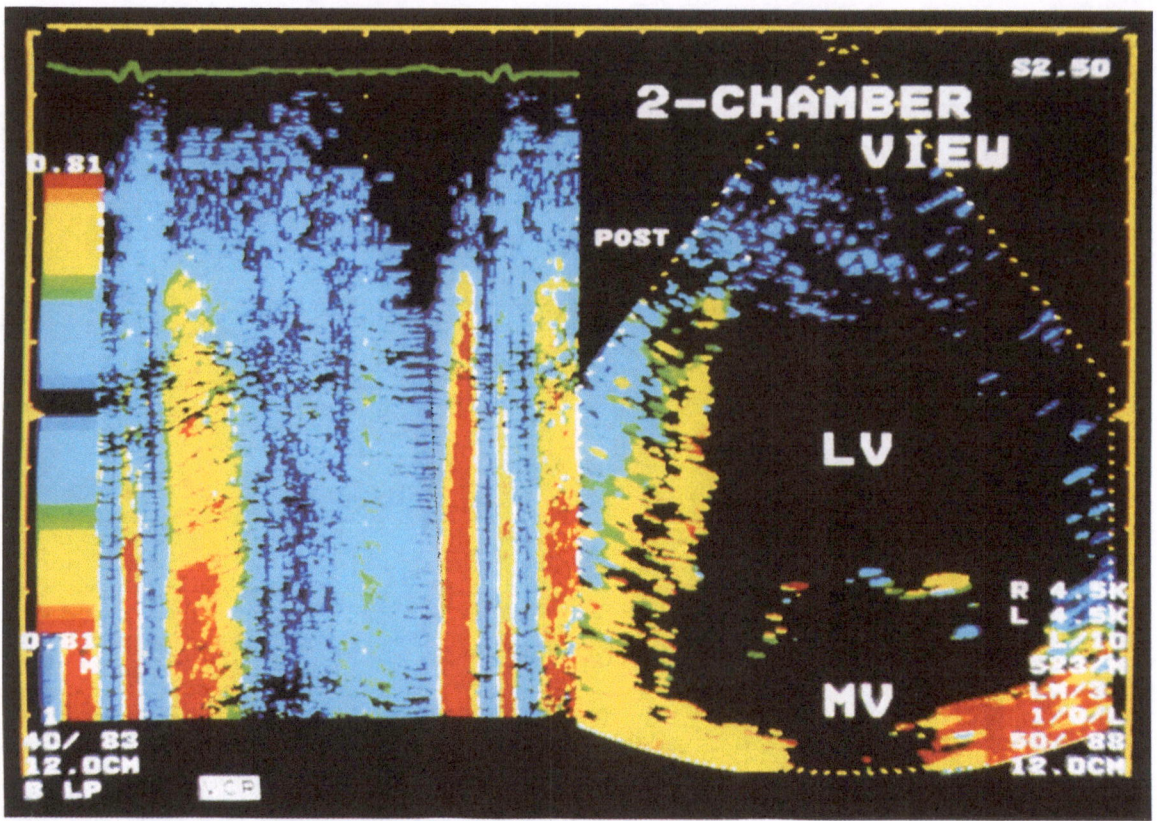

Fig. 8.12. Coronary artery disease. Left ventricular posterior wall velocities in the same patient with coronary artery disease as in Figs. 8.10–8.11. Different color scale is used; the velocities are coded by color independent of velocity direction: blue-coded velocities to up 1.15 cm/s, green-coded velocities up to 1.45 cm/s yellow-coded velocities to 4.6 cm/s, and red-coded velocities over 4.6 cm/s. At this machine setting the peak velocity during the cardiac cycle is clearly visualized in the late-diastole after the P-wave on the ECG. (LV = left ventricle, MV = mitral valve, POST = left ventricular posterior wall)

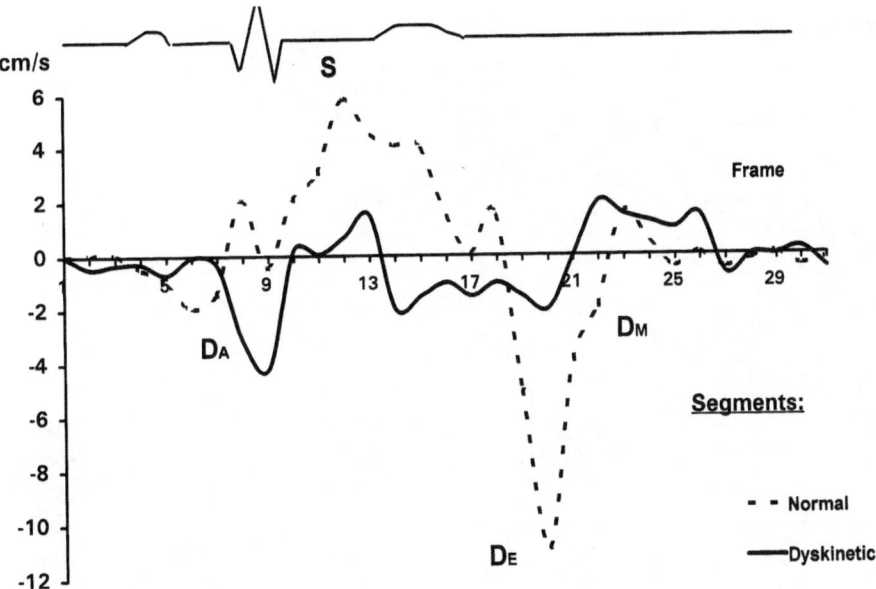

Fig. 8.13. Interventricular septum (segment 2) velocities in subsequent frames from the apical view in a patient with coronary artery disease and dyskinesis in comparison with a representative healthy subject. (S=peak systolic velocity, D_E=peak early-diastolic velocity, D_M=peak mid-diastolic velocity, D_A=peak late-diastolic velocity)

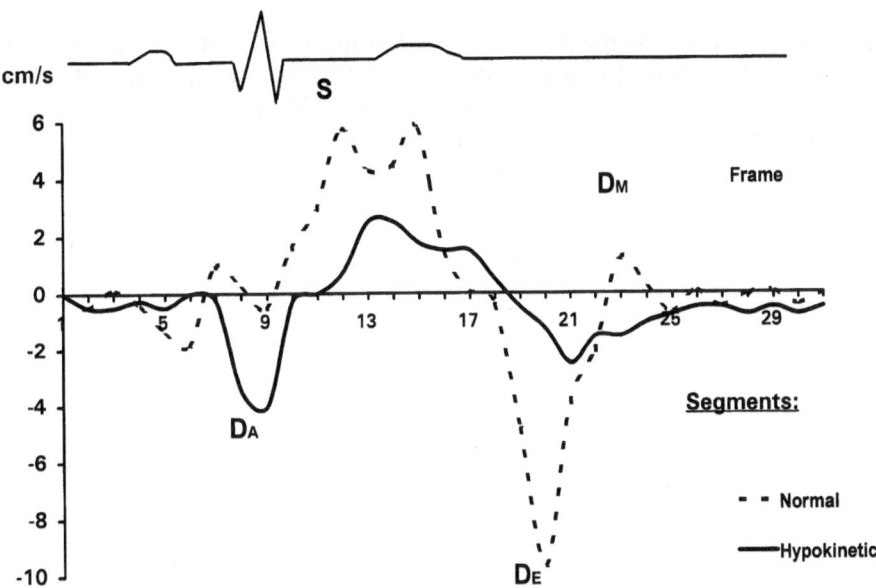

Fig. 8.14. Left ventricular posterior wall (segment 6) velocities in subsequent frames from the parasternal view in a patient with coronary artery disease and posterior wall hypokinesis in comparison with a representative healthy subject. (S=peak systolic velocity, D_E=peak early-diastolic velocity, D_M=peak mid-diastolic velocity, D_A=peak late-diastolic velocity)

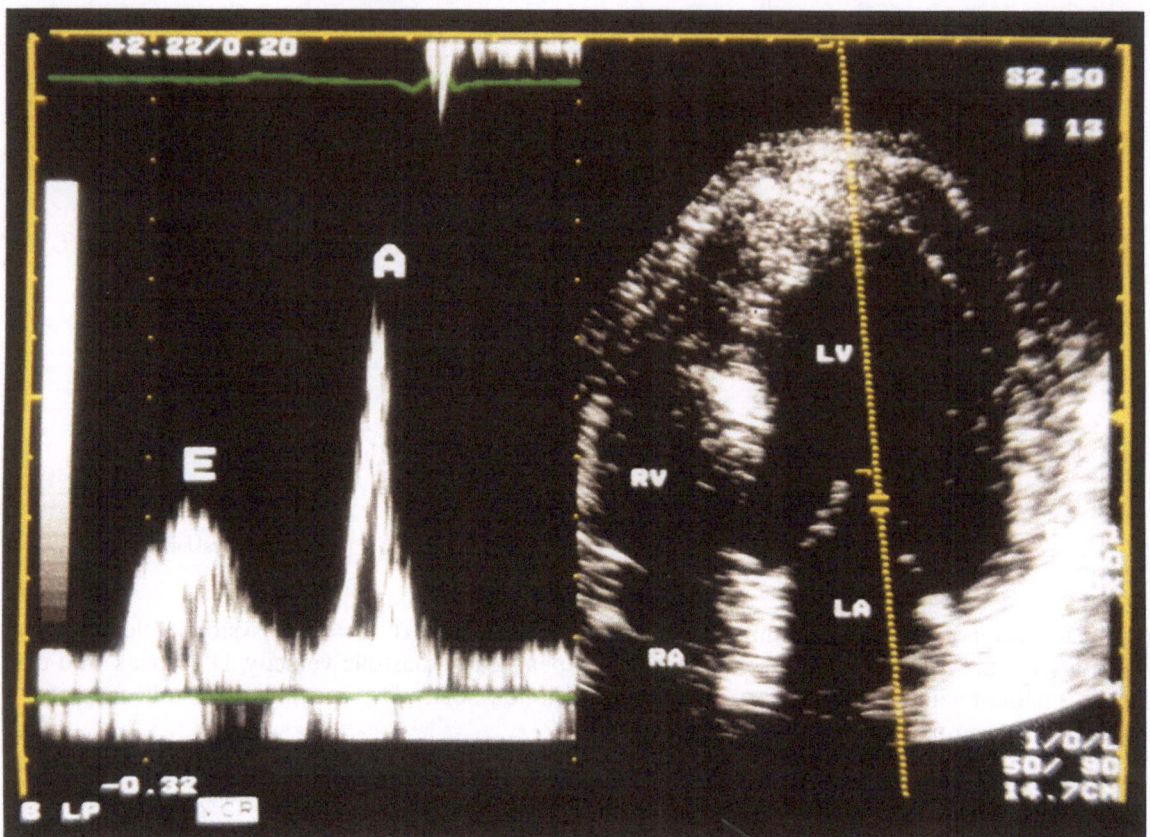

Fig. 8.15. Coronary artery disease. Disturbance of diastolic function. Mitral inflow in the same patient with coronary artery disease as in Figs. 8.10–8.12. Peak atrial velocity of the mitral inflow is higher than peak early-diastolic velocity. (A = atrial wave of the mitral inflow, E = early-diastolic wave of the mitral inflow, LA = left atrium, LV = left ventricle, RA = right atrium, RV = right ventricle)

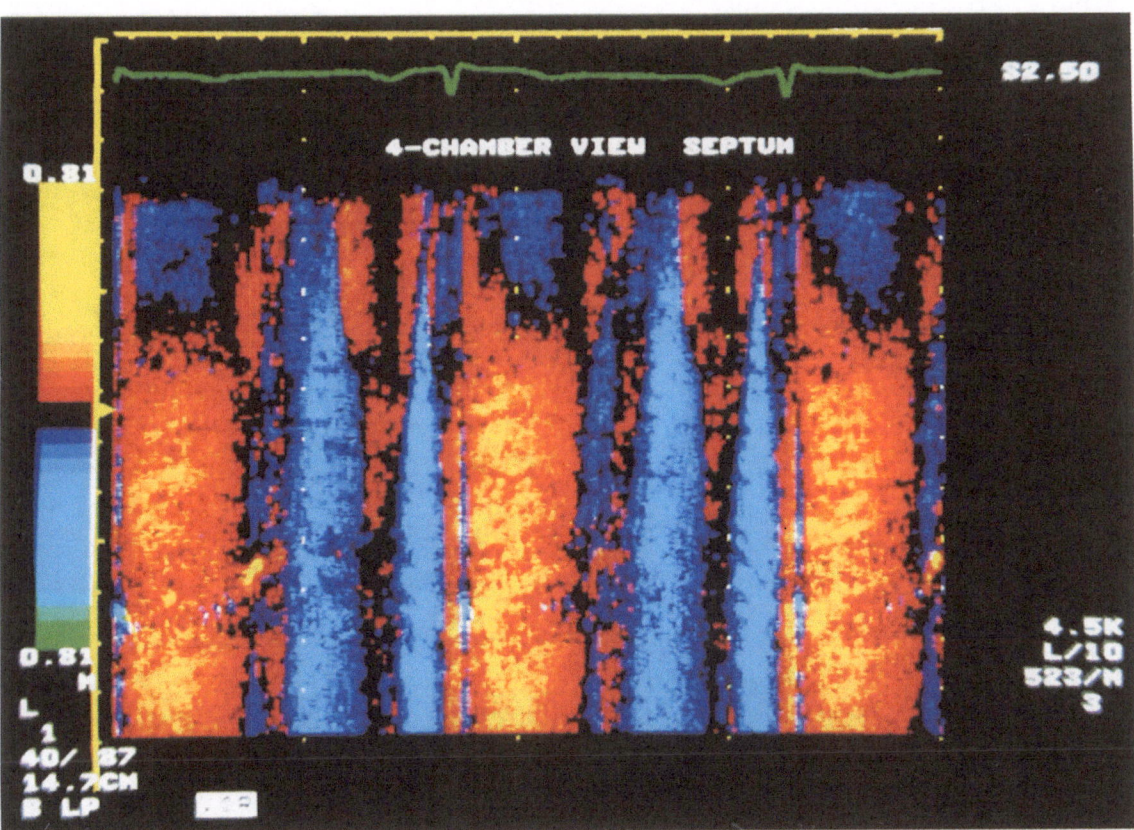

Fig. 8.16. Coronary artery disease. Interventricular septum velocities in a patient with coronary artery disease. TDE M-mode recordings from apical four-chamber view using a 2.5 MHz transducer. Machine settings are: non-color-coded velocities up to 0.61 cm/s, red- or dark blue-coded velocities up to 2.5 cm/s, yellow- or bright blue-coded velocities over 2.5 cm/s, green-coded backward velocities over 8.3 cm/s. The interventricular septum is moving toward the transducer during systole and away from the transducer during diastole, as found in normal subjects. However, TDE M-mode recordings show the abnormal septal velocities. During early diastole the velocity is in the posterior wall is 2.63 cm/s, and lower than the peak systolic velocity (3.17 cm/s). The highest velocities during the cardiac cycle occur at the atrial filling phase (7.42 cm/s). Note the high reproducibility of the tissue Doppler M-mode recording from beat to beat

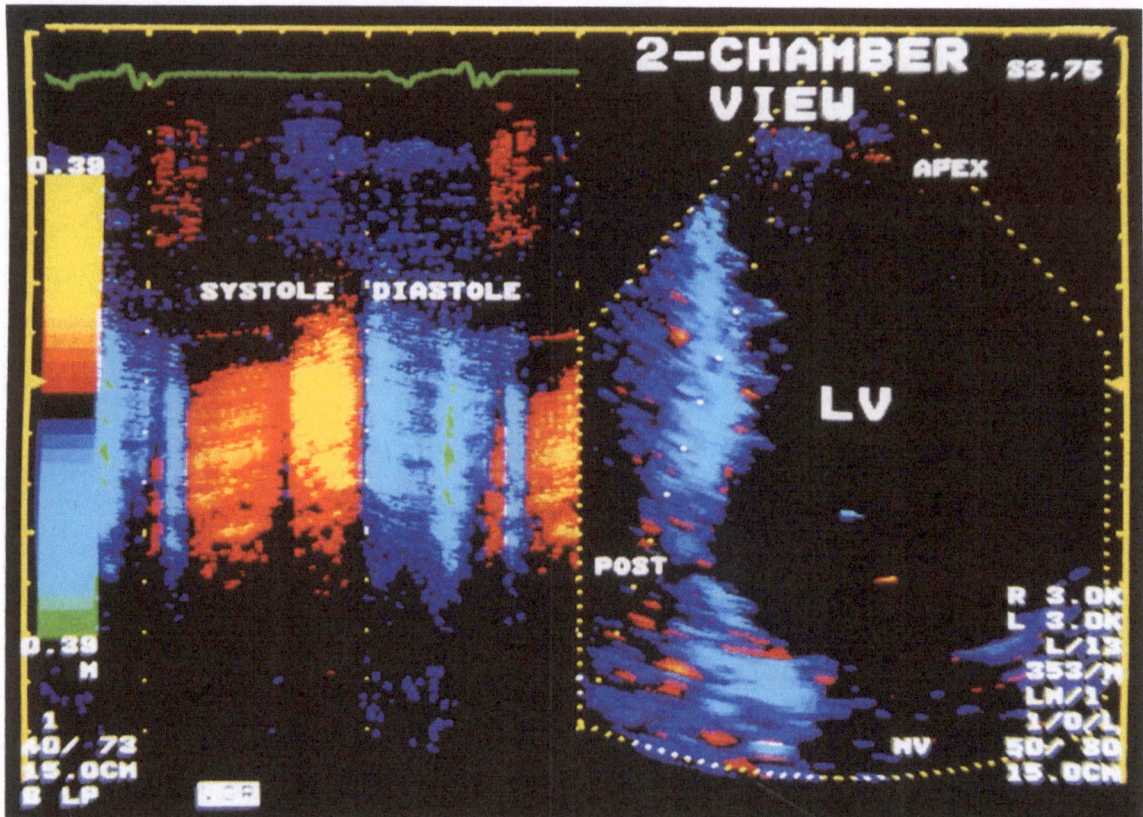

Fig. 8.17. Coronary artery disease. Left ventricular posterior wall velocities in a patient with coronary artery disease. Apical two-chamber view using a 3.75 MHz transducer with tissue Doppler M-mode recording. Machine settings are: non-color-coded velocities up to 0.30 cm/s, red- or dark blue-coded velocities up to 1.25 cm/s, yellow- or bright blue-coded velocities over 1.25 cm/s, green-coded backward velocities over 4.1 cm/s. Diastolic frame in two-dimensional image. The left ventricular posterior wall is moving toward the transducer during systole and away from the transducer during diastole, as found in normal subjects. However, TDE M-mode shows the abnormality of the posterior wall velocities. In early- and mid-systole the left ventricular posterior wall is moving toward the transducer with relatively low velocities of about 1.0–1.5 cm/s. The peak systolic velocity occurs in late systole in sharp contrast to findings in healthy subjects. Asynchrony is present. The time between onset and peak of systolic velocity is prolonged as a new marker for coronary artery disease. (LV = left ventricle, MV = mitral valve, POST = left ventricular posterior wall)

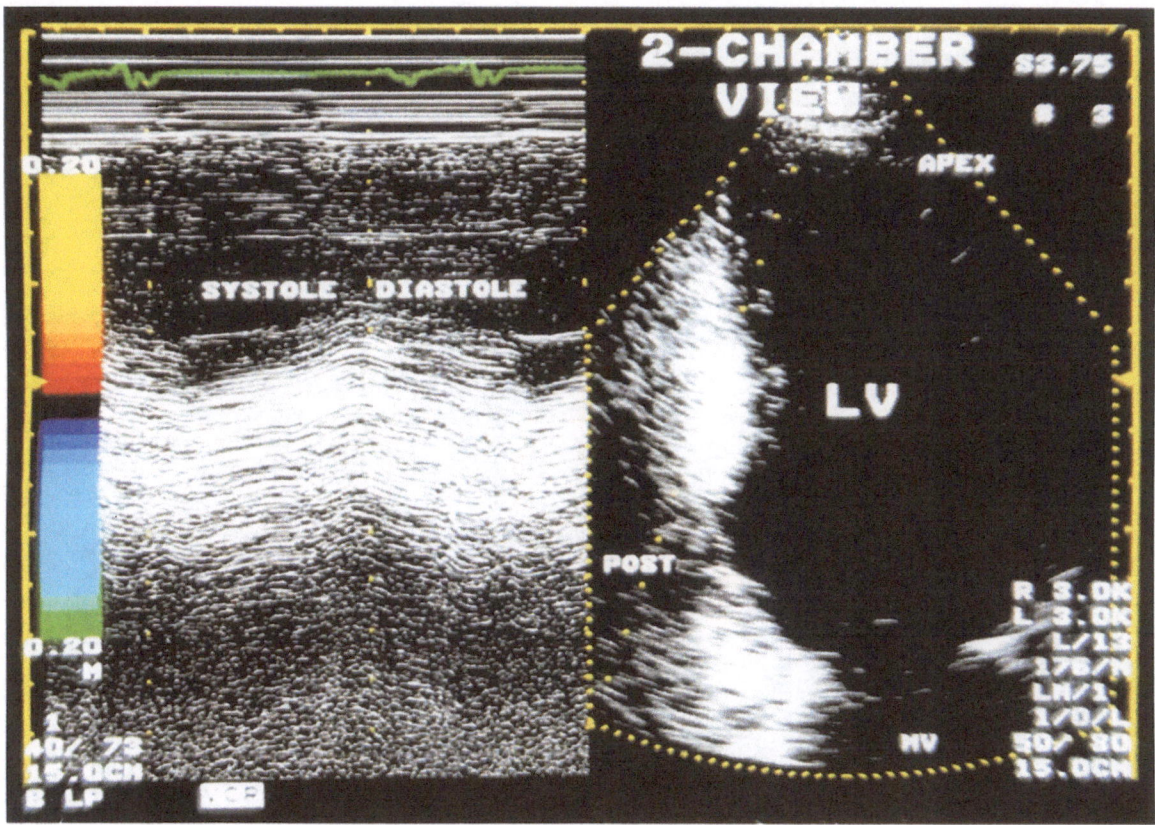

Fig. 8.18. The same recordings as in Fig. 8.15 without TDE information

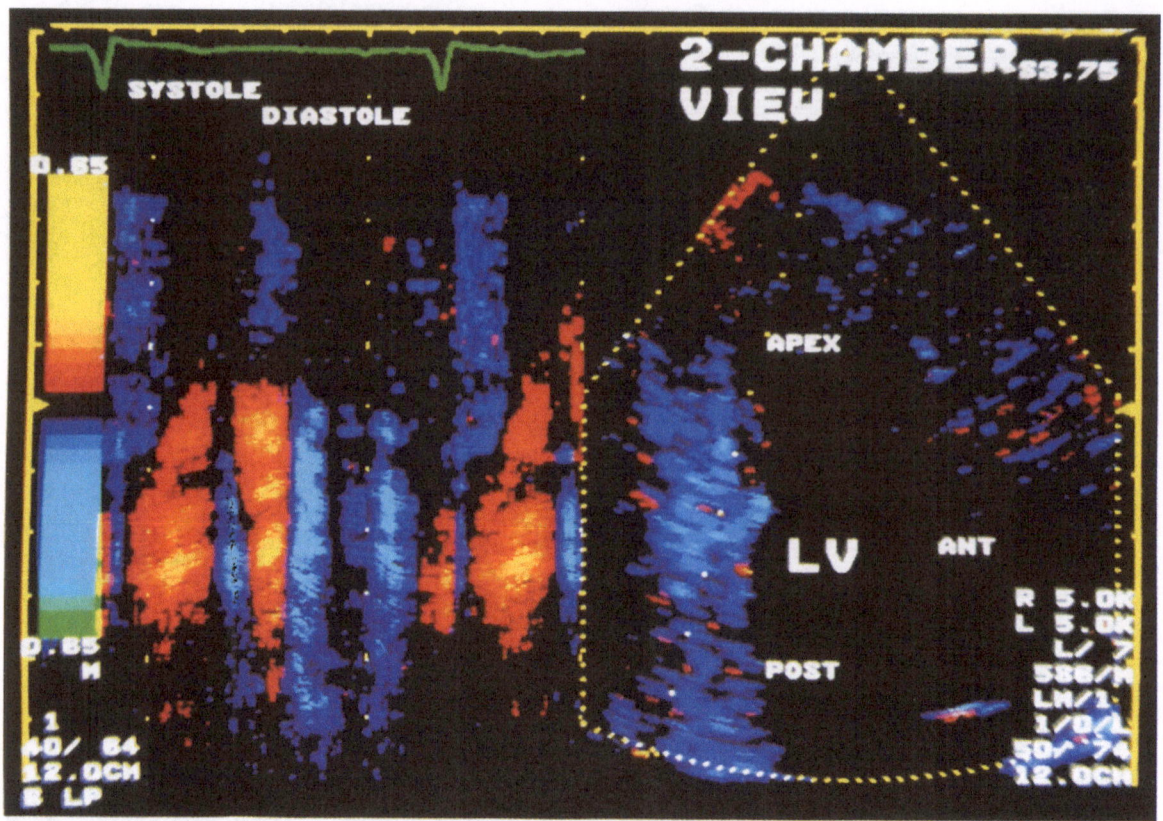

Fig. 8.19. Coronary artery disease. Left ventricular posterior wall velocities in a patient with coronary artery disease. Apical two-chamber view using a 3.75 MHz transducer with TDE M-mode recording. Machine settings are: non-color-coded velocities up to 0.50 cm/s, red- or dark blue-coded velocities up to 2.0 cm/s, yellow- or bright blue-coded velocities over 2.0 cm/s, green-coded backward velocities over 6.7 cm/s. Diastolic two-dimensional image. Similar wall motion abnormality as shown in Fig 8.18. The peak systolic velocity does not occur until late systole, which is indicated by yellow color-coding. Two phases of diastolic motion with higher peak velocity at early diastole. (ANT = left ventricular anterior wall, LV = left ventricle, POST = left ventricular posterior wall)

Chapter 9 TDE and Stress Echocardiography

T. Buck

Color-coded "tissue Doppler echocardiography" (TDE) is a new noninvasive imaging technique which provides further knowledge about regional myocardial function, which can be revealed by stress echocardiography. Thus it is important to describe the myocardial function by TDE under resting conditions, but especially during stress testing, in order to discover early signs of myocardial ischemia.

Stress Echocardiography

Stress echocardiography provides the assessment of left ventricular function, regional wall motion and wall thickening, both at rest and during increasing myocardial oxygen consumption. Experimental studies demonstrate a close relation between coronary perfusion and wall thickening [13]. Decrease of coronary perfusion causes impairment of systolic and diastolic ventricular function [15]. Exercise-induced impairment of ventricular function is more sensitive in the detection of ischemia than electrocardiographic stress testing and angina [8]. The primary indication for stress echocardiography is the diagnosis of coronary heart disease. The number of vessels involved, the functional integrity and follow-up examinations after coronary interventions are of great clinical relevance. Stress echocardiography is helpful for evaluating myocardial and ventricular function, also for hypertrophic, dilative and restrictive cardiomyopathy [4].

Stress echocardiography will mainly be performed by dynamic exercise (bicycle/treadmill) or by pharmacological stimulation of the myocardium. In combination of stress echocardiography with new imaging techniques, as for example TDE, pharmacological stress will be preferred in order to avoid artefacts due to the patient's body motion during dynamic stress. Pharmacological stress is normally produced with either dobutamine and arbutamine or other catecholamine derivates with positive inotropic and chronotropic effects, or with dipyridamole, a vasodilator producing "coronary steal". Dobutamine and enoximone [9] provide additional information about inotropic reserve as an indicator of myocardial viability [12].

Diagnostic Importance of Stress Echocardiography

Impairment of regional and global left ventricular function during myocardial stimulation is induced by myocardial ischemia. Myocardial ischemia develops under stress by well defined steps as shown in an "ischemic cascade" (Fig. 9.1). For the

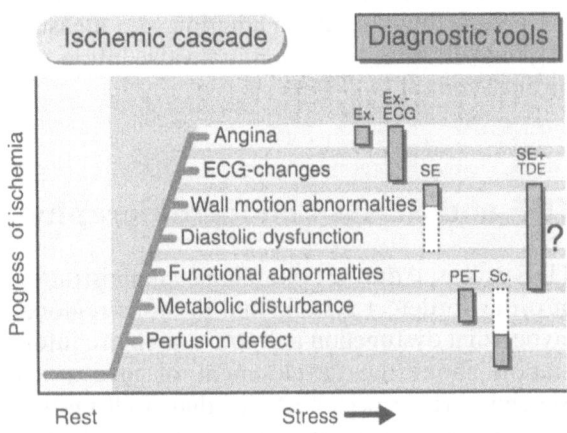

Fig 9.1. Development of ischemia under increasing myocardial stress and diagnostic tools to detect changes (modified from Picano 1992, Hendrickx 1978). Abbreviations: Ex. = dynamic exercise; Ex.-ECG = exercise-ECG; SE = stress echocardiography; PET = positron emission tomography, Sc. = myocardial scintigraphy; SE + TDE = stress echocardiography and tissue Doppler-echocardiography

diagnosis of coronary heart disease it is important to detect early stages of the ischemia process, because therefore angina and ST-T changes in the ECG are not sensitive enough.

Left ventricular function is often normal at rest and impairment of left ventricular function only develops under stimulation of oxygen consumption [1]. On the other hand, coronary stenoses documented by angiography do not conclusively lead to regional or global wall motion abnormalties, for example, in case of sufficient collateralization. Stress echocardiography has two main applications to patients with coronary heart disease: Verification of the diagnosis and assessment of the functional significance of coronary stenoses demonstrated at angiography [10, 11].

Conventionally, stress echocardiography assesses regional wall motion using a 16-segment division of the left ventricle, and it classifies wall motion and wall thickening as either normokinesia, hypokinesia, akinesia, or dyskinesia [2, 14]. Semiquantitative measurement of wall motion is performed by the centerline- and radiant-methods. Additionally, changes of global ventricular function are measured as enddiastolic and endsystolic volumes, and ejection fraction. In case of severe regional wall motion abnormalties already at rest, for example with "hibernating" and "stunned" myocardium, dobutamine stress echocardiography is able to provide information about the viability of the myocardium [6, 12]. In addition, as a measure of global diastolic function mitral valve inflow can be analyzed [3].

TDE and Stress Echocardiography

TDE was used during dobutamine administration in order to detect systolic and diastolic regional myocardial dysfunction and to obtain more information about the development of myocardial ischemia, which occurs earlier than wall motion abnormalties, for instance, regional diastolic dysfunction (see Fig. 9.1).

Beyond the assessment of regional wall motion and wall thickening by standard two-dimensional (2-D) echocardiography, TDE provides an accurate detection of direction and velocity of the myocardium by color-coding cardiac tissue [5] (Fig 9.2). Thereby abnormal wall motion induced by stress and often not detected by standard 2-D-echocardiography can by described and exactly analyzed [6] (Fig. 9.3).

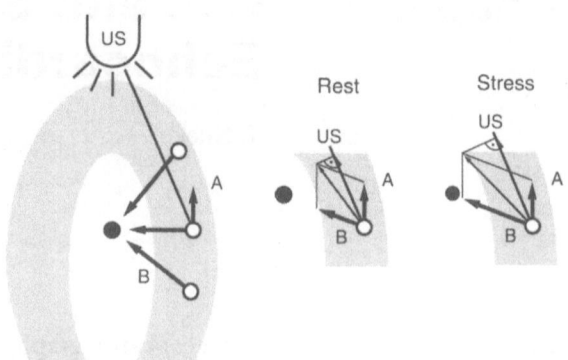

Fig. 9.2. Diagram showing the principles of composition of wall motion vectors. The two focusing figures are demonstrating different cases of wall motion. The left figure examplifies resting condition and the right figure documents the changes on vector-length under increasing inotropy. The vector of wall motion each time is, a composition of two vectors, one representing the movement of the heart (vector A) and one representing wall motion in direction to the heart's center of gravity (vector B). However, we can each time only measure a vector different from the composed vector, as shown in the diagrams

By encoding velocity of wall motion by color-brightness, it is possible to monitor myocardial velocities during increasing myocardial stimulation (Fig. 9.4). Thus, quantification of left ventricular function during stress might include assessment of regional changes in myocardial velocities. A further diagnostic advantage may be the ability to analyze changes in the duration of the different components of systole and diastole, information that has previously been available only by invasive techniques.

Therefore, TDE seems to be a new valuable method to provide further information about ventricular and regional myocardial functions and ventricular physiology (see Fig. 9.1), especially under conditions of myocardial stress.

References

1. Bach DS, Armstrong WF (1992) Dobutamine stress echocardiography. Am J Cardiol 69:90H–96H
2. Bourdillon PD, Broderick TM, Sawada SG, Armstrong WF, Ryan T, Dillon JC, Fineberg NS, Feigenbaum H (1989) Regional wall motion index for infarct and non-infarct regions after reperfusion in acute myocardial infarction: comparison with global wall motion index. J Am Soc Echocardiogr 2:398–407

3. Buck Th, Baumgart D, Schön F, Erbel R (1994) Significant relation of E/A-ratio according to severity of coronary artery disease during dobutamine-stress-echocardiography [abstract]. Eur J Appl Physiol 69:23

4. Buck Th, Aly F, Baumgart D, Schön F, Leischik R, Görge G, Haude M, Erbel R (1995) Inotropic reserve in presence of dilated and ischemic cardiomyopathy during dobutamine-stress-echocardiography [abstract]. First International Meeting of the Working Group on Heart Failure, Amsterdam, European Society of Cardiology

5. Buck Th, Drozdz J, Schön F, Leischik R, Baumgart D, Ge J, Görge G, Haude M, Erbel R (1995) Use of color-coded tissue Doppler for dobutamine stress echocardiography [abstract]. J Am Coll Cardiol [24, 2] Spec. Iss.

6. Buck Th, Wallbridge DR, Drozdz J, Zamorano J, Bruch Ch, Görge G, Haude M, Erbel R (1995) Tissue Doppler echocardiography improves the detection of regional myocardial ischemia during dobutamine stress [abstract]. Eur Heart J (1995)

7. Cigarroa CG, Filippi de CR, Brickner E, Alvarez LG, Wait MA, Grayburn PA (1993) Dobutamine stress echocardiography identifies hibernating myocardium and predicts recovery of left ventricular function after coronary revascularisation. Circulation 88:430–436

8 Hendrickx CR, Baic H, Nelkins P, Leusen K, Fishbein MC, Vatner SF (1978) Depression of regional blood flow and wall thickening after brief coronary occlusion. Am J Physiol 234:H653–660

9. Leischik R, Baumgart D, Buck Th, Zeppelini R, Oelert H, Erbel R (1994) Enoximon – Belastungsechocardiographie – ein neuer Test zum Nachweis des vitalen Myokards [abstract]. Z Kardiol 83 (Suppl):64

10. Mc Neill AJ, Fioretti PM, El-Said EM, Salustri A, DeFeyter PJ, Roelandt JRTC (1992) Dobutamine stress echocardiography before and after coronary angioplasty. Am J Cardiol 69:740–745

11. Mertes H, Erbel R, Nixdorff U, Mohr-Kahaly S, Krüger S, Meyer J (1993) Exercise echocardiography for the evaluation of patients after nonsurgical coronary artery revascularisation. J Am Coll Cardiol 21:1087–1093

12. Piérard LA, De Landsheere CM, Berthe C, Rigo P, Kulbertus HE (1990) Identification of viable myocardium by echocardiography during dobutamine infusion in patients with myocardial infarction after thrombolytic therapy: comparison with positon emmission tomography. J Am Cardiol 15:1021–1031

13. Ross J Jr (1991) Myocardial perfusion-contraction matching. Implications on coronary heart disease and hibernation. Circulation 83:1076–1083

14. Schiller NB, Shak PM, Crawford M, DeMaria A, Devereux R, Feigenbaum H, Gutgesell H, Reichek N, Salm D, Schnittger J, Silverman AH, Tajik AJ (1989) Recommendations for quantitation of the left ventricle by two-dimensional echocardiography. J Am Soc Echocardiogr 2:358–367

15. Segar DS, Brown SE, Sawada SG, Ryan T, Feigenbaum H (1992) Dobutamine stress echocardiogarphy: correlation with coronary lesion severity as determined by quantitative angiography. J Am Coll Cardiol 19:1197–1202

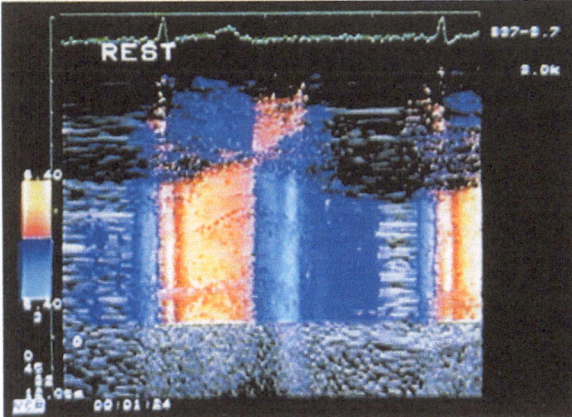
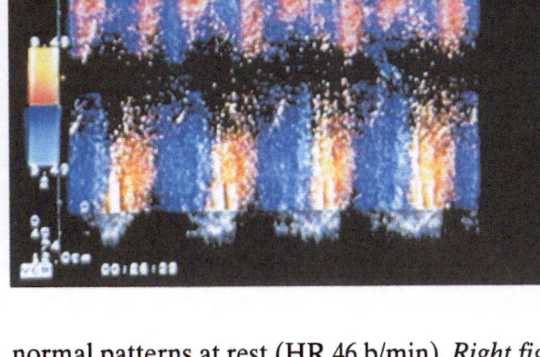

Fig. 9.3. M-mode description of a "fluttering" of the left ventricular apex. The lower colored M-mode band of the picture shows the lower part of the posterior wall in an apical two-chamber view. The upper colored M-mode band represents the movement of the apex. *Left figure:* M-mode with normal patterns at rest (HR 46 b/min). *Right figure:* M-mode showing the "fluttering" of the apex at peak stimulation (HR 144 b/min) with changing the direction of its movement twice as well as the posterior wall

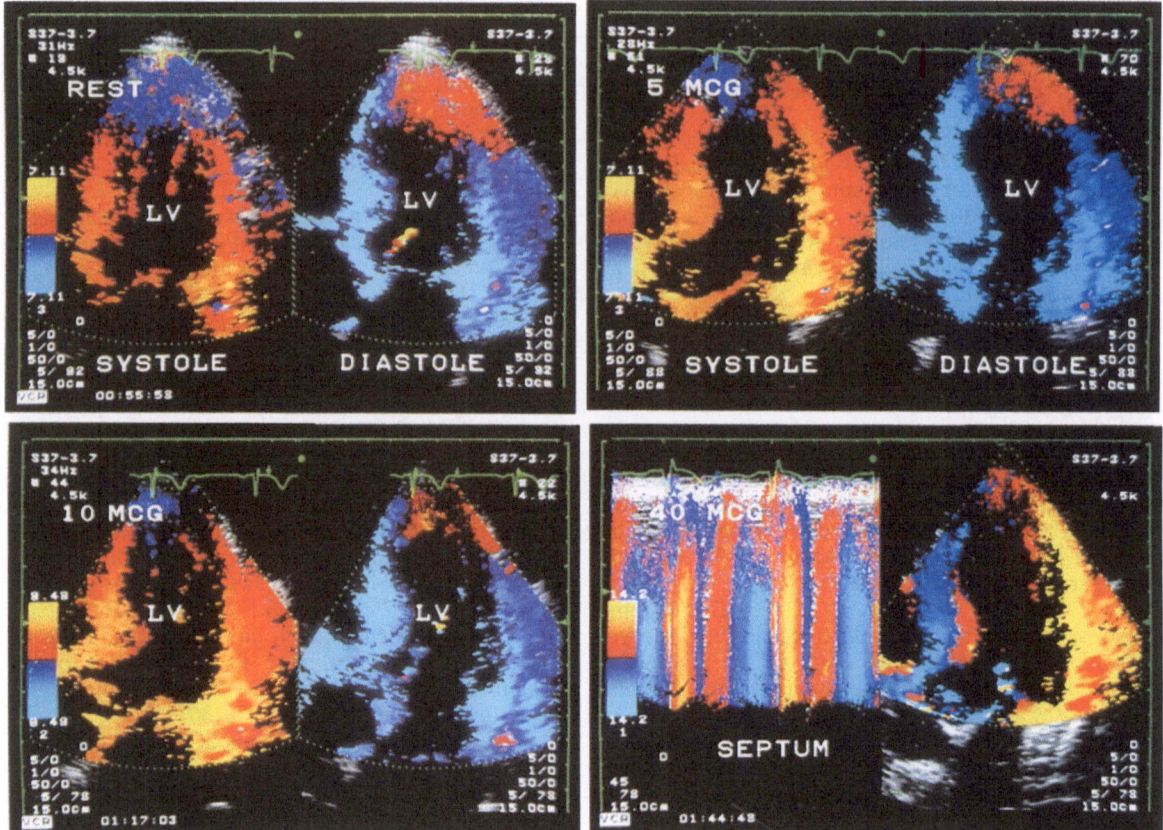

Fig. 9.4. Development of abnormal wall motion of the lateral left ventricular wall induced by dobutamine stress echocardiography as a sign of ischemia. *Left, upper figure:* Left ventricular wall function detected by TDE in a typical five-chamber view showing normal patterns with low velocities (2–4 cm/s) and the same direction of wall motion of the septum and lateral wall with an opposite direction of the apex. *Right, upper figure:* At the dose of 5 µg/kg/min Dobutamine with similar patterns as at rest but higher wall motion velocities (2–7 cm/s). *Left, lower figure:* At the dose of 10 µg/kg/min dobutamine further normal patterns at increasing wall motion velocities (4–9 cm/s). *Right, lower figure:* At the right side showing at diastole an abnormal movement of the lateral wall with an opposite direction to the septal movement. Overall, there are high velocities (6–14 cm/s) at peak stimulation (HR 123 b/min). Also, there seems to be a sign of subendocardial ischemia at the septum

Chapter 10 Hypertrophic Cardiomyopathy

D. R. Wallbridge

Background: Abnormal Diastolic Function

Hypertrophic cardiomyopathy is a primary myocardial disease characterised by left ventricular hypertrophy, involving the interventricular septum and also the ventricular free wall to varying degrees, and by normal or supernormal systolic ejection performance. Impaired left ventricular relaxation and filling has a major pathophysiological role, together with reduced chamber compliance. These changes contribute to increased left ventricular end-diastolic and left atrial pressures and thus to the development of cardiac symptoms ("diastolic heart failure"). For this reason, determination of the severity of left ventricular diastolic dysfunction has important implications for the management of patients with hypertrophic cardiomyopathy.

Diastolic function has been extensively studied in hypertrophic cardiomyopathy. Prolongation of the isovolumic relaxation period has been demonstrated by digitized contrast ventriculography [14], M-mode echocardiography [1], digitized M-mode echocardiography [7, 15–17], radionuclide ventriculography [2], and by pulsed Doppler echocardiography [13]. The rate of rapid filling is either normal [10] or reduced [16], and as a consequence, the atrial contribution to ventricular filling is increased [6].

Noninvasive evaluation of diastolic filling is problematical, because left ventricular dynamics are influenced by many factors. The importance of loading conditions in patients with non-obstructive hypertrophic cardiomyopathy is reported by *Hausdorf* [8]. An increase in afterload by infusion of angiotensin II improves early diastolic dysfunction, with a reduction in isovolumic relaxation time and an increase in rapid diastolic filling. The application of new techniques for assessing diastolic function, such as the pattern of left ventricular posterior wall motion by M-mode echocardiography, has also been limited by the influence of afterload and preload [18]. A further difficulty, highlighted by *Hanrath* [7], is that abnormal early diastolic function is not specific to hypertrophic cardiomyopathy, and a similar pattern is seen in patients with concentric left ventricular hypertrophy secondary to hypertension or aortic stenosis.

Regional Differences in Cardiac Function

Left ventricular relaxation has been considered to be influenced by regional nonuniformity as well as by myocardial inactivation and loading conditions ("triple control of relaxation") [5]. It is well known that in coronary artery disease regional nonuniformity of left ventricular wall motion is associated with abnormal ventricular relaxation [11]. In patients with hypertrophic cardiomyopathy, because of the broad heterogeneity in the distribution of left ventricular hypertrophy, it is reasonable to expect that spatial and temporal nonuniformity is present and might play a role in left ventricular diastolic dysfunction.

Bonow [4] showed that patients with hypertrophic cardiomyopathy have a higher than normal degree of rapid ventricular filling asynchrony as well as heterogeneity in the regional distribution of the amount of early versus late filling. The region of augmented filling during atrial systole involved the septum in 38 of 48 patients, but was concordant with the localisation of hypertrophy by echocardiography in only 18 of 33 patients. Administration of verapamil was associated with more uniform regional diastolic performance and improvement in global diastolic filling. In a further study, the time constant of regional wall stress decrease was significantly correlated with isovolumic relaxation time and tended to be more prolonged in regions with increased wall thickness [9]. More recently, *Betocchi* [3] showed that diastolic asynchrony is not increased in the majority of patients with hypertrophic cardiomyopathy, but in those in whom it is present, an impairment in peak filling rate can be observed. In contrast, asynergy is a very common finding in patients with hypertrophic cardiomyopathy due to inhomogeneity of regional wall motion: normal wall motion but increased stiffness of the septum, combining with hyperkinesia of the free wall.

Whilst magnetic resonance myocardial tagging has demonstrated abnormal segmental wall motion in hypertrophic cardiomyopathy, at this time, the image quality is insufficient to document the diastolic filling period of the left ventricle [12].

Mechanisms Underlying Regional Variation in Diastolic Function

Whilst the precise mechanisms are unclear at present, there are some possible explanations:

1. *Heterogeneous myocardial hypertrophy:* In hypertrophied regions, not only impaired myoplasmic calcium removal but also excessively reduced contraction load may contribute to the slower relaxation. But factors other than hypertrophy itself must also contribute to impaired regional diastolic function, because one-third of patients manifest reduced rapid filling in segments of the left ventricle that are not hypertrophied [11].
2. *Regional foci of myocardial fibrosis:* may affect relaxation
3. *Outward wall motion during isovoluminc contraction:* is more pronounced in hypertrophied regions [4, 7]. Because outward wall thickness increases the regional area and reduces wall thickness, the rate of decrease in wall stress during isovolumic relaxation decreases, leading to impaired relaxation in the hypertrophied regions.
4. *Regional myocardial ischaemia:* particularly subendocardial ischaemia may cause slow and asynchronous regional relaxation.

TDE Experience

From the above discussion it will be apparent that there is a requirement for regional assessment of myocardial contraction and relaxation in subjects with hypertrophic cardiomyopathy. Tissue Doppler echocardiography may be used to advantage in this condition because of the unique ability of this imaging technique to demonstrate the magnitude, direction and timing of changes in myocardial velocity. (See figure legends.)

References

1. Alvares RF, Shaver JA, Gamble WH, Goodwin JF (1984) Isovolumic relaxation period in hypertrophic cardiomyopathy. J Am Coll Cardiol 3:71–81
2. Betocchi S, Bonow RO, Bacharach SL, Rosing DR, Maron BJ, Green MV (1986) Isovolumic relaxation period in hypertrophic cardiomyopathy: assessment by radionuclide angiography. J Am Coll Cardiol 7:74–81
3. Betocchi S, Hess OM, Losi MA, Nonogi H, Krayenbuehl HP (1993) Regional left ventricular mechanics in hypertrophic cardiomyopathy. Circulation 88:2206–2214
4. Bonow RO, Vitale DF, Maron BJ, Bacharach SL, Frederick TM, Green MV (1987) Regional left ventricular asynchrony and impaired global left ventricular filling in hypertrophic cardiomyopathy. J Am Coll Cardiol 9:1108–1116
5. Brutsaert DL, Rademakers FE, Sys SU (1984) Triple control of relaxation: implications in cardiac disease. Circulation 96:190–196
6. Grossman W, McLaurin LP (1976) Diastolic properties of the left ventricle. Ann Intern Med 84:316–326
7. Hanrath P, Mathey DG, Siegert R, Bleifeld W (1980) Left ventricular relaxation and filling pattern in different forms of left ventricular hypertrophy. Am J Cardiol 45:15–23
8. Hausdorf G, Siglow V, Nienaber CA (1988) Effects of increasing afterload on early diastolic dysfunction in hypertrophic cardiomyopathy. Br Heart J 60:240–246
9. Hayashida W, Kumada T, Kohno F, Noda M, Ishikawa N, Kojima J, Himura Y, Kawai C (1991) Left ventricular regional relaxation and its nonuniformity in hypertrophic cardiomyopathy. Circulation 84:1496–1504
10. Hess OM, Murakami T, Krayenbuehl HP (1986) Does verapamil improve left ventricular relaxation in patients with myocardial hypertrophy. Circulation 74:530–543
11. Ludbrook PA, Byrne JD, Tiefenbrunn AJ (1981) Association of asynchronous protodiastolic segmental wall motion with impaired left ventricular relaxation. Circulation 64:1201–1211
12. Maier SE, Fischer SE, McKinnon GC, Hess OM, Krayenbuehl H-P, Boesiger P (1992) Evaluation of left ventricular segmental wall motion in hypertrophic cardiomyopathy with myocardial tagging. Circulation 86:1919–1928
13. Maron BJ, Spirito P, Green KJ, Wesley YE, Bonow RO, Arce J (1987) Noninvasive assessment of left ventricular diastolic function by pulsed Doppler echocardiography in patients with hypertrophic cardiomyopathy. J Am Coll Cardiol 10:733–742

14. Sanderson JE, Gibson DG, Brown DJ, Goodwin JF
(1977) Left ventricular filling in hypertrophic cardiomyopathy. An angiographic study. Br Heart J
39:661–670
15. Sanderson JE, Traill TA, St John-Sutton MG,
Brown DJ, Gibson DG, Goodwin JF (1978) Left
ventricular relaxation and filling in hypertrophic
cardiomyopathy: an echocardiographic study. Br
Heart J 40:596–601
16. St John Sutton MG, Tajik AJ, Gibson DG, Brown
DJ, Seward JB, Giuliani ER (1978) Echocardiographic assessment of left ventricular filling and
septal and posterior wall dynamics in idiopathic

hypertrophic subaortic stenosis: an echocardiographic study. Circulation 57:512–520
17. Upton MT, Gibson DG (1973) Measurement of
instantaneous left ventricular dimension and filling
rate in man, using echocardiography. Br Heart J
35:1141–1149
18. Yoneda Y, Suwa M, Hanada H, Hirota Y, Kawamu-
ra K (1992) Noninvasive detection of left ventricular
diastolic dysfunction using M-mode echocardiography to assess left ventricular posterior wall kinetics
in hypertrophic cardiomyopathy. Am J Cardiol
70:1583–1588

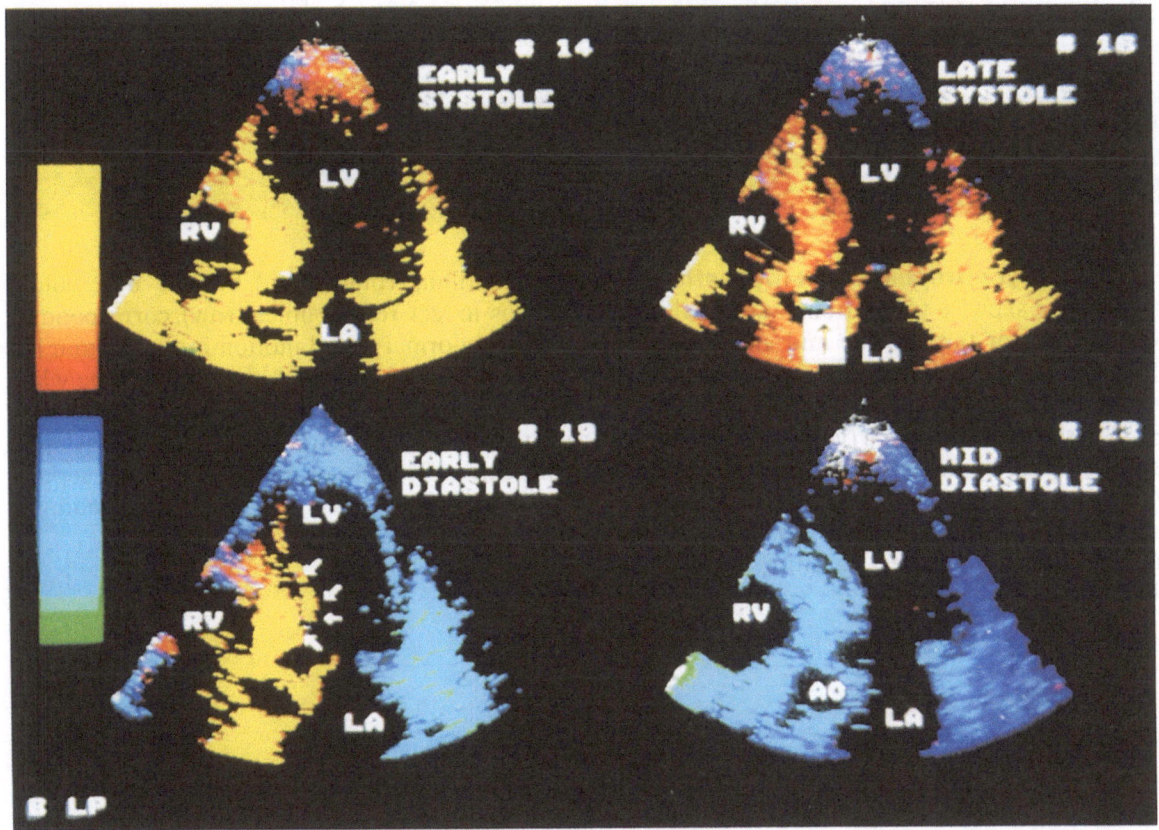

Fig. 10.1. Hypertrophic cardiomyopathy. A typical apical five-chamber view showing asymmetrical septal hypertrophy. The upper frames show normal patterns of colour myocardial velocity during systole, with the left ventricular septum and lateral wall coloured yellow (movement towards the transducer), and the apex blue (movement away from the transducer). The normal diastolic pattern (bottom right) is the reverse of the systolic pattern, with the septum and lateral walls coloured blue, and the apex yellow. However, the bottom left frame shows events early in diastole, when both the septum (yellow) and apex (blue) show abnormal colour related to abnormal myocardial motion. Asynchrony of the heart

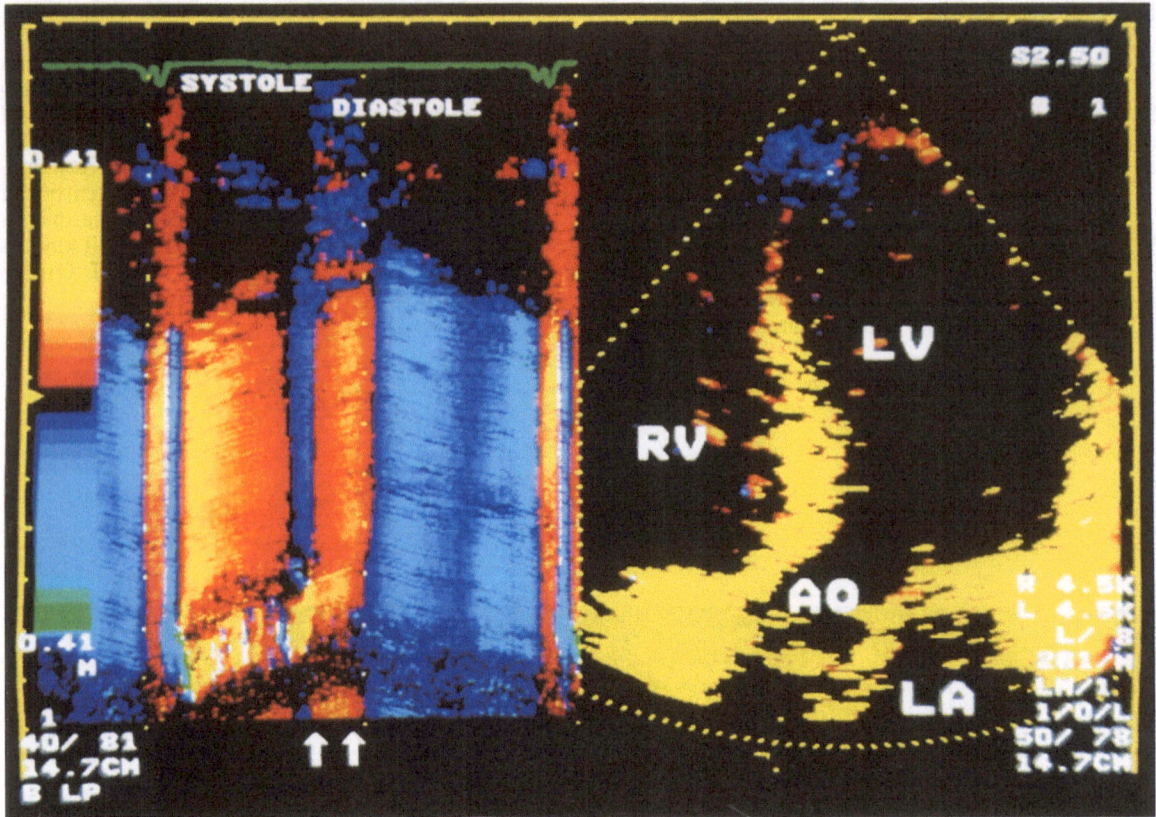

Fig. 10.2. Hypertrophic cardiomyopathy. The right image shows a frame from systole, with the M-mode cursor through the mid and basal septum. The temporal relation of myocardial colour velocities may be appreciated by reference to the ECG in the M-mode image (left). Systolic ejection is represented by the broad yellow/red band, and is normal. Diastole commences with isovolumic relaxation (short dark blue band). The expected normal pattern would be a transition to rapid ventricular filling (blue/white) but the next colour band is, in fact, red (double arrow), corresponding to the abnormal septal motion in the bottom left image of Fig. 10.1. In fact, the normal blue/white band appears to be delayed. The second blue/white band at the end of diastole represents atrial contraction. This abnormal motion of the septum and apex early in diastole is a common finding in hypertrophic cardiomyopathy

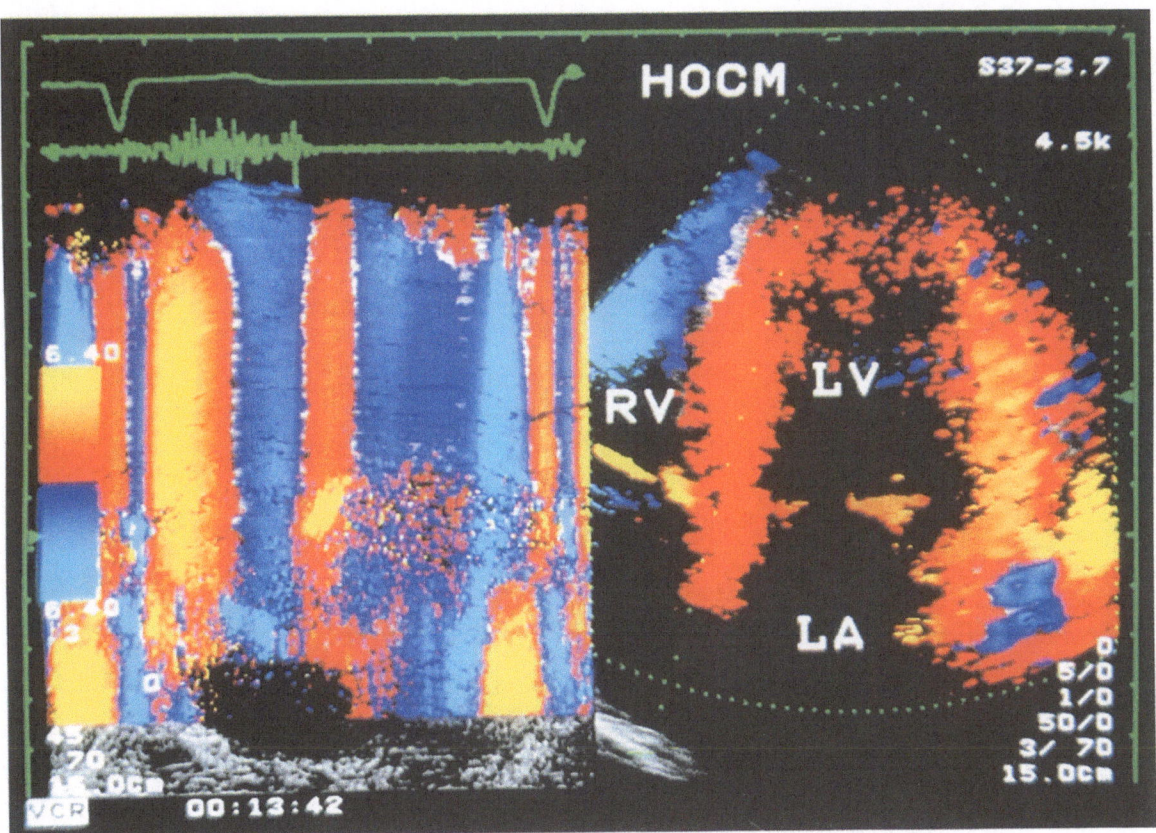

Fig. 10.3. Hypertrophic cardiomyopathy. Left-hand frame. The inclusion of the phonocardiogram with the M-mode image of the septum shows that the abnormal red band (Fig. 10.2) occurs after opening of the mitral valve: that is, during rapid ventricular filling. Due to the increased dependence of the septum on atrial contraction for diastolic filling, the blue/white band at the end of diastole is particularly prominent in this image

Chapter 11 **Cardiac Amyloidosis**

J. Drozdz, R. Erbel

Amyloid infiltration of the heart often occurs in patients with systemic amyloidosis and is recognized as the leading cause of death [4]. Echocardiography has been used as a noninvasive diagnostic method in symptomatic and asymptomatic patients with cardiac amyloidosis [2, 5, 6]. Characteristic echocardiographic features of advanced disease have been described. Progression of amyloid infiltration of the heart in serial M-mode, two-dimensional, and Doppler echocardiographic examinations were reported [1, 3]. TDE was used in patients with known amyloidosis in order to obtain a new insight into the disease as the amyloid infiltration of the myocardium was thought to induce changes of myocardial velocity. It should be expected that the peak systolic and diastolic velocities of the left ventricular myocardium in cardiac amyloidosis are lower than in normal subjects. This was previously reported using computerized M-mode echocardiography in parasternal long axis views by analyzing the rate of left ventricular diameter changes [5].

Velocity Pattern in Cardiac Amylodosis

For measurement of the velocity of the myocardium the sample-volume was placed within the left ventricular walls. In normal subjects (see chapter 5) four peaks of the left ventricular velocity pattern are detected: peak systolic velocity, peak early-diastolic, mid-diastolic, and late-diastolic velocity. The velocity pattern in cardiac amyloidosis differs from that of normal subjects in several aspects (Fig. 11.1).

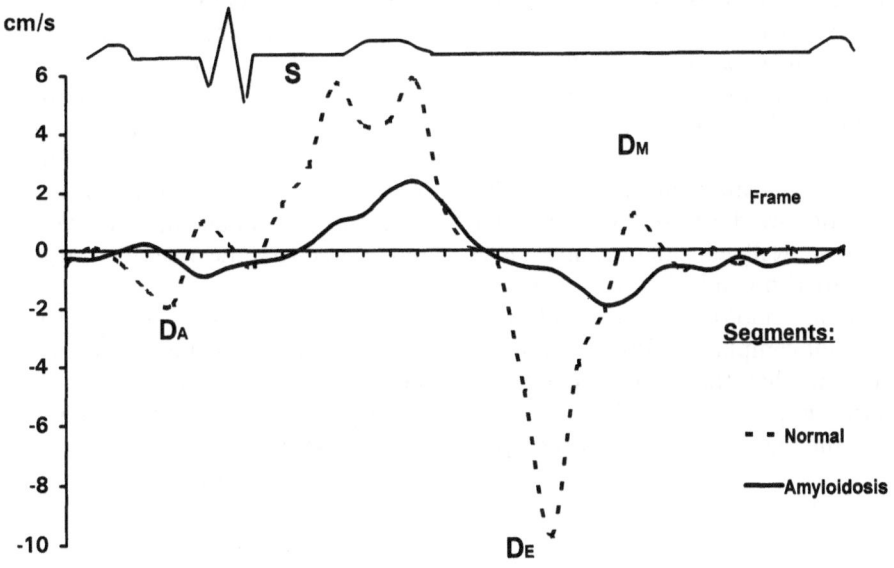

Fig. 11.1. Left ventricular posterior wall (segment 6) velocities in subsequent frames from the parasternal view in a patient with advanced cardiac amyloidosis in comparison with a representative healthy subject. (S = peak systolic velocity, D_E = peak early-diastolic velocity, D_M = peak mid-diastolic velocity, D_A = peak late-diastolic velocity)

First of all, the velocity pattern of cardiac amyloidosis is flattened, in contrast to the peaking pattern in normal subjects (Figs. 11.2–11.8). The changes of myocardial velocities are diminished, and both acceleration and deceleration of myocardial velocities are reduced.

Peak systolic and early diastolic velocities of the left ventricular wall in cardiac amyloidosis are decreased in comparison to the normal subject. In advanced cardiac amyloidosis more pronounced changes are related to the peak diastolic velocity. Subsequently, peak early-diastolic (D_E) to peak systolic velocity (S) ratio was found to be below -1.3, in sharp contrast to the ratio in normal subjects ($D_E/S = -1.5 - -2.0$) (Fig. 11.3).

The peak early-diastolic to peak systolic velocity ratio of the left ventricular wall segments may describe the diastolic dysfunction in patients with cardiac amyloidosis. The regional diastolic dysfunction evaluated by studying the ratios of the velocities of some parts of the myocardial wall may be of clinical value.

The mid-diastolic wall velocities in normal subjects show a short phase immediately following the early-diastolic ventricular expansion. The velocity direction at mid-diastole is opposite to the direction of velocity of early diastolic phase.

In patients with amyloidosis this mid-diastolic velocity pattern with opposite velocity direction to the early-diastolic phase cannot be seen. There is a lowered level of velocity of the left ventricular wall in diastole with only one phase of myocardial wall velocity. This may be explained by an increased myocardial stiffness due to amyloid infiltration and low early-diastolic velocities (Figs. 11.6, 11.7).

In patients with cardiac amyloidosis the late-diastolic wall velocities are decreased. Low late-diastolic left ventricular wall velocities in amyloidosis can be related to a possible left atrial systolic function disturbance and/or decreased left ventricular myocardial compliance. But it has to be taken into account that the velocity pattern is different at different phases of the disease, as has been shown for the mitral inflow pulsed Doppler signals [2].

invasively, giving insight into left ventricular mechanisms in cardiac amyloidosis.

The time delay between electrical activation and mechanical response of the left ventricular walls can be estimated as preejection period (PEP) and isovolumic contraction time (ICT). The time intervals can be estimated by calculating the time between the Q-wave on the ECG and the peak systolic wall velocity, as the brightest color on the TDE M-mode recording.

The time from Q-wave to the diastolic time intervals depends strongly on the heart rate. A new reference point should therefore be designated. This point can be determined as the end of systole, visualized as the color reversal at the end of T-wave on the ECG. The time could also be estimated from the end of systole to the peak diastolic wall velocity, visualized as the brightest TDE color-coding.

Finally, a time delay exists between electrical activation of the left atrium and the filling of the left ventricle visualized as a myocardial color-coded map similar to that during early relaxation. This can be estimated from the M-mode TDE recording by measuring time between the P-wave on the ECG to the onset of left ventricular filling.

In cardiac amyloidosis the PEP time was comparable to that of normal subjects (66 ± 15 ms), but the time between electrical activation and the peak systolic velocity was prolonged (over 150 ms vs. 129 ± 23 ms in normal subjects). This prolonged time may represent disturbances of the left ventricular systolic function.

The time from color reversal to peak diastolic velocity was prolonged in patients with cardiac amyloidosis in comparison to healthy subjects (over 120 ms vs. 94 ± 36 ms in healthy subjects). This may be dependent on myocardial stiffness and related to reduced acceleration of myocardial velocity.

The time delay between P-wave to left ventricular filling is found to be longer in amyloidosis than in the control group (over 50 ms vs. 31 ± 12 ms in healthy subjects). This could be related to the left myocardial stiffness and/or to the prolonged time from atrial electrical activation to atrial mechanical response.

Time Analysis in Cardiac Amyloidosis

Apart from peak velocities of the myocardial wall, new TDE parameters could be estimated non

New Signs of Cardiac Amyloidosis

All moving structures that reflect ultrasonic beams can generate a Doppler shift, which represents the difference between transmitted and received frequencies. The Doppler shift allows measurement of the velocities of a target reflecting the ultrasonic beam. The measured velocity of the cardiac tissue can be displayed as a color map superimposed onto the conventional black and white two-dimensional echocardiographic image. Theoretically, all parts of the moving cardiac tissue should be coded by color in TDE. However, this depends on its velocity and the gain setting. The lowest tissue velocity coded by color may be set to be very low (below 0.1 cm/s) (Figs. 11.6, 11.8). The gain setting should be adjusted to the actual examination conditions. In general, using optimal tissue Doppler velocity scale and gain setting, nearly all parts of the cardiac tissue are coded by color during systolic and diastolic motion in healthy subjects.

In contrast, in some patients with cardiac amyloidosis a non-color-coded region within the interventricular septum ("sandwich-pattern") was detected in TDE recording in the parasternal and apical view (Fig. 11.2). The borders of the cardiac tissue are coded by the same colors, red during systole and blue during diastole. The non-color-coded region moves in the same direction with similar velocities. This illustrates that absent color-coding depends not on low tissue velocity, but on low amplitude of the received ultrasonic signal.

The low amplitude of the received ultrasonic signal can also be demonstrated on the conventional black and white echocardiographic image. The visualization of this region is improved using the new method of TDE. Measurement of the area of non-color-coded region can be performed.

Low velocity peaks of left ventricular wall in cardiac amyloidosis give the particular possibility to study interdependence between motion of the myocardial walls and total heart movement (Fig. 11.8). We previously described (see chapter 6) that the net wall velocity measured by TDE in the parasternal view depends mainly on two velocities: one is related to wall motion during the cardiac cycle, and the second is related to total heart movement within the chest.

During the main part of systole the velocity of total heart movement plays a minor role in healthy subjects. Consequently, there is only a short phase at endsystole (30–60 ms), when the velocity of the heart exceeds the velocity of the interventricular septum motion. At this time both the interventricular septum and the posterior left ventricular wall move toward the transducer.

The total heart movement in patients with cardiac amyloidosis seems to be similar in direction to that of normal subjects. Surprisingly, the contribution of the whole heart movement to the net TDE velocity is higher than in healthy subjects. Amyloid infiltration of the heart principally changes the wall velocity during the cardiac cycle. In advanced cardiac amyloidosis, the net velocity of the interventricular septum seems to depend greatly on the total heart movement in contrast to findings in healthy subjects.

Consequently, in early amyloidosis the phase at end-systole, when the velocity exceeds the velocity of the interventricular septum motion during the cardiac cycle is longer than in healthy subjects (>60 ms). In advanced cardiac amyloidosis, during the major part of systole, both the interventricular septum and the posterior left ventricular wall move in the same direction, toward the transducer (Fig. 11.9). This may be misdiagnosed as abnormal septum motion. However, in the apical view there is a characteristic normal velocity pattern of the interventricular septum. Furthermore, there is no septum motion abnormality in conventional black and white, two-dimensional echocardiography, and there is normal septum thickening during systole. Analysis of the aortic wall velocity may also be helpful as the depressed ventricular function and possible amyloid infiltration of the wall change the normal TDE pattern (Fig. 11.10).

Conclusion

TDE offers supplementary diagnostic information in cardiac amyloidosis. There are characteristic abnormalities in the velocity pattern concerning both velocity values and time intervals. Low velocities of the left ventricular walls during the cardiac cycle change the contribution of different velocity components. This may change the TDE color-coding. Furthermore, abnormal color-coding distribution within the myocardial wall, with non-color-coded regions in the middle of the myocardium can be demonstrated ("sandwich phenomenon").

References

1. Cueto Garcia L, Tajik AJ, Kyle RA, Edwards WD, Greipp PR, Callahan JA, Shub C, Seward JB (1984) Serial echocardiographic observations in patients with primary systemic amyloidosis: an introduction to the concept of early (asymptomatic) amyloid infiltration of the heart. Mayo Clin Proc 59:589–97
2. Klein AL, Hatle LK, Taliercio CP, Oh JK, Kyle RA, Gertz MA, Bailey KR, Seward JB, Tajik AJ (1991) Prognostic significance of Doppler measures of diastolic function in cardiac amyloidosis. A Doppler echocardiography study. Circulation 83:808–16
3. Klein AL, Hatle LK, Taliercio CP, Taylor CL, Kyle RA, Bailey KR, Seward JB, Tajik AJ (1990) Serial Doppler echocardiographic follow-up of left ventricular diastolic function in cardiac amyloidosis. J Am Coll Cardiol 16:1135–41
4. Kyle RA, Greipp PR (1983) Amyloidosis (AL): clinical and laboratory features in 229 cases. Mayo Clin Proc 58:665–83
5. Martin G, Sutton SS, Reichek N, Kastor JA, Giuliani ER (1982) Computerized M-mode echocardiographic analysis of left ventricular dysfunction in cardiac amyloid. Circulation 66:790–9
6. Siqueira-Filho AG, Cunha CL, Tajik AJ, Seward JB, Schattenberg TT, Giuliani ER (1981) M-mode and two-dimensional echocardiographic features in cardiac amyloidosis. Circulation 63:188–96

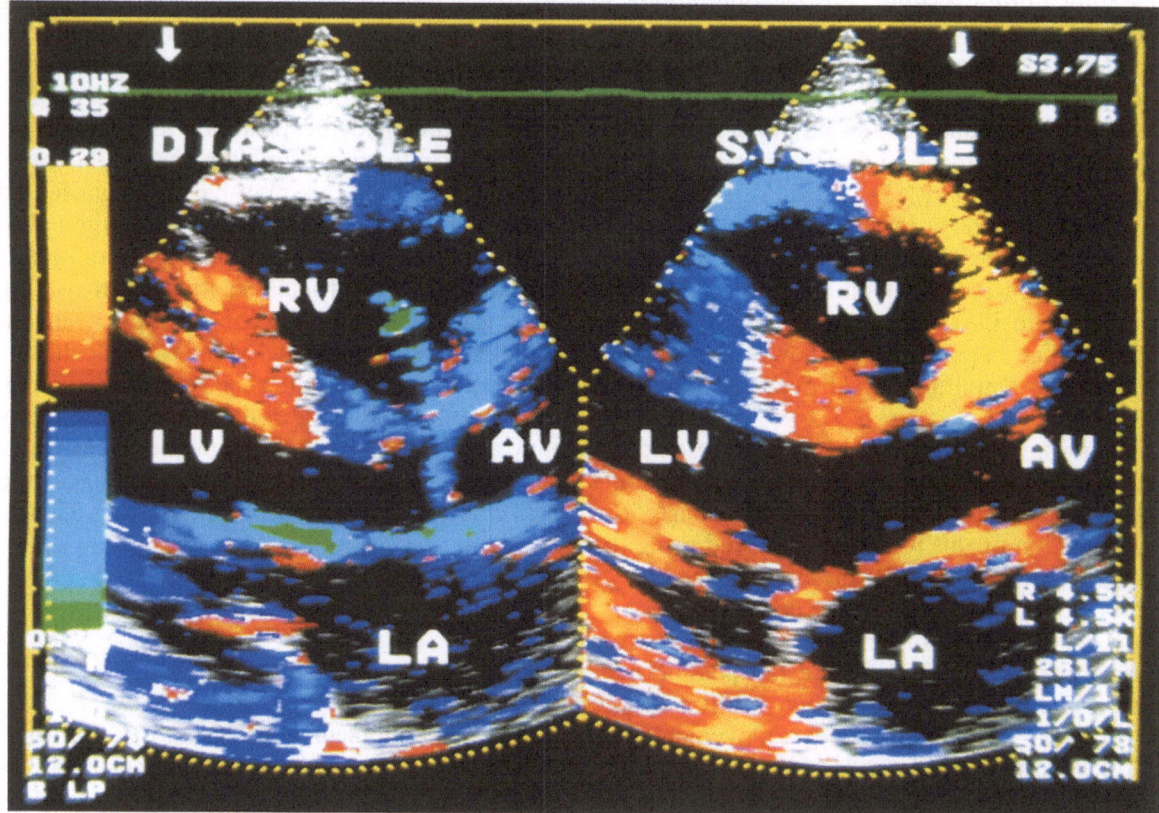

Fig. 11.2. Cardiac amyloidosis. Systolic and diastolic frame in the parasternal long axis view. The lowest color-coded velocity is set to be 0.12 cm/s. The highest measurable velocity is set to be 1.8 cm/s. The forward velocities are coded by red up to 0.4 cm/s, and by yellow above 0.4 cm/s. The backward velocities are coded by dark blue up to 0.4 cm/s, by bright blue up to 1.5 cm/s, and by green above 1.5 cm/s. Typical direction of the velocities of left ventricular walls. A non-color-coded region within the interventricular septum is presented. Good definition of the right ventricular anterior wall. During systole right ventricular anterior wall is moving toward the apex. Color-coding corresponds to wall movement direction in regard to the transducer position. As a result, the apical part of the right ventricular wall is coded by blue and the basal part is coded by red-yellow. Note the difference between systolic and diastolic right ventricular wall thickness. (AO = aortic root, LA = left atrium, LV = left ventricle, RV = right ventricle)

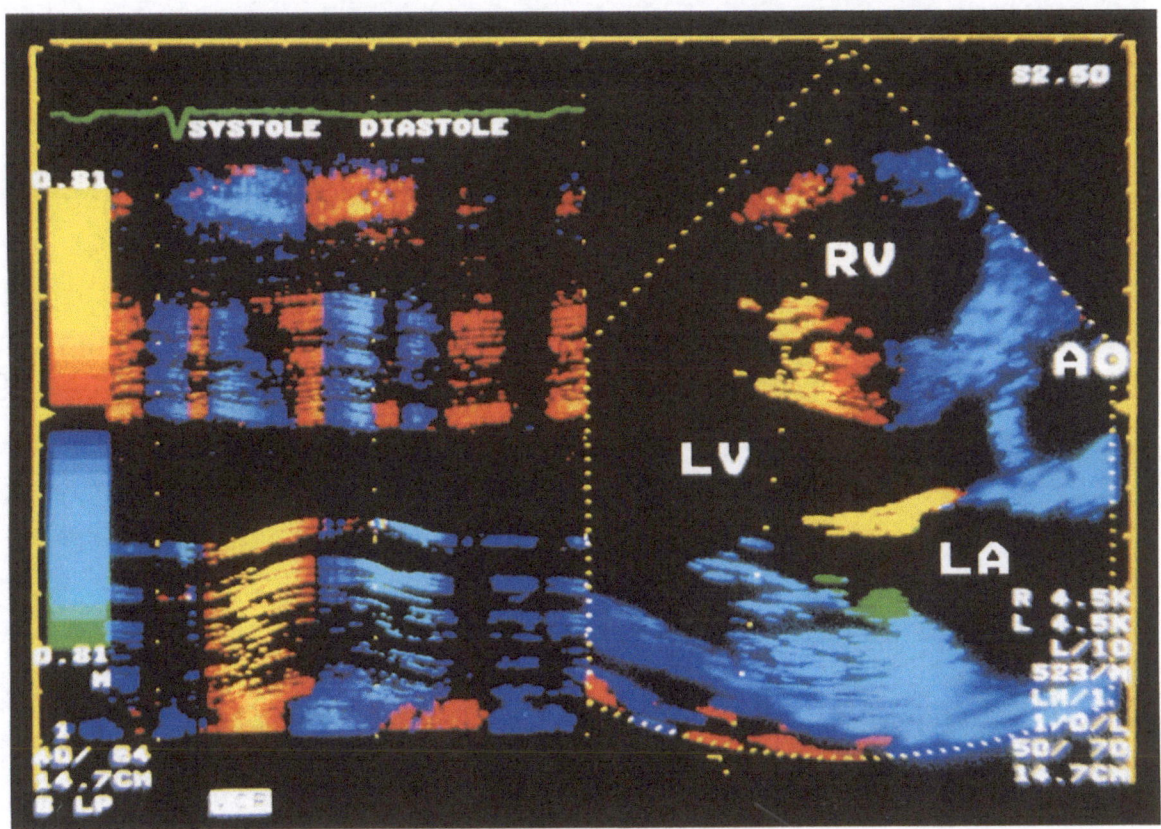

Fig. 11.3. Cardiac amyloidosis. 11.3 a. Early stage of amyloidosis (see legend of Fig. 11.3 b, page 106)

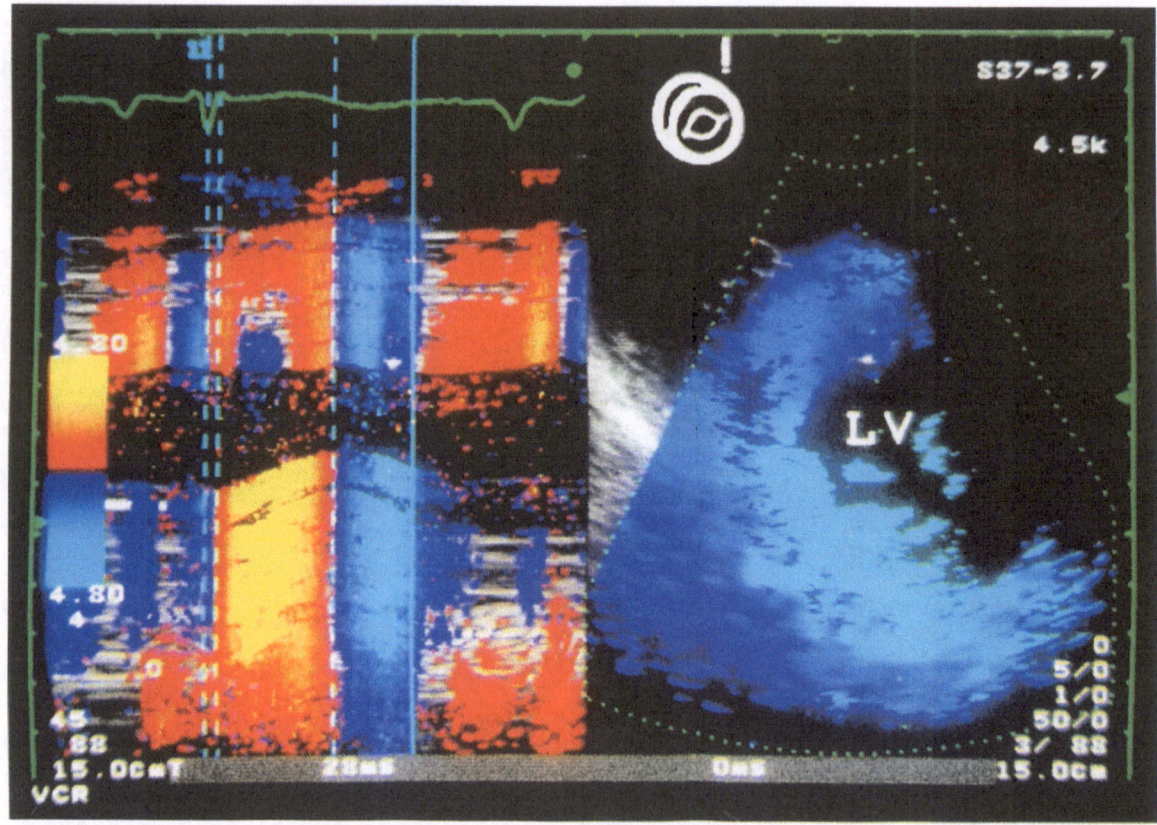

Fig. 11.3. Cardiac amyloidosis. Page 105 Fig. 11.3a: early stage of amyloidosis; page 106 Fig. 11.3b: late stage of amyloidosis in same patient [male, 53 years old]. M-mode tissue Doppler echocardiography in the parasternal long axis view using a 3.75 MHz transducer. Machine settings are: non-color-coded velocities up to 0.2 cm/s, red- or dark blue-coded velocities up to 0.9 cm/s, yellow-coded forward velocities above 0.9 cm/s, bright blue-coded backward velocities from 0.9 cm/s up to 3.0 cm/s, and green-coded backward velocities above 3.0 cm/s. Good visualization of interventricular septum and left ventricular posterior wall movement. In the early stage of amyloidosis the diastolic posterior wall velocity exceeds the systolic velocity. Within the interventricular septum non-color-coded region is visualized in both modalities: two-dimensional and M-mode color-coded tissue Doppler echocardiography. All borders of this region are coded with red-yellow color showing movement toward the transducer. The non-color-coded region is moving toward the transducer as well. Missing color-coding depends also on low amplitude of the signal received. The two-dimensional image represents an early diastolic frame. Enlarged left atrium with clear definition of the left atrial posterior wall moving with high velocity toward the transducer. Right ventricular anterior wall is visualized by TDE in both M-mode and two-dimensional images. However, the ultrasonic beam is not perpendicular to the right ventricular wall and the M-mode measurement overestimate the right ventricular wall thickness. The measurement of the right ventricular wall thickness can be performed by M-mode TDE after medial angulation of the ultrasonic beam. (AO = aortic root, LA = left atrium, LV = left ventricle, RV = right ventricle)

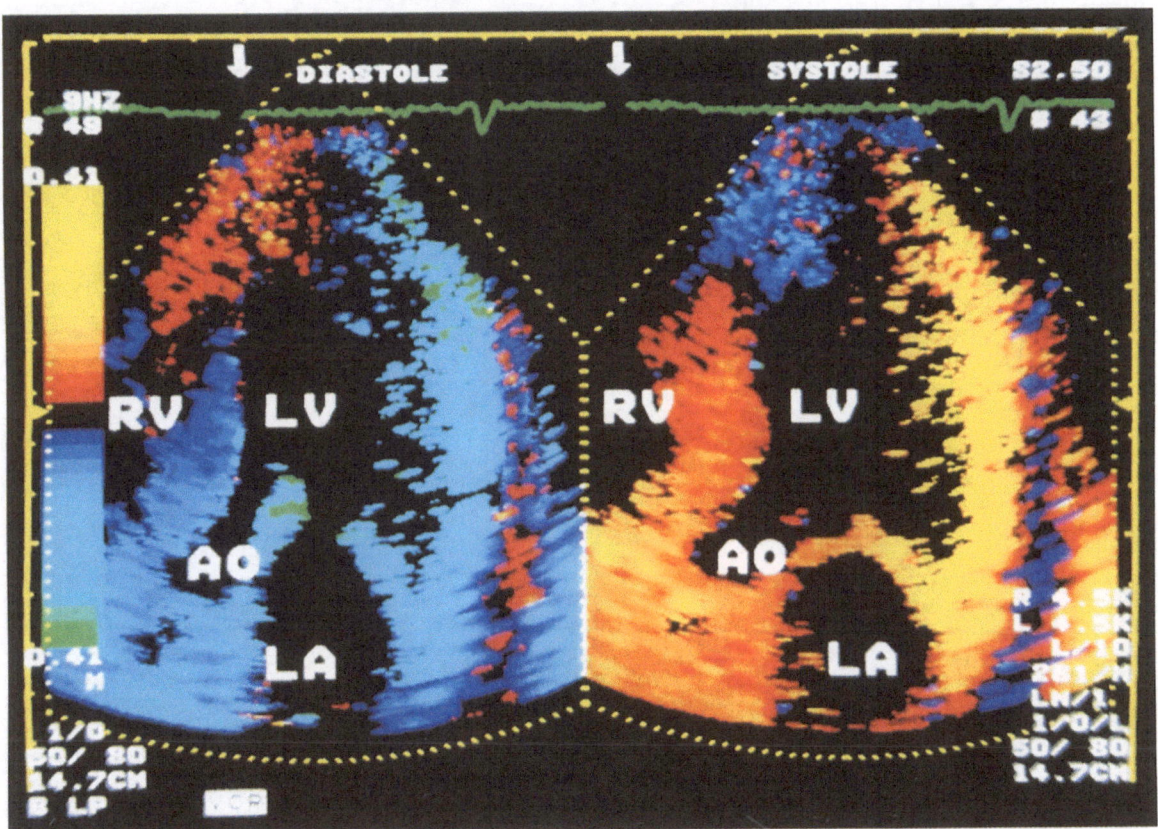

Fig. 11.4. Cardiac amyloidosis. Apical long axis view of the left ventricle in systole and early diastole using a 2.5 MHz transducer. Machine settings are: non-color-coded velocities up to 0.14 cm/s, red- or dark blue-coded velocities up to 0.44 cm/s, yellow- or bright blue-coded velocities above 0.44 cm/s. Both interventricular septum and posterior wall are moving toward the transducer during systole and away from the transducer during early diastole. In contrast, the apex is moving in the opposite direction with the corresponding color-coding. Good definition of the epicardial border of the left ventricular posterior wall. (AO = aortic root, LA = left atrium, LV = left ventricle, RV = right ventricle)

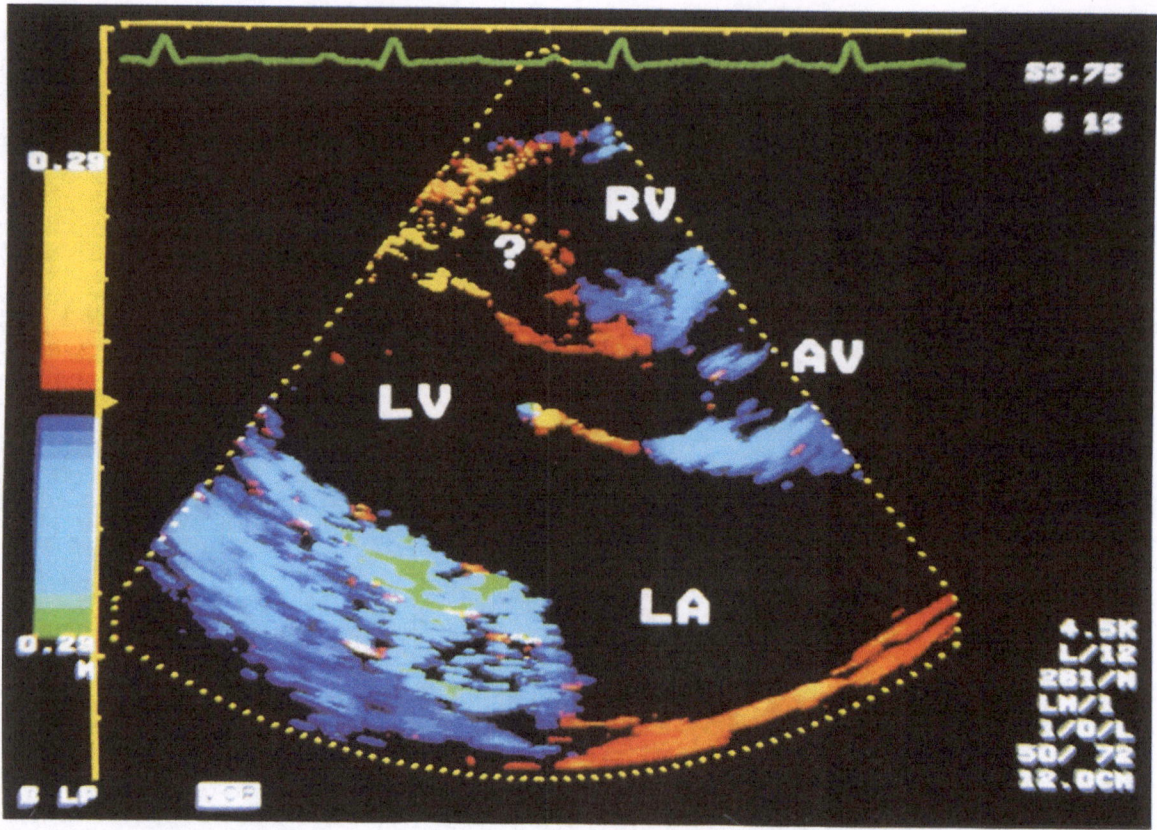

Fig. 11.5. Cardiac amyloidosis. Parasternal long axis view using a 3.75 Mhz transducer. "Sandwich" pattern of the IVS. Diastolic frame. The lowest color-coded velocity is set to be 0.12 cm/s. The highest measurable velocity is set to be 1.8 cm/s. The forward velocities are coded by red up to 0.4 cm/s, and by yellow above 0.4 cm/s. The backward velocities are coded by dark blue up to 0.4 cm/s, by bright blue up to 1. 5 cm/s, and by green above 1.5 cm/s. The posterior wall of the left ventricle moves away from the transducer, the interventricular septum moves toward the transducer. Within the interventricular septum the non-color-coded region is demonstrated. Enlarged left atrium. The posterior wall of the left atrium is moving toward the transducer indicating atrial emptying during early diastole. Good definition of the epicardial border of the posterior left ventricular wall. The anterior mitral leaflets moving toward the transducer during early diastole. Note aliasing effect. Closed aortic valve. The aortic root moves away from the transducer. Good definition of the right ventricular anterior wall. (AO = aortic root, LA = left atrium, LV = left ventricle, RV = right ventricle, *IVS* = interventricular septum)

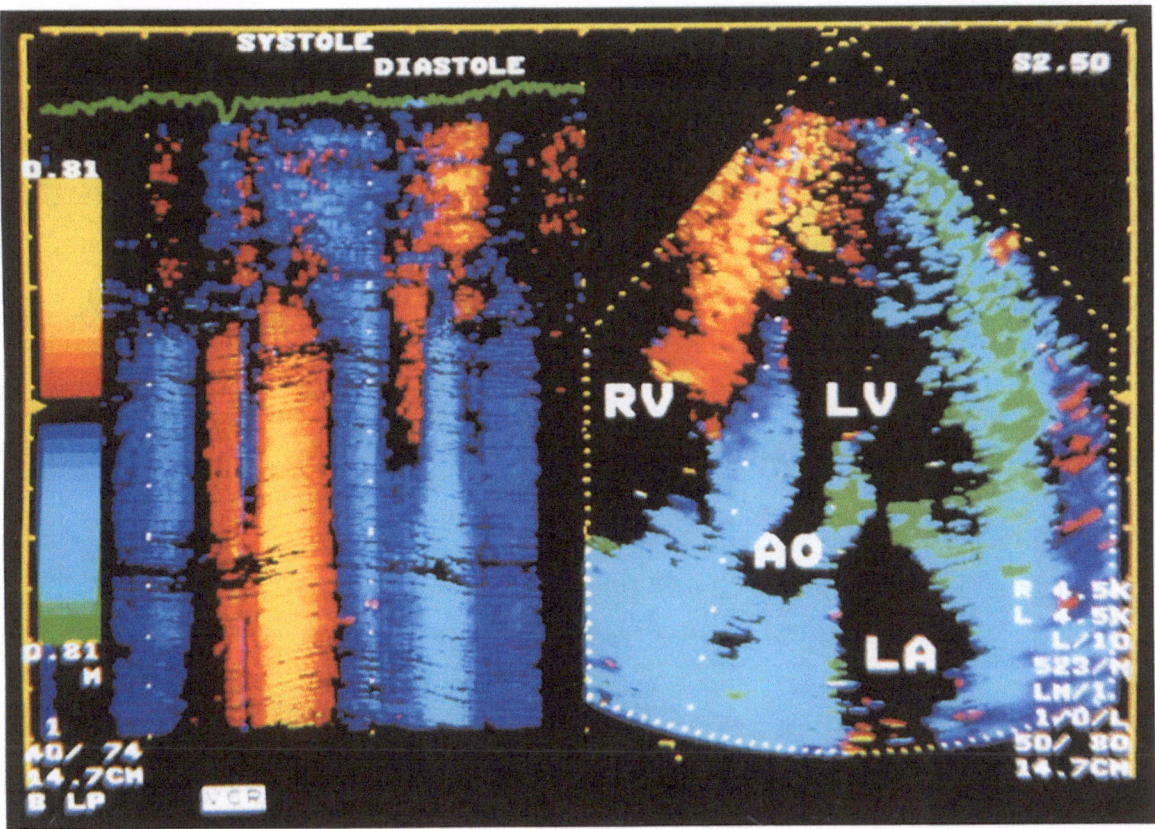

Fig. 11.6. Cardiac amyloidosis. M-mode cursor position through the interventricular septum in apical long axis view. Machine settings are: non-color-coded velocities – up to 0.33 cm/s, red- or dark blue-coded velocities up to 1.1 cm/s, green-coded backward velocities above 4.4 cm/s. After Q-wave on the ECG the systolic motion starts with corresponding red-yellow coding. Short duration of the forward septum motion and following longer backward motion coded by blue. The peak systolic velocity occurs in the first phase of systole, as visualized by yellow color-coding. No mid-diastolic forward motion of the interventricular septum is seen corresponding to the disturbed compliance of the myocardium in amyloidosis. Flat velocity pattern in contrast to peaking in healthy subjects. The apex shows reversed movement directions which is indicated by opposite color-coding. (AO = aortic root, LA = left atrium, LV = left ventricle, RV = right ventricle)

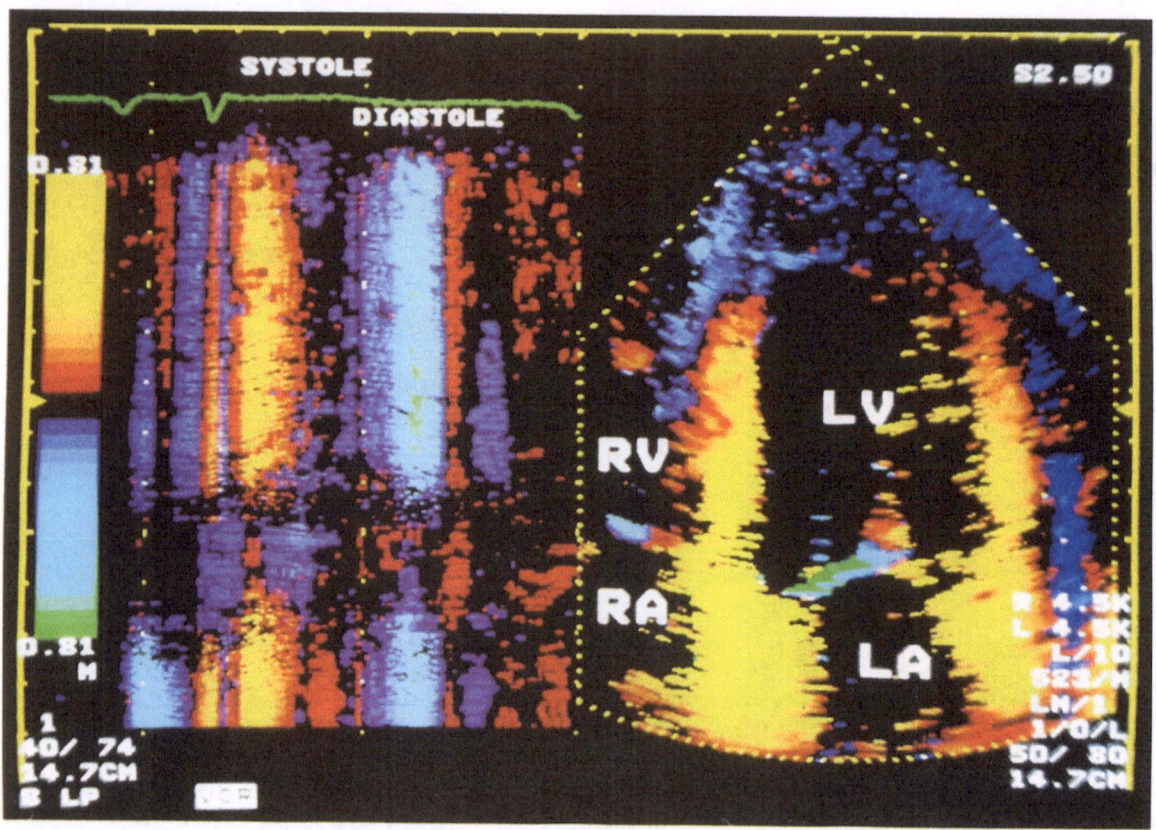

Fig. 11.7. Cardiac amyloidosis. M-mode cursor position through the lateral left ventricular wall. Early systolic frame on the 2-D image. The machine settings are the same as in Fig. 11.6. After the Q-wave on the ECG the systolic forward motion starts. The peak forward velocity indicated by bright-yellow coding occurs in early-systole. After color reversal in early diastole relatively low tissue velocities are recorded. The peak backward velocity in diastole occurs later than in normal subject. During late diastole low forward velocities are recorded. The time delay after start of the P-wave on the ECG and the backward motion of the lateral left ventricular wall exceeds 170 ms. Very low wall velocities are recorded at this phase indicated by dark blue color-coding. (A = left atrium, LV = left ventricle, RA = right atrium, RV = right ventricle)

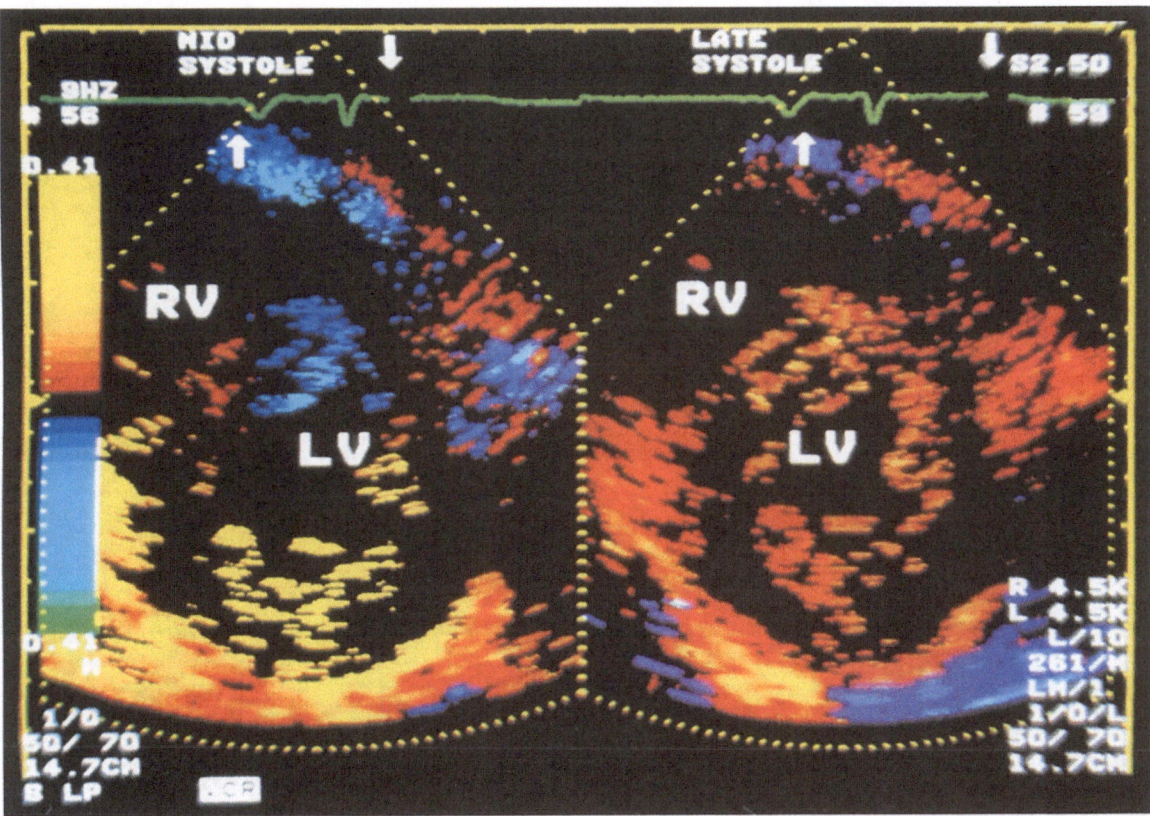

Fig. 11.8. Cardiac amyloidosis. Parasternal short axis view at the papillary muscle level. Amyloidosis with "sandwich" pattern of the LV walls. Mid-systolic *(left)* and late-systolic frame *(right)*. The left ventricle is moving toward the anterior chest wall during late systole indicated by red color-coding of the entire visualized left ventricular walls. Apart from the wall velocity during the cardiac cycle, the velocities of whole left ventricular movement within the chest must be taken into consideration. Both components, the veloc-ities of the cardiac wall motion during cardiac cycle, and the velocity of whole left ventricular movement within the chest, yield the net TDE velocity. The net velocity of the posterior wall is an addition of both velocities, whereas for the inter-ventricular septum the net velocity is a subtrac-tion of both velocities. Consequently, not only the value, but also the direction of the velocity of the interventricular septum depends on contribution of both velocities. (LV = left ventricle, RV = right ventricle)

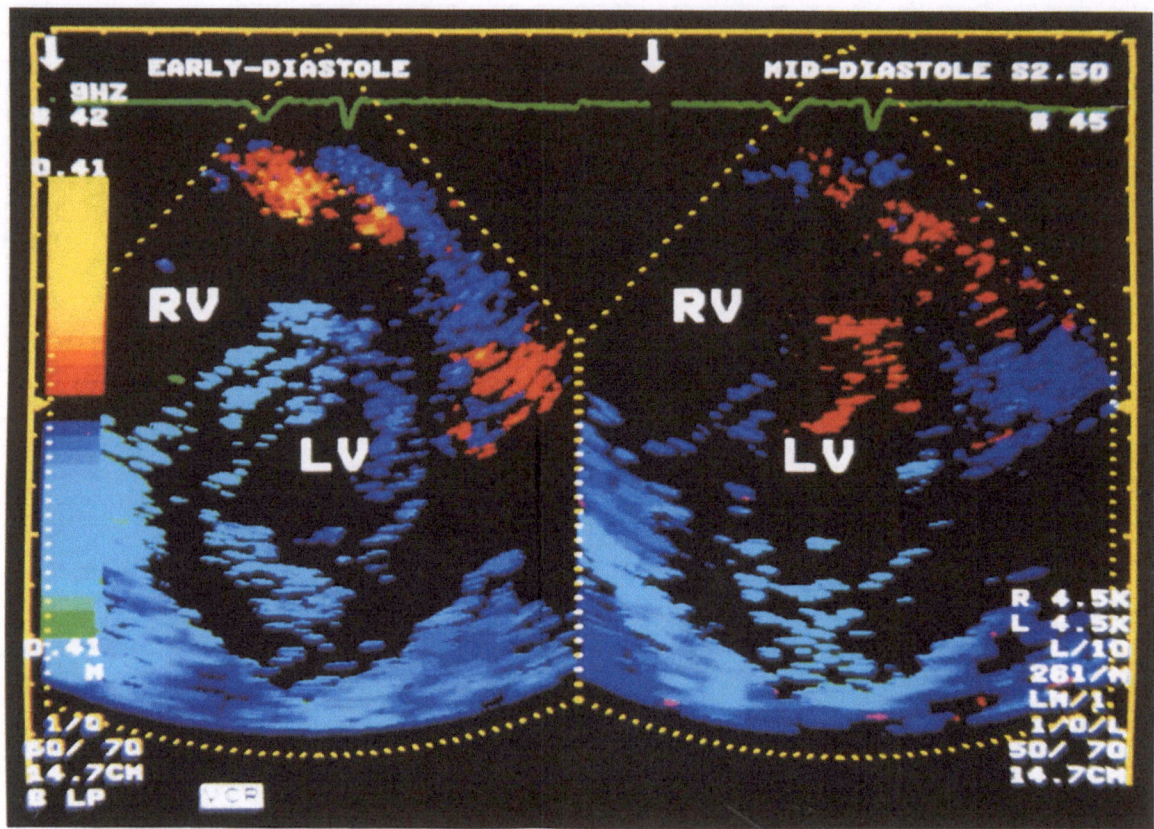

Fig. 11.9. Cardiac amyloidosis. Parasternal short axis view at the papillary muscle level. Early-diastolic *(left)* and mid-diastolic frame *(right)*. The entire heart is moving away from the anterior chest wall during early diastole, which is indicated by blue color-coding of the visualized left ventricular walls. In the next frames the velocity of the diastolic motion of the interventricular septum exceeds the heart velocity. This is indicated by red-coding of the antero-septal region. (LV = left ventricle, RV = right ventricle)

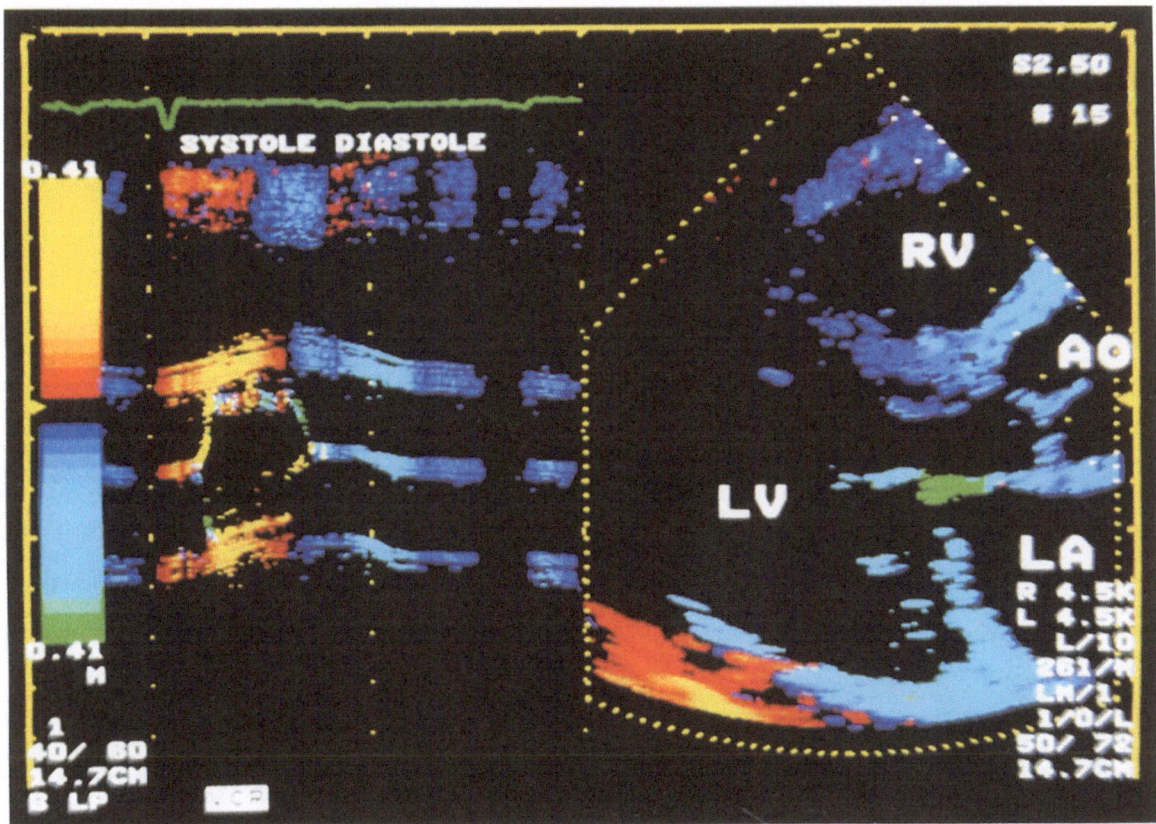

Fig. 11.10. Cardiac amyloidosis. M-mode recording of the aortic root motion in the parasternal long axis view using a 2.5 MHz transducer. The machine settings are: non-color-coded velocities up to 0.17 cm/s, red- or dark blue-coded velocities up to 0.48 cm/s, green-coded backward velocities above 2.24 cm/s. The only visualized structures which velocities exceeding the 2.24 cm/s are the leaflets of the mitral and aortic valve. The velocity of the aortic root mainly depends on heart motion. Other contributing factors include left and right ventricular shape changes and left atrial function. The forward aortic root velocity during systole exceeds the backward velocity during diastole. The time delay between start of the P-wave on the ECG to backward aortic root motion velocity is short and does not exceed 50 ms, in sharp contrast to the 150 ms time delay recorded over the left ventricular wall at the same machine settings. (AO = aortic root, LA = left atrium, LV = left ventricle, RV = right ventricle)

Chapter 12   Aortic Wall Velocity

J. Drozdz, R. Erbel, J. Zamorano

Echocardiography allows to study the anatomy of the aortic root and other parts of the aorta in parasternal, apical, suprasternal, and subcostal views. Using the transesophageal approach, nearly all parts of the thoracic aorta can be analyzed with high accuracy [3, 10].

Tissue Doppler Echocardiography (TDE) provides morphological and functional information by estimation of aortic wall velocities. First, the velocities of the aortic wall as a moving uniform structure within the chest are analyzed, and the mechanism of the motion is discussed, as well as potential clinical implications. The velocity differences between both aortic walls in the parasternal long axis view are described. This difference exists as a consequence of aortic diameter changes (aortic pulsation) during the cardiac cycle. The clinical usefulness of these findings is discussed.

Systole

The aortic root moves during systole toward the transducer in the parasternal view. This motion is induced by the ejection of blood into the aorta.

The aortic root velocity direction during this phase is similar to that of the left ventricular posterior wall and opposite to that of the interventricular septum.

Parameter of Left Ventricular Systolic Function

The aortic root excursion has been studied using M-mode in the parasternal view. The aortic wall excursion can be measured as a distance between end-diastolic and end-systolic aortic wall position. This has been used as a parameter of left ventricular systolic function [7, 13]. Poor left ventricular systolic function resulted in decreased aortic wall excursion compared to the healthy subjects.

The TDE examination offers a new parameter: aortic wall velocity. The aortic wall velocities in the parasternal long axis view are diminished in patients with poor left ventricular function. Peak anterior wall velocity in early systole of the ascending aorta in healthy subjects is above 6 cm/s. Peak aortic wall velocity in patients with slightly decreased left ventricular function was measured 4 to 6 cm/s, and in patients with markedly decreased left ventricular function it was below 4 cm/s. The potential role of TDE can be seen in on-line estimation of left ventricular systolic function by measuring aortic wall velocity.

Late Systole

During early- and mid-systole the interventricular septum and the anterior aortic wall move in opposite directions. During late systole the aortic root still moves in the anterior direction. During this phase both the interventricular septum and the aortic root move in the same direction: toward the transducer.

Early Diastole

In early diastole the direction of the velocity vector of both aortic walls is backward with high velocity.

Mid- and Late Diastole

In the next phase of diastole the rapid posterior movement of the aorta is interrupted, but usually not reversed.

After the P-wave on the ECG a second rapid backward motion of the aortic root is present. For the first time not only the systolic but also the diastolic function of the aorta can be studied non-invasively. Its relationship to hysteresis remains to be established.

Systole

From the transthoracic approach the normal aorta shows the highest wall velocities in early systole (normal values: peak anterior aortic wall velocity 5.1 ± 1.4 cm/s, peak posterior aortic wall velocity 4.9 ± 1.4 cm/s). Velocity drops during the second and third third of systole. These findings reflect the foreward movement of the aorta and the expansion. The higher velocity in early systole reflects the fact that 70% of the stroke volume is ejected by the ventricle in the first third of the systole (Fig. 12.10).

Systolic Time Intervals

The recorded ECG and echocardiogram reveal the clear separation of important systolic time intervals such as left ventricular ejection time (LVET) and the isovolumic contraction period. Taking into acount the ECG also the preejection period (PEP) can be calculated. Thus the very important ratio

PEP/LVET (normal range as 0.4–0.5)

can be assessed in only one scan plane, without necessity to record aortic and mitral valve motion or the pulse tracings (Fig. 12.10). This will have important applications for clinical pharmacology as well as assessment of cardiac toxicity of cytotoxic agents like adriamycine.

Interesting is also the change of the wall velocity pattern in the preejection period. In the normals there is a short foreward and a little longer backward movement during the isovolumetric contraction period, this pattern is significantly changed in hypertension as the foreward motion period is longer and the backward motion period shorter. This may indicate a prolongation of the preejection period.

Also, the most reliable parameter for estimating left ventricular contractility (Q-S2) can be determined without any difficulty and with high accuracy. The recorded ECG and the end of the foreward movement of the aorta (the beginning of the second heart sound) are demarcated by TDE with a short interruption of the forward movement.

Determination of pulse wave velocity is also possible in the ascending aorta, the aortic arch and the descending aorta (Fig. 12.10). As M-mode recordings have a very high time resolution, the assessment of the time difference between the onset of foreward movement (red color-coded) in the different aortic parts gives the velocity between the scanning areas – the pulse wave velocity can be determined taking into account the distance between both aortic segments.

Velocity Ratios

The peak systolic velocity of the aortic wall is similar to that of the left ventricular posterior wall. Peak early-diastolic velocity is lower than that of the posterior left ventricular wall. As a consequence, the peak early-diastolic to peak systolic velocity ratio is lower than described for left ventricular myocardium ($D_E/S = 1.0$–1.5 for aorta vs. 1.5–2.0 for myocardium).

The peak late-diastolic velocity to peak early-diastolic velocity ratio is for the aortic walls approximately four times higher than for the left ventricular posterior wall ($D_A/D_E = 1.0$–1.8 for aorta vs. 0.25–0.4 for myocardium).

Coronary Artery Disease

In patients with coronary artery disease the velocity patterns of the aortic wall differ from that of healthy subjects. The peak systolic velocities are diminished proportional to disturbed global left ventricular function.

There is also abnormal velocity distribution during diastole. The peak early-diastolic velocities are decreased. This seems to be dependent on diminished rapid filling. In some patients with good left ventricular function and diastolic disturbances the peak early-diastolic velocity is markedly decreased. In these patients the peak late-diastolic velocities are increased and the ratio peak late-diastolic to peak early-diastolic velocity is higher than in healthy subjects.

Poor left ventricular function usually results in decreased peak systolic and early- and late-diastolic velocity. More pronounced is the decrease of early-diastolic velocities. The ratio of peak late-diastolic to peak early-diastolic velocity is higher than 2.0. Often, the ratio of peak early-diastolic velocity to peak systolic velocity is decreased (< 1.0). The sensitivity and specificity of these signs for the detection of coronary heart disease have to be established.

Congestive Heart Failure

In congestive heart failure the velocities of the aortic root during all cardiac phases are decreased. There is also an abnormal velocity distribution. The peak systolic velocity is decreased due to a reduced left ventricular function. The early-diastolic velocities are markedly decreased, and the ratio peak early-diastolic velocity to peak systolic velocity is decreased. The late-diastolic velocities are reduced. The ratio of peak late-diastolic velocity to peak early-diastolic velocity, however, is often normal.

Arteriosclerosis/Hypertension

As an exciting field for the new echocardiographic method, TDE allows the noninvasive estimation of the aortic compliance. Atherosclerotic vascular disease is the most common cause of death in the Western World. The diagnostic methods for morphological assessment of arterial atherosclerotic disease include transthoracic and transesophageal echocardiography, carotid Duplex sonography, tonometry, intravascular ultrasound, magnetic resonance imaging and catheterization techniques. Evaluation of aortic anatomy by the imaging techniques and demonstration of arteriosclerotic lesions are provided by today's invasive and noninvasive methods. However, there is still a need of functional information. This includes the aortic "Windkessel".

"Windkessel" Model of the Aorta

The aortic "Windkessel" model consists of resistance, compliance, and characteristic impedance. The highest accuracy for estimation of aortic "Windkessel" is provided by invasive methods [5]. However, noninvasive methods may also provide information about aortic "Windkessel". Long-term follow-up of patients at a high risk of atherosclerosis can be done. The influence of therapy on aortic compliance has to be analyzed, particularly in relation to ACE inhibitors.

Background

During the development of arteriosclerosis, the aortic wall forms fatty streaks, later atheromas, and complex lesions with calcification and thrombosis. This results in aortic stiffness increase, which has been demonstrated both in animals and in humans [1, 2, 12, 18]. Arteriosclerosis produces a loss of elastin and an increase of collagen. Both components are closely linked and both are affected by many factors, for example by age, hypercholesterolemia, hypertension, diabetes, and connective tissue diseases [1, 2, 8, 12, 14].

Aortic Distensibility

The compliance and elasticity of an arterial wall is determined by the ratio of elastin, and collagen in the wall [8, 18]. Aortic compliance (or distensibility, as a term more often used today) is the volume per unit change in relation to pressure [8, 9, 15]. In other words, distensibility means that the volume of a structure can be enlarged by force. The aortic distensibility also depends on ejection of blood [16]. Since only part of the energy produced by the left ventricle during systole results in forward systolic flow in the aorta, the remaining energy is stored in the distended aorta. During diastole, this energy is converted into diastolic aortic forward flow [12, 15].

Aortic Elasticity

This term is used to describe the stored energy in the aortic wall during systole [15, 16]. This energy is used to exert force in aortic contraction during diastole. The aortic contraction provides the power for the generation of diastolic pressure and is significant in maintaining stable peripheral flow in spite of the cycle of cardiac ejections [12]. Elasticity of the aorta can also be understood as an auxiliary mechanism to cardiac function in terms of preserving peripheral circulation [11, 15, 16]. It is of great interest, for example, in coronary circulation. During systole flow within the myocardium is minimal. Flow in the coronary arteries takes place mainly during diastole. This is influenced by the diastolic pressure in the aortic "Windkessel". Thus, blood supply to the heart in part depends on the elasticity of the aorta.

Current Techniques for Estimation of Aortic Distensibility

Current methodology for the noninvasive determination of aortic and large artery distensibility involves two approaches: the estimation of distensibility from the fractional diameter change of a given aortic segment by imaging techniques against the pressure change (pulse pressure), and the estimation of the distensibility by pulse wave velocity measurement [5, 6].

In clinical practice the first method has been used, but only in a small group of patients [6, 17]. For calculation of the distensibility of the ascending aorta the following formula has been validated [4]:

$$\text{distensibility} = \frac{(\text{systolic} - \text{diastolic aortic diameter})}{(\text{diastolic aortic diameter}) \times (\text{pulse pressure})}$$

For the noninvasive estimation of distensibility of the ascending aorta, the end-diastolic and end-systolic diameters of the studied vessel to estimate the diameter change, and the end-diastolic and end-systolic pressures, to estimate the pulse pressure is used [1, 17].

The diastolic diameter and diameter change of the ascending aorta and aortic arch can be obtained by means of conventional transthoracic echocardiography. The noninvasive measurement of pressure change has several limitations. First, using the sphygmomanometer by applying the Korotkov sound method, we can estimate the pressure in the brachial artery, but not in the aorta. Second, the acquired pressure slightly underestimates the systolic blood pressure, but markedly overestimates the diastolic blood pressure [17]. Consequently, the net result underestimates the pressure change. The calculated aortic distensibility will be overestimated [17].

The best noninvasive method for calculating aortic distensibility is the applanation tonometer. In order to assess the effect of vascular structured abnormalities of the aorta on pulsatile load in humans this instrument was developed [19]. The arterial pulse contour can be visualized. An augmentation index was determined, representing the fraction of the pulse pressure contributed by a reflected wave [20]. With age the waveforms increase. Patients with increased load and left ventricular mass have an increased dominant late systolic peak [21, 22, 23]. The calculation of the pulse wave velocity can be used to estimate aortic distensibility by recording the pressure pulse at the carotid artery and the femoral artery and determining the time delay between both waves. But it has be taken into account that the reflected pressure wave is superimposed on the forward pulse wave. This explains, why the pulse pressure is better correlated with left ventricular mass in patients than the systolic or diatolic blood pressure.

New Technique of TDE

A new method for determining aortic distensibility based on the measurement of aortic wall velocities is proposed.

The velocities of the anterior aortic wall in young, healthy subjects differ from that of the posterior aortic wall. The difference between velocity of the anterior and posterior aortic wall is, in general, positive during systole and negative during diastole. This is expected, because there is a change of the aortic diameter during the cardiac cycle. The aorta becomes larger during systole and smaller during diastole. The typical maximal differences in young, healthy subjects with long-term arterial hypertension, marked coronary artery disease, and in aged subjects the velocities of both aortic walls were similar. The velocity difference between both aortic walls was diminished. These findings may be consistent with increased aortic stiffness due to atherosclerosis in this groups of individuals.

Timing of Aortic Pulsation

By TDE of the aortic wall, the pattern of anterior and posterior aortic wall velocity are received (Fig. 12.1). Using a high frame-rate, the velocity values during the cardiac cycle can be obtained. By subtraction of both anterior and posterior wall velocities in the same frame, the velocity pattern of aortic enlargement and diminution can be estimated (Fig. 12.2). Also, the mean acceleration and deceleration of the aortic pulsation can be computed, providing new information.

In hypertension a change of the systolic foreward wall velocity pattern is detected (Fig. 12.11). The measured velocity of forward motion is high in early systole as in normals, but the velocity in the mid- and late systole is significantly higher than in normals (Fig. 12.11). In mid- and late systole, it is up to 10 times higher than in normals. In the M-mode tracing a yellow color pattern not only in early systole but also in late systole can be seen. In normals, however, a yellow color pattern is found only in early systole.

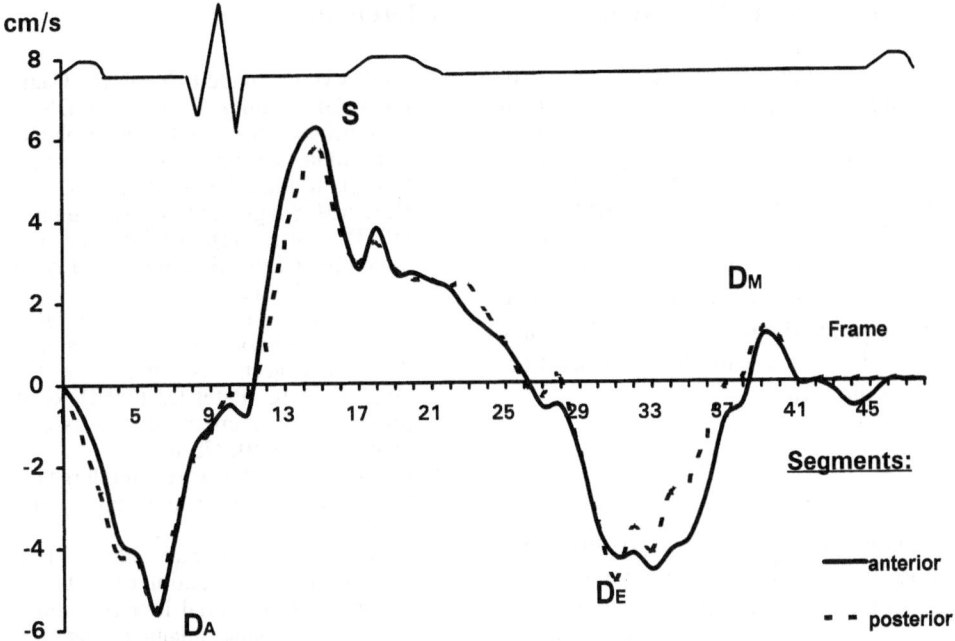

Fig. 12.1. Velocities of anterior and posterior aortic wall in subsequent frames in the parasternal view in a representative healthy young subject. (S = peak systolic velocity, D_E = peak early-diastolic velocity, D_M = peak mid-diatolic velocity, D_A = peak late-diastolic velocity)

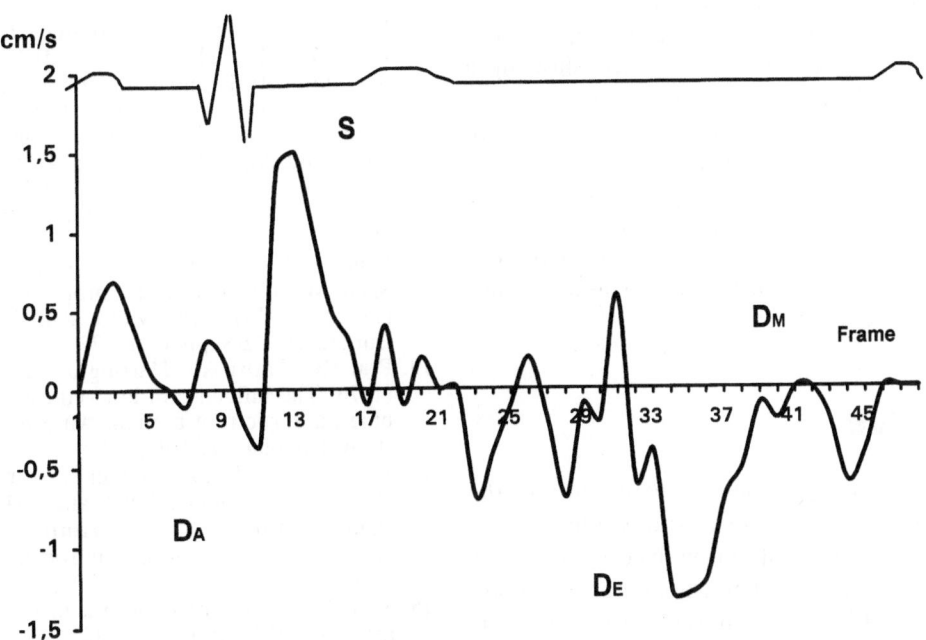

Fig. 12.2. Velocities of aortic pulsation in subsequent frames in the parasternal view in a representative healthy, young subject. The velocity of aortic pulsation is reached as a result of the subtraction of anterior and posterior aortic wall velocity. (Velocities of whole aorta for time correlations: S = peak systolic velocity, D_E = peak early-diastolic velocity, D_M = peak mid-diatolic velocity, D_A = peak late-diastolic velocity)

Other Parts of the Arterial System

The estimation of function of other parts of the aorta is possible by transthoracic, subcostal and suprasternal views. The new window to the heart and great vessels by the transesophageal approach has provided new, valuable morphological information [3]. Also, functional information can be obtained using TDE. Application of higher frequencies to the systems and proximity to the structures is of great advantage. The evaluation of other superficial arteries using linear transducers will be done in the future.

Diastole

In diastole TDE shows a backward movement coded blue in the normal ascending and descending aorta as well as the abdominal aorta. Interestingly, the velocity calculated showed the highest values at the end of the diastolic period (normal values 6.0 ± 1.3 cm/s). After the P-wave an additional signal coded blue, backward movement, was found (Fig. 12.10).

In patients with hypertension, the diastolic wall velocity is quite different. Two separate backward movements can be seen. One can be related to the rapid return of the aorta reflecting the increased stiffness, representing increased hysteresis. The second part begins after the P-wave, showing a short, reversed wall movement and more intense backward movement. The quantitative analysis of the TDE images shows an enhanced velocity in early diastole up to 7 cm/s in hypertension. As the aortic diameter is decreasing during this period, the velocity of the anterior wall is higher than of the posterior wall (about 1.0 cm/s). This difference was also found at late diastole.

Conclusion

TDE of the aorta provides a new insight into the pathophysiology of the aorta and will have great impact on studies of patients with coronary artery disease and hypertension in whom the aortic compliance is reduced. In addition, the new method has become available for determination of systolic time intervals in only one scan plane, without the necessity of recording the phonocardiogram and carotid pulse. Also, the pulse wave velocity can be determined in different parts of the aorta with high accuracy.

References

1. Dart AM, Lacombe F, Yeoh JK, Cameron JD, Jennings GL, Laufer E, Esmore DS (1991) Aortic distensibility in patients with isolated hypercholesterolemia, coronary artery disease, or cardiac transplant. Lancet 338/8762:270–3
2. Dart AM, Silagy C, Dewar E, Jennings G, McNeil J (1993) Aortic distensibility and left ventricular structure and function in isolated systolic hypertension. Eur Heart J 14:1465–70
3. Erbel R, Engberding R, Daniel W, Roelandt JRTC, Visser C, Rennollet H (1989) Echocardiography in diagnosis of aortic dissection. Lancet 457–61
4. Greenfield JC, Patel DJ (1962) Relation between pressure and diameter in the ascending aorta of man. Circ Res 10:778–81
5. Hickler RB (1990) Aortic and large artery stiffness: Current methodology and clinical correlations. Clin Cardiol 13:317–22
6. Honda T, Yano K, Matsuoka H, Hamada M, Hiwada K (1994) Evaluation of aortic distensibility in patients with essential hypertension by using cine magnetic resonance imaging. Angiology 45:207–12
7. Kasper W, Meinertz T, Heppert V, Kersting F (1980) Die Bewegung der Aortenhinterwand im M-mode-Echokardiogramm: ein Parameter der linksventrikulären Funktion. Z Kardiol 69:573–6
8. Lehmann ED, Gosling RG, Parker JR, DeSilva T, Taylor MG (1993) A blood pressure independent index of aortic distensibility. Br J Radiol 66:126–31
9. Li JK, Zhu (1994) Arterial compliance and its pressure dependence in hypertension and vasodilation. Angiology 45:113–7
10. Mugge A, Daniel WG, Niedermeyer J, Hausmann D, Nikutta P, Lichtlen PR (1992) Usefulness of a new automatic boundary detection system (acoustic quantification) for assessing stiffness of the descending thoracic aorta by transesophageal echocardiography. Am J Cardiol 70:1629–31
11. O'Rourke M (1991) Arterial compliance and wave reflection. Arch Mal Coeur Vaiss 84/Spec. Iss. III: 45–8
12. Pannier BM, London GM, Cuche JL, Girerd X, Safar ME (1990) Physical properties of the aorta and cardiac hypertrophy in essential hypertension. Eur Heart J 11/Suppl G:17–23
13. Prat RC, Parisi AF, Harrington JJ, Sasahara AA (1976) The influence of left ventricular stroke volume on aortic root motion. An echocardiographic study. Circulation 53:947–53
14. Savolainen A, Keto P, Hekali P, Nisula L, Kaitila I, Viitasalo M, Poutanen VP, Standertskjold-Nordenstam CG, Kupari M (1992) Aortic distensibility in children with the Marfan syndrome. Am J Cardiol 70:691–3
15. Seely S (1989) Atherosclerosis or hardening of the arteries? Int J Cardiol 22:5–12
16. Seely S (1991) Aortic distensibility (letter). Lancet 338:696–7
17. Stefanadis C, Stratos C, Boudoulas H, Kourouklis C, Toutouzas P (1990) Distensibility of the ascending aorta: comparison of invasive and noninvasive techniques in healthy men and in men with coronary artery disease. Eur Heart J 11:990–6

18. Underwood SR, Mohiaddin RH (1993) Magnetic resonance imaging of atherosclerotic vascular disease. Am J Hypertens 6/II Suppl:335S–9S

19. Kelly R, Hayward C, Avolio A, O'Rourke M (1989) Noninvasive determination of age-related changes in the human arterial pulse. Circulation 80:1652–59

20. Murgo JP, Westerhof N, Giolma JP, Altobelli SA (1980) Aortic input impedance in normal man: relationship to pressure wave forms. Circulation 62:105–16

21. Saba PS, Roman MJ, Pini R, Spitzer M, Ganau A, Devereux RB (1993) Relation of arterial pressure waveform to left ventricular and carotid anatomy in normotensive subjects. J Am Coll Cardiol 22:1873–80

22. Marchais SJ, Guerin AP, Pannier BM, Levy BI, Safar ME, London GM (1993) Wave reflections and cardiac hypertrophy in chronic uremia: influence of body size. Hypertension 22:876–83

23. Safar ME, Toto-Moukouo JJ, Bouthier JA, Asmar RE, Levenson JA, Simon AC, London GM (1987) Arterial dynamics, cardiac hypertrophy, and anti-hypertensive treatment. Circulation 75 (suppl 1): I-156–I-161

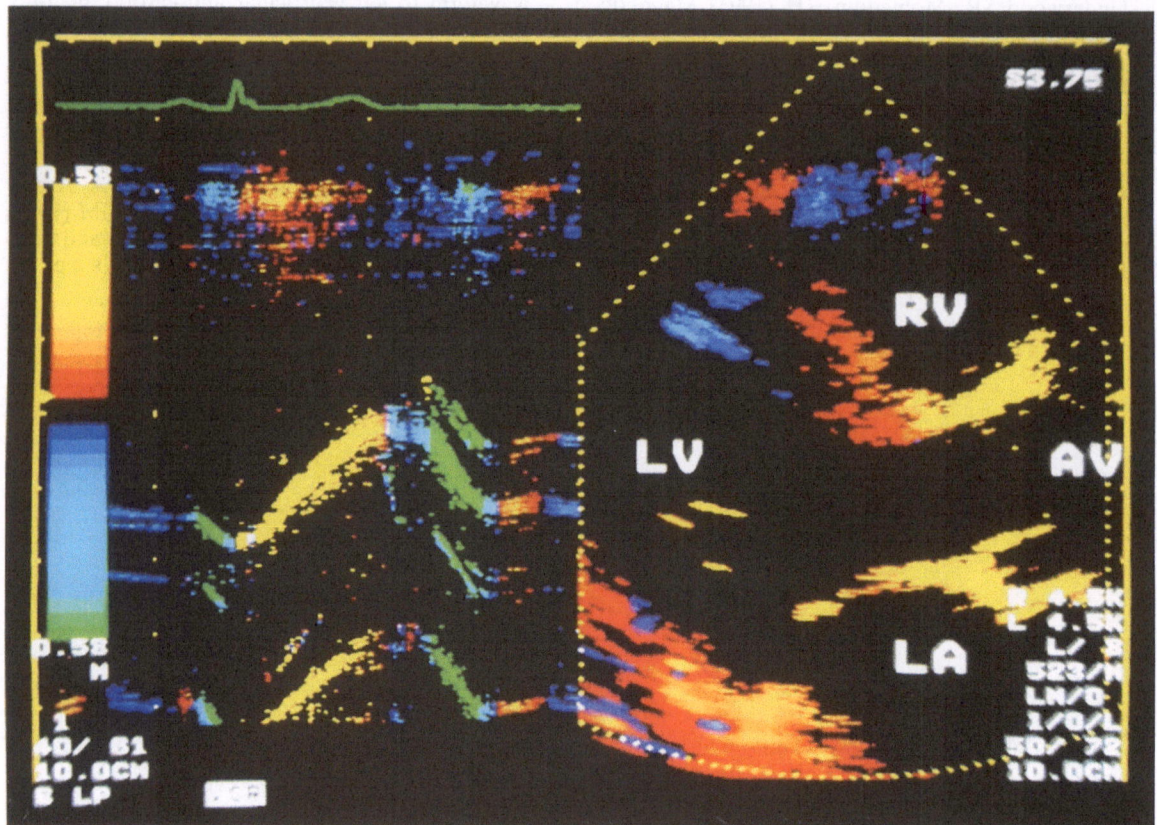

Fig. 12.3. Normal aorta. Parasternal long axis view using a 3.75 MHz transducer. Two-dimensional tissue Doppler echocardiographic image during systole. M-mode registration through the aortic root. Machine settings are: non-color-coded velocities up to 0.21 cm/s, red or dark blue coded velocities up to 1.0 cm/s, yellow coded forward velocities above 1.0 cm/s, bright blue coded backward velocities from 1.0 cm/s up to 3.0 cm/s, and green coded backward velocities above 3.0 cm/s. Aortic root is moving toward the transducer during systole and away from the transducer during early and late diastole. After the early-diastolic phase of the aortic root velocity the opposite velocity direction occurs. This is indicated by red color-coding in mid-diastole. The aortic root velocity directions during the cardiac cycle are opposite to those of the interventricular septum and similar to those of the left ventricular posterior wall and right ventricular anterior wall in this view. Normal velocity distribution during the cardiac cycle: the peak systolic velocity of the anterior aortic wall measured by tissue Doppler achieves 5.75 cm/s, peak early diastolic velocity: 6.75 cm/s, and peak late diastolic velocity after P-wave on the ECG: 7.50 cm/s. Typical aortic root velocity ratios: $D_E/S = 1.17$, $D_A/D_E = 1.11$. The peak systolic velocity of the aortic root is similar to that of the ventricular wall. In contrast, the peak early-diastolic velocity is lower, and the peak velocity in late diastole is higher than corresponding velocity of ventricular walls. (AV = aortic valve, LA = left atrium, LV = left ventricle, RV = right ventricle)

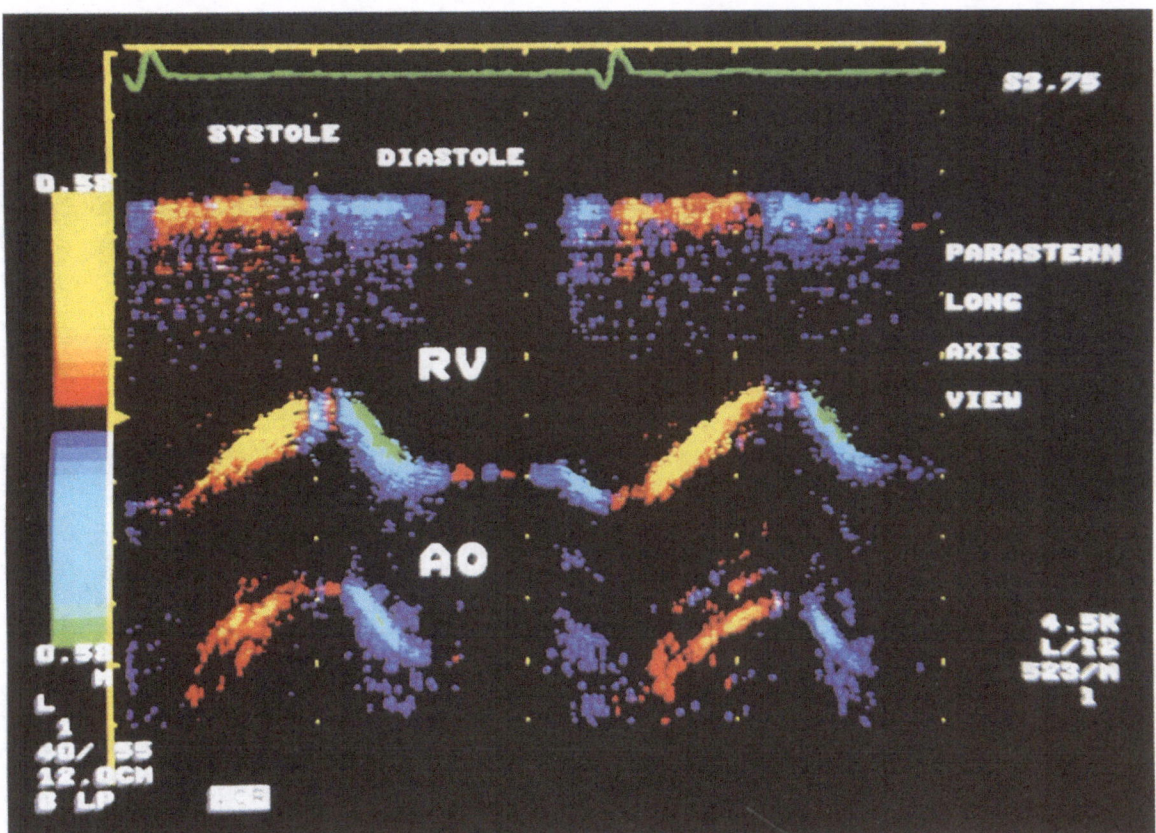

Fig. 12.4. Acromegaly. M-mode registration of the aortic root in the parasternal long axis view. Machine settings are: non color-coded velocities up to 0.42 cm/s, red or dark blue coded velocities up to 2.0 cm/s, yellow coded forward velocities above 2.0 cm/s, bright blue coded backward velocities from 2.0 cm/s up to 6.0 cm/s, and green coded backward velocity above 6.0 cm/s. Typical velocity directions of the aortic root. The peak systolic velocity of the anterior aortic wall is 5.25 cm/s as estimated by TDE. The ejection fraction estimated by two-dimensional echocardiography is 69%. Abnormal velocity distribution during diastole. The peak late-diastolic velocity 3.25 cm/s (coded by blue) is lower than peak early-diastolic velocity 6.75 cm/s (coded by green). This may be an early sign of left ventricular diastolic dysfunction in acromegaly. (AO = aortic root, RV = right ventricle)

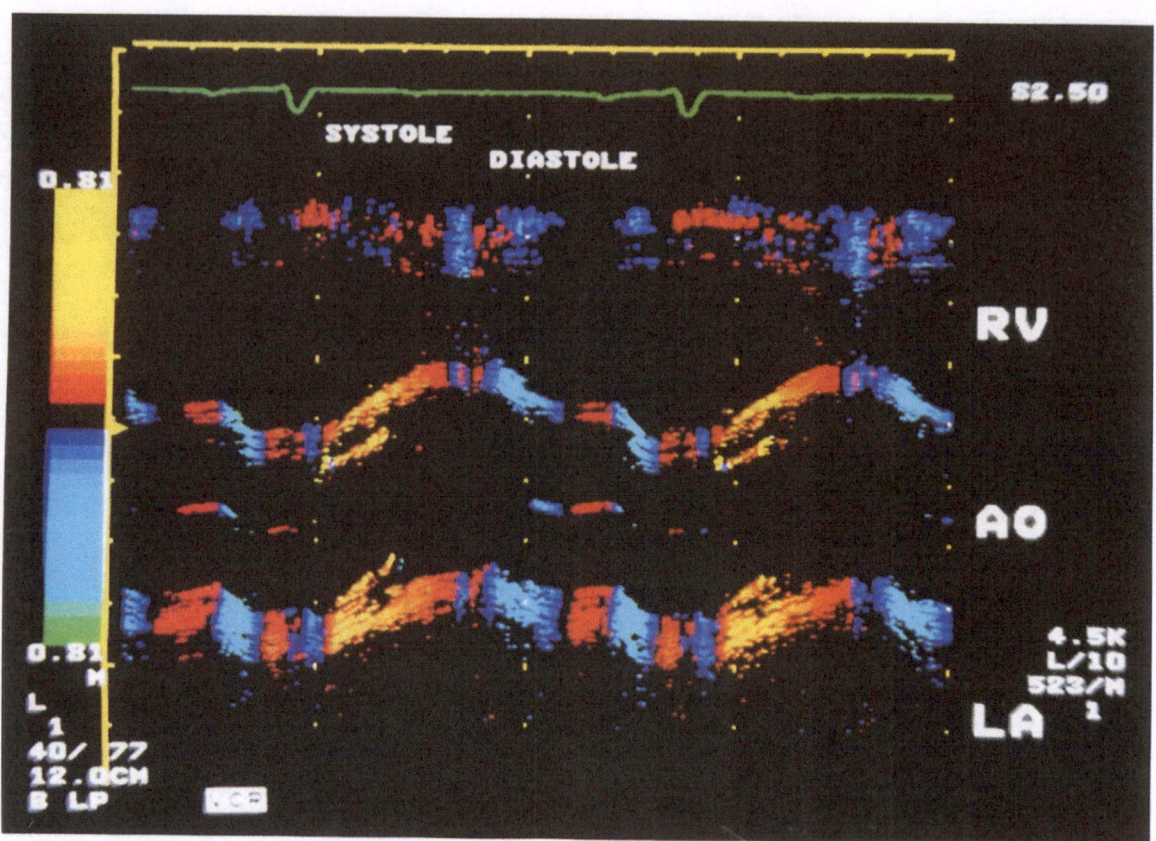

Fig. 12.5. Coronary artery disease. M-mode registration of the aortic root in the parasternal long axis view using a 2.5 MHz transducer. The machine settings are: non-color-coded velocities up to 0.31 cm/s, red or dark blue coded velocities up to 1.4 cm/s, yellow coded forward velocities above 1.4 cm/s, bright blue coded backward velocities from 1.4 cm/s to 4.1 cm/s, and green coded backward velocities above 4.1 cm/s. Typical directions of aortic root velocities during the cardiac cycle. Abnormal velocity distribution during the cardiac cycle. Decreased systolic velocities of the anterior aortic wall (peak systolic velocity: 3.75 cm/s). Ejection fraction determined by echocardiographic disc method 51%. Decreased early-diastolic velocities (peak early-diastolic velocity: 3.25 cm/s). Decreased early-diastolic to systolic velocity ratio: 0.87 (in healthy subjects: $D_E/S = 1.0–1.5$). Increased peak late-diastolic velocity: 7.75 cm/s. The peak late-diastolic velocity is higher than peak early-diastolic velocity and ratio of peak late-diastolic to peak early-diastolic velocity is increased: 2.38 (in healthy subjects: $D_A/D_E = 1.0–1.8$). (AO = aortic root, LA = left atrium, RV = right ventricle)

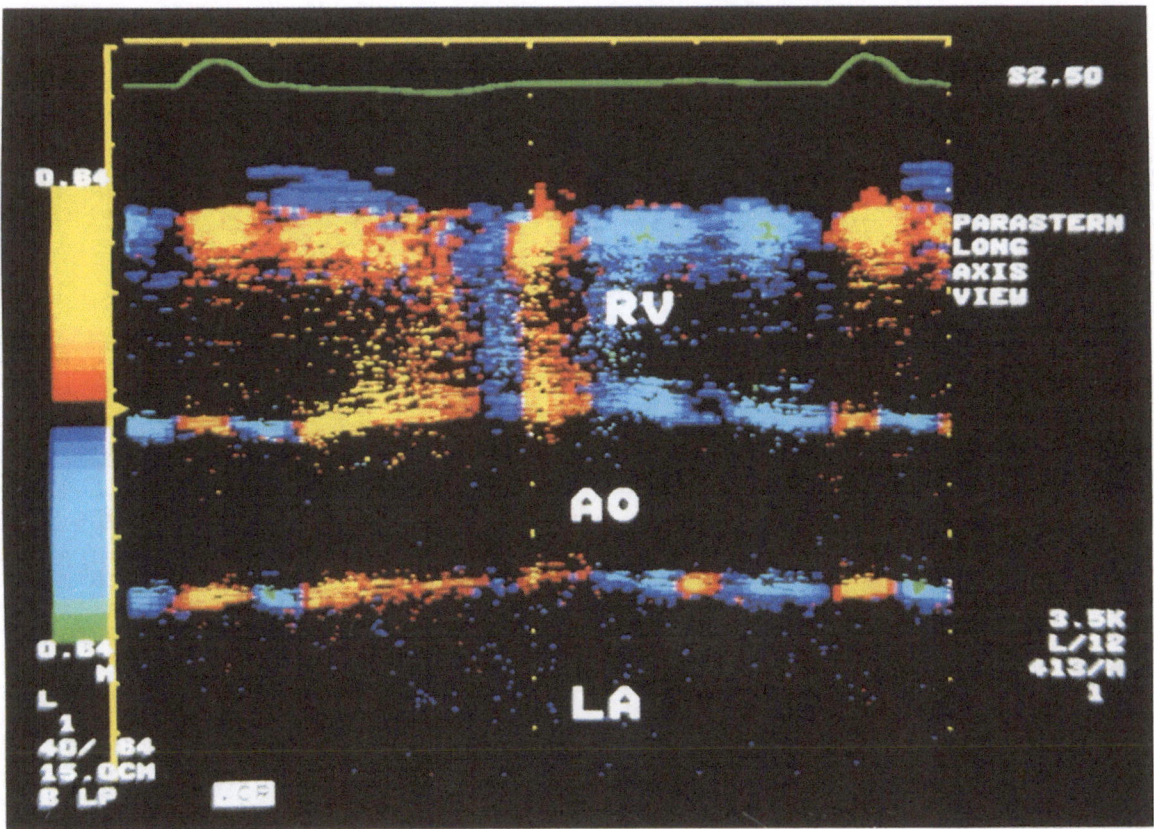

Fig. 12.6. Congestive heart failure. M-mode registration of the aortic root in the parasternal long axis view using a 2.5 MHz transducer. The machine settings are: non-color-coded velocities up to 0.12 cm/s, red or dark blue coded velocities up to 0.6 cm/s, yellow coded forward velocities above 0.6 cm/s, bright blue coded backward velocities from 0.6 cm/s up 1.6 cm/s, and green coded backward velocities above 1.6 cm/s. Low velocities of the aortic root during the cardiac cycle due to poor ventricular function. The ejec-tion fraction estimated by echocardiography is 21%. The peak systolic velocity of the anterior wall of the aorta: 1.75 cm/s, the peak early-diastolic velocity: 1.50 cm/s, and the peak late-diastolic velocity: 1.00 cm/s. Abnormal velocity distribution. The peak early-diastolic to peak systolic velocity ratio $D_E/S = 0.86$. The peak late-diastolic velocity to early-diastolic velocity ratio $D_A/D_E = 0.67$. (AO = aortic root, LA = left atrium, RV = right ventricle)

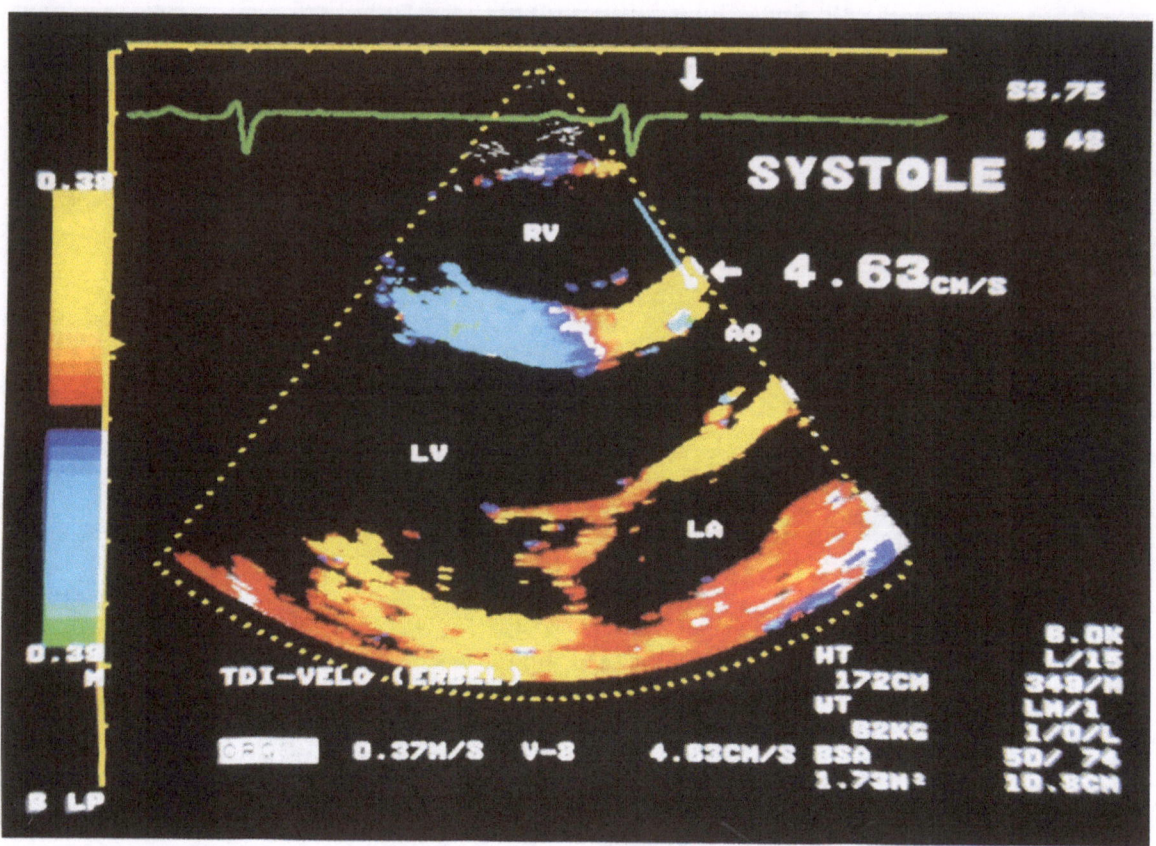

Fig. 12.7. Normal heart. Parasternal long axis view with anterior aortic wall velocity measurements. Machine setting: non-color-coded velocities up to 0.29 cm/s, red or dark blue coded velocities up to 1.3 cm/s, yellow coded forward velocities above 1.3 cm/s, bright blue coded backward velocities from 1.3 cm/s up to 4.0 cm/s, and green coded backward velocities above 4.0 cm/s. During systole the aortic root moves toward the transducer with the velocity direction and velocity values are similar to those of posterior left ventricular wall. Aortic wall velocity direction is opposite to the interventricular septum. Opened aortic valve leaflets moving in the same direction as the aortic root. Measured velocity of the anterior aortic wall is 4.63 cm/s (left). The posterior wall is moving in the same frame with the velocity 4.13 cm/s. The velocity difference between both aortic walls represents the aortic enlargement during systole. Posterior wall of the left atrium moves toward the transducer as a consequence of heart movement. (AO = aortic root, LA = left atrium, LV = left ventricle, RV = right ventricle)

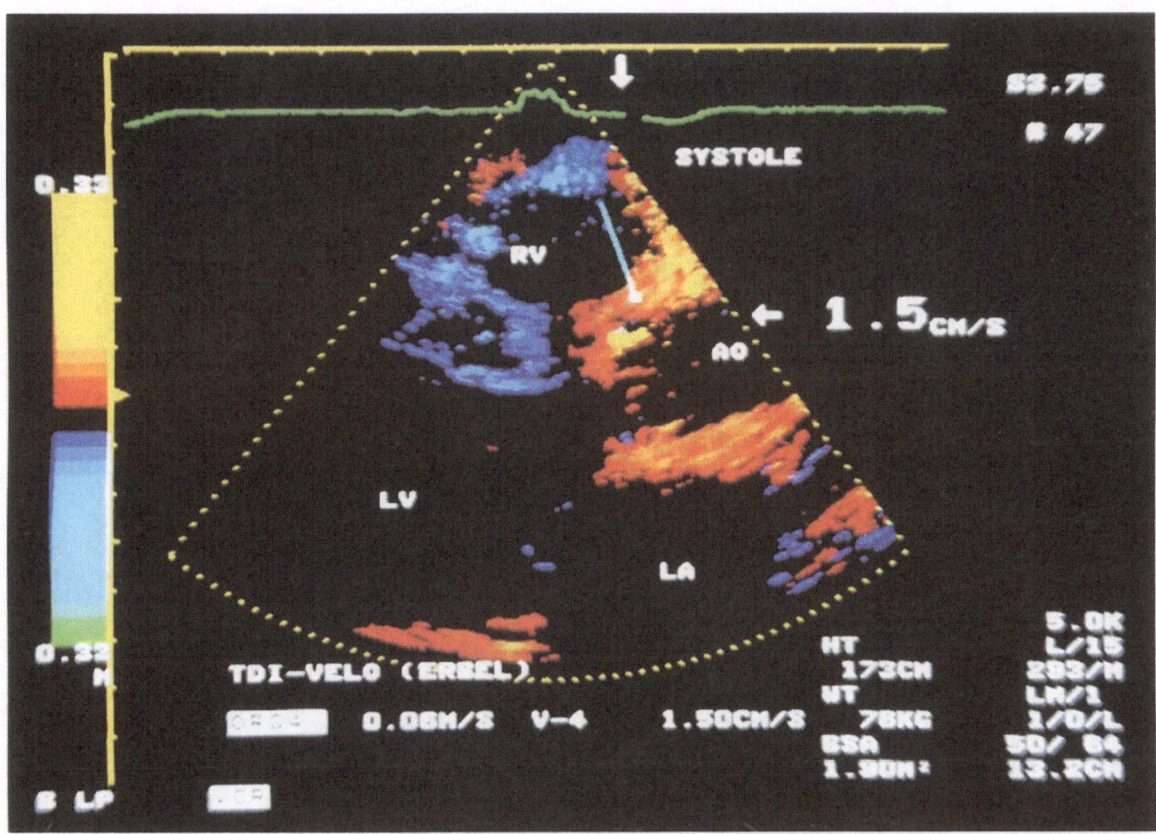

Fig. 12.8. Coronary artery disease. Parasternal long axis view with aortic wall velocity measurements during systole. Machine settings are: non-color-coded velocities up to 0.49 cm/s, red or dark blue coded velocities up to 2.3 cm/s, yellow coded forward velocities above 2.3 cm/s, bright blue coded backward velocities from 2.3 cm/s up to 4.0 cm/s, and green coded backward velocities above 6.8 cm/s. Typical direction of aortic root velocity during systole. The same velocity of both aortic walls (1.50 cm/s) as an abnormal finding. Absent difference between both aortic wall velocities due to aortic stiffness. (AO = aortic root, LA = left atrium, LV = left ventricle, RV = right ventricle)

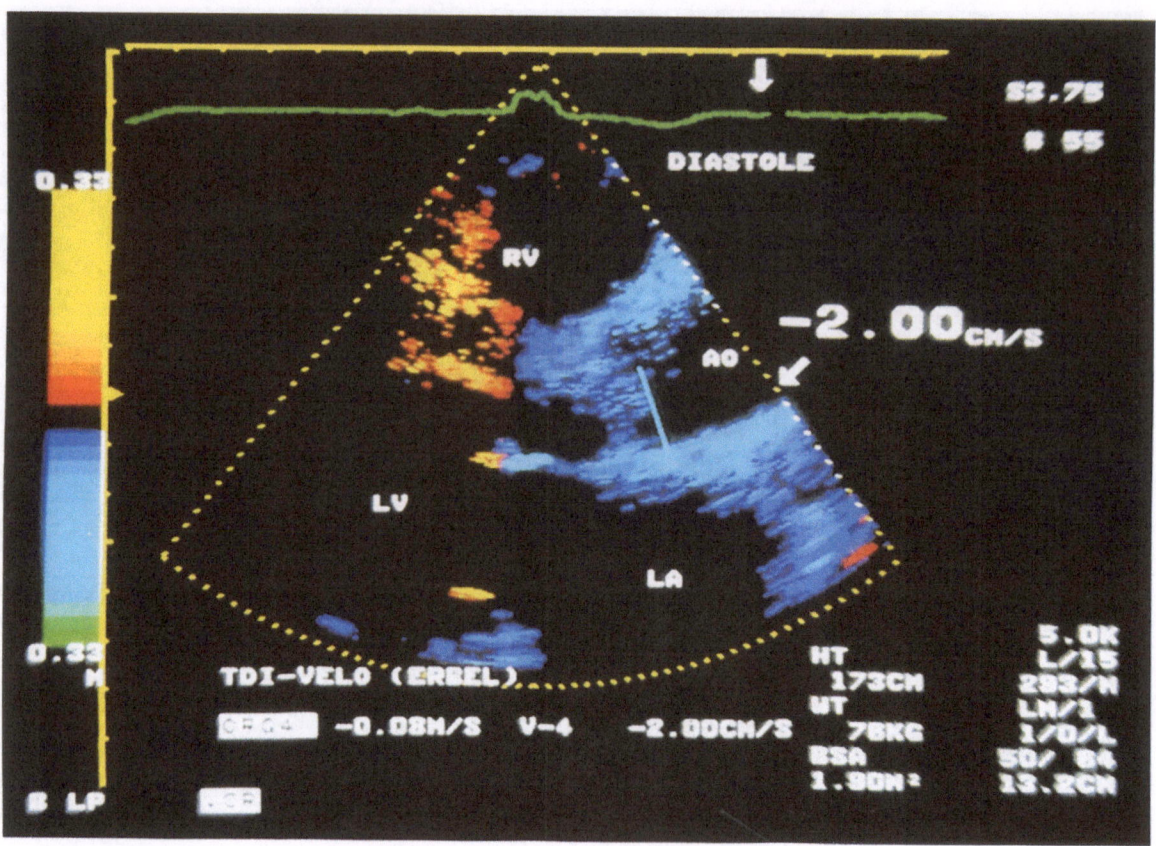

Fig. 12.9. Coronary artery disease. The same patient and the same machine settings as in Fig. 12.8. Aortic wall velocity measurements during diastole. Typical direction of aortic root velocity during diastole. Lack of difference between the two aortic walls (–2.00 cm/s) is an abnormal finding. (AO = aortic root, LA = left atrium, LV = left ventricle, RV = right ventricle)

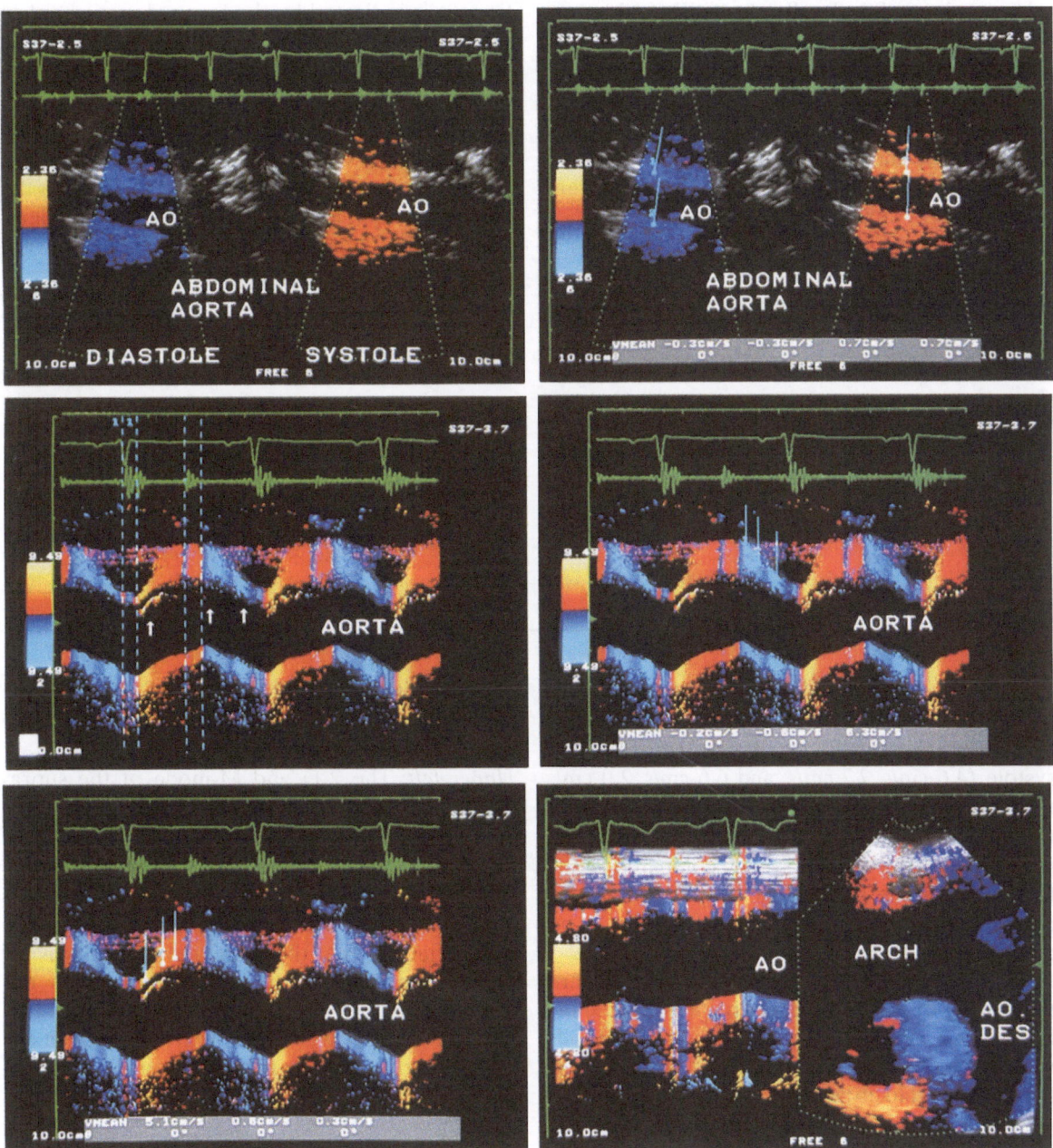

Fig. 12.10. Normal TDE values of the aorta in M-mode recorded at the level of the aortic root, TDE two-dimensional echocardiographic image of the aortic arch and abdominal aorta.

Upper part of the abdominal aorta in the long axis scanned in diastole and systole demonstrating forward motion during systole and backward motion during diastole. The calculated velocity in systole is 0.7 cm/s for the anterior and posterior wall and in diastole 0.3 cm/s for both walls.

Middle part and *lower left* M-mode TDE of the aortic root simultaneously recorded with the ECG and the phonocardiogram showing forward movement during systole and backward movement during diastole. Indicated with time markers in the middle left figure is the start and end of the isovolumetric contraction period, the left ventricular ejection time (LVET), and time of isovolumetric relaxation. Starting with the measurement before the short anterior movement at the beginning of the QRS complex the preejection period (PEP) can be measured. During systole there is a yellow color-coding meaning high velocity in the first third and red color in mid- and late systole meaning reduced wall velocity. The values are 5.1 cm/s in the first third, 0.6 cm/s in the second and 0.3 cm/s in the third third *(lower left)*.

In diastole *(middle right)* the velocity is low in the early and mid third with 0.2 and 0.6 cm/s, and highest at the end of the diastole after the P wave 6.3 cm/s. During diastole continuous backward movement is visualized.

Lower right: 2-D and M-mode of suprasternal scanning in TDE mode with ECG and phonocardiogram. The increase of the diameter of the aor-

tic root is indicated by the forward movement of the upper *(red)* and backward movement of the lower *(blue color)* aortic wall. In diastole there is a backward movement of both walls with a shrinking of the diameter and forward motion of the aortic inferior wall in mid diastole. During late diastole both walls are moving forward, again the diameter of the aorta is shrinking, which is demonstrated by yellow color of the upper and red color of the inferior wall of the aorta

---

▷

Fig. 12.11. Hypertension. M-mode in TDE of the aortic root. The velocity of the anterior wall is higher than the posterior wall in the early and late systole (4.6 cm/s, 2.7 cm/s, and 6.6 cm/s, 2.9 cm/s respectively). In contrast to the normal pattern, the velocity of the aortic wall is increased in the mid- and late third of the systole compared to the first third of the systole (6.6 cm/s, 5.0 cm/s, 2.8 cm/s). Compared to the normal values it is increased up to 10 times.

In diastole *(middle left)* the continuing backward movement of the aorta is interrupted by a short forward motion. This pattern is enhanced. A lower velocity can be recorded in normals, but in hypertension the velocity signals are positive and not negative. Therefore the color is *red*. In addition,

the velocities in early and mid diastole are increased compared to the normal controls (5.5 cm/s, 2.3 cm/s, 6.0 cm/s).

Upper left: The 2-D and M-mode of the suprasternal scanning demonstrated in TDE mode. The velocity pattern is strikingly different from the normal pattern, showing a shortened systolic forward movement of the cranial aortic wall as well as disturbed pattern of the inferior aortic wall reflecting that the pulse wave velocity is increased. In diastole the normal pattern is not found. In hypertension there is a continuous forward movement which means cranial movement of the aortic arch in the suprasternal scanning plane. The shortening of the aortic diameter can be seen

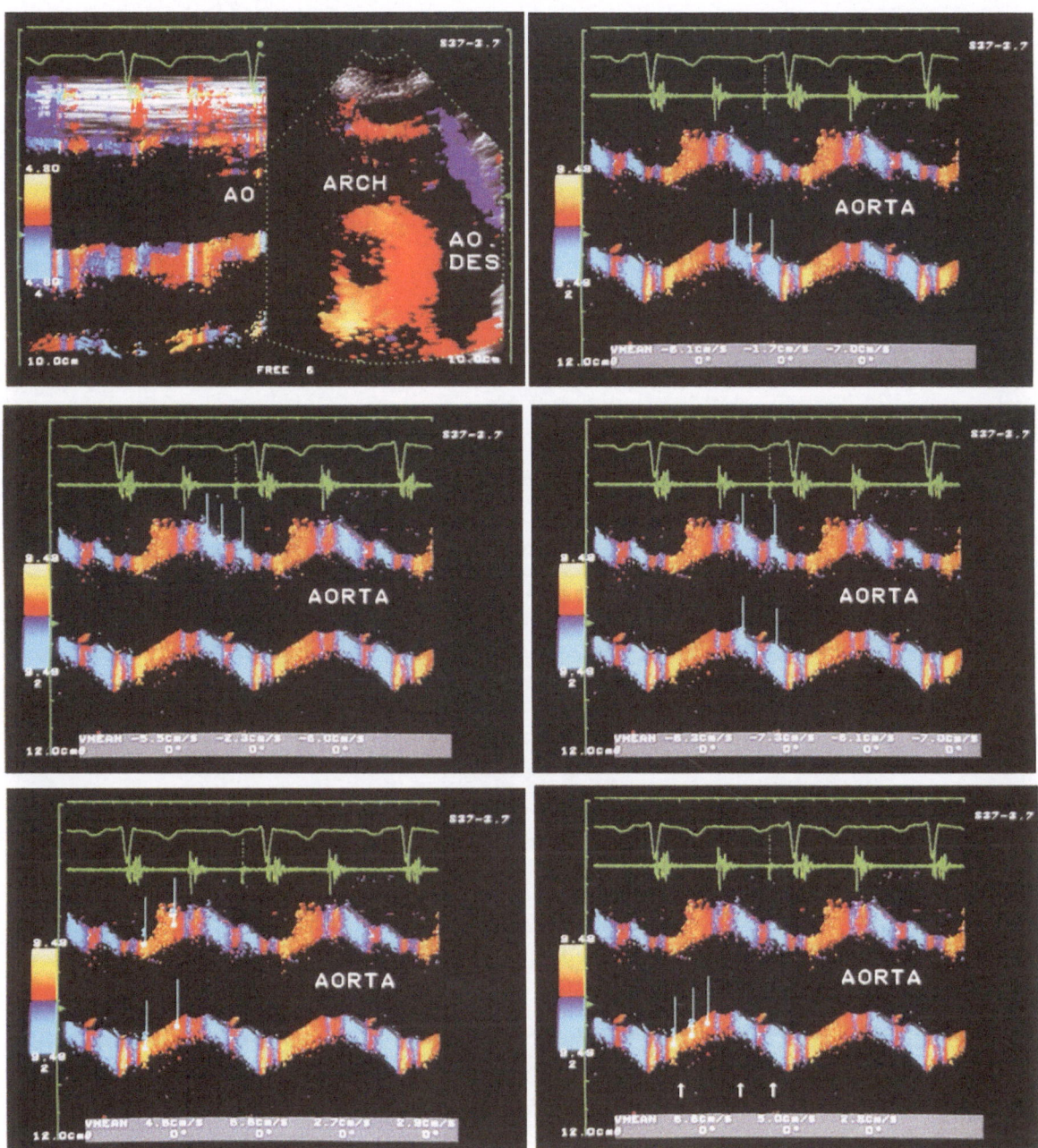

Fig. 12.11. Hypertension

Chapter 13   **Hemodynamics by TDE**

J. Zamorano

The assessment of the different phases of the cardiac cycle may be useful in different clinical settings, clinical pharmacology and clinical research. Diastole starts with closure of the aortic valve, ends with mitral valve closure, and is classically divided into four phases (isovolumic relaxation, rapid filling, diastasis and atrial contraction). Systole commences with the opening of the aortic valve, and is divided into three different phases (isovolumic contraction, rapid ejection and slow ejection).

The current understanding of the different phases of the cardiac cycle is based on hemodynamic studies. However, these techniques are invasive, time consuming, and unsuitable for serial evaluations. Because of this, efforts have been made to try to determine the cardiac cycle by noninvasive methods [3]. However, similar, precise, noninvasive assessment of cardiac hemodynamics has not been available up to now, despite the application of M-mode, pulsed Doppler, phonocardiographic, and radionuclide techniques [2, 7–9]. The diversity of these non-invasive approaches reflects the complexity of the problem, and the absence of a standard method to fully assess cardiac physiology.

Of all the noninvasive techniques, echocardiography has been the most common method to assess both systolic and diastolic function [6]. However, current echocardiographic techniques assess global systolic and diastolic function, but are unable to distinguish the individual phases of contraction (isovolumic ejection, rapid ejection, late ejection) and relaxation (isovolumic filling, rapid filling, diastasis, atrial contraction) [1, 4, 5].

Potentials of TDE

Tissue Doppler echocardiography allows the measurement of myocardial velocities (according to the pulse Doppler principle) and the identification of the direction of the moving tissue according to the color M-mode and two-dimensional (2D) patterns [9]. Tissue velocity towards the transducer is coded in red, and that away from the transducer in blue. A semiquantitative way of estimating tissue velocities is possible with different color codings, so high forward velocities are colored red-yellow and high backward velocities are coded in white-blue.

With the use of TDE it is possible not only to detect different systolic and diastolic tissue velocities, but even different velocity patterns during systole and diastole. From the technical point of view, the different patterns observed in color M-mode TDE studies require an appropriate gain setting to maintain optimal coloring of the myocardium. Also, Doppler velocity range must be set as low as possible, depending on the maximum velocity of the myocardium, to encompass all myocardial color velocities.

In normal subjects, a cyclic pattern of myocardial velocities is seen during most cardiac cycles. While the velocity pattern appears to be consistent between different myocardial segments, the precise color coding (red or blue) will depend on the echocardiographic view.

With reference to the ECG, several distinct phases of color M-mode TDE are apparent. In normal subjects, from the apical four-chamber view, the septum is colored in red during systole and in blue during diastole (Fig. 13.1). Higher velocities within systole are represented as yellow-red and within diastole as white-blue. Systole starts with a red band, followed by a yellow-red one during early systole, and ends with a dark-red during late systole. The relationship between these different velocity phases within the systole and the different systolic phases (isovolumic ejection, rapid ejection and late ejection) of the cardiac cycle remains to be established. In diastole two negative (colored in blue, away from the transducer) peak velocities separated by an area of slow velocity are found in normal subjects. As with systole, these four different velocity interfaces seen during diastole may correspond with the different phases of diastole (isovolumic relaxation, rapid filling, diastasis and atrial contraction).

In summary, with the use of TDE different myocardial velocities are found throughout the cardiac cycle. This typical pattern is strongly consistent with physiologic changes that occur in cardiac physiology as assessed by hemodynamics. Not only systolic but also diastolic time intervals at any given localization can be assessed. Regional time intervals can be determined. Further studies that confirm the hypothesis of a non-invasive assessment of cardiac physiology by TDE are needed. However, a noninvasive reproducible examination of the different phases of the cardiac cycle is an attractive potential of TDE [10].

References

1. Appleton C, Hatle L, Popp R (1988) Relation of transmitral flow velocity patterns to left ventricular diastolic function: New insight from a combined hemodynamic and Doppler echocardiographic study. J Am Coll Cardiol 12:426–440
2. Burwash I, Otto C, Pearlmann A (1993) Use of Doppler derived left ventricular time intervals for non-invasive assessment of systolic function. Am J Cardiol 72:1331–1333
3. Erbel R, Brennecke R, Görge G, Meyer J (1989) Accuracy and limitations of two dimensional echocardiography in quantitative evaluation of left ventricular function. Z Kardiol 78:131–142
4. Hanrath P, Mathey DG, Kremer P, Sonntag F, Bleifeld W (1980) Effect of verapamil on left ventricular isovolumic relaxation time and regional left ventricular filling in hypertrophic cardiomyopathy. Am J Cardiol 45:1258–1264
5. Lawson WE (1986) A new use of M-mode echocardiography in detecting left ventricular diastolic dysfunction in coronary artery disease. Am J Cardiol 58:210
6. Lewis R, Rittgers S, Forester W, Boudoulas H (1977) A critical rewiew of the systolic time intervals. Circulation 56:146–158
7. Shapiro SM, Bersohn MM, Laks MM (1991) In search of the holy grail: the study of diastolic ventricular function by the use of Doppler echocardiography. J Am Coll Cardiol 17:1517–1519
8. Spirito P, Maron B, Belloti P, Chapella F, Vecchio C (1986) Noninvasive assessment of left ventricular diastolic function: Comparative analysis of pulsed Doppler ultrasound and digitized M-mode echocardiography. Am J Cardiol 68:337–348
9. Sutherland GR, Stewart J, Groundstroem WE, Moran CM, Fleming A, Guell F, Riemersma RA, Fenn LN, Fox A, McDicken WN (1994) Color Doppler myocardial imaging: A new technique for the assessment of myocardial function. J Am Soc Echocardiogr 7:441–458
10. Zamorano J, Wallbridge D, Ge J, Drozdz J, Buck T, Baumgart D, Haude M, Erbel R (1995) Assessment of cardiac physiology by tissue Doppler echocardiography. Comparison with pressure recordings during heart catheterisation. Z Kardiol 84 (Suppl 1):170

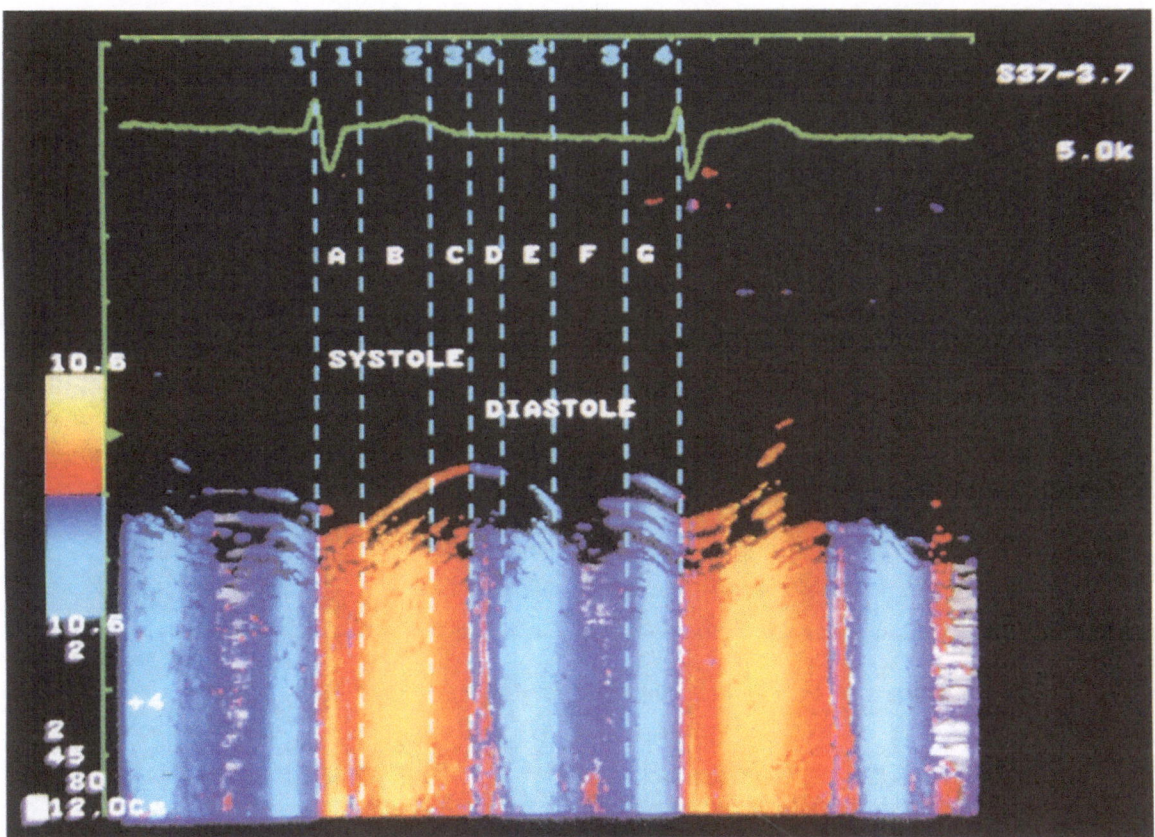

Fig. 13.1. M-mode TDE image of the septum from the apical view in a normal subject. Systole is represented by a red band and diastole by a blue one. Different velocities are found within systole (A–C) and diastole (D–G). Systole starts with slow velocity phase (A, colored in red), is followed by a high velocity one (B, colored in yellow-red), and ends with another low velocity phase (C, colored in red). During diastole two phases of low velocity (colored in blue, D, F) separated by an area of high velocity (colored in white-blue, E, G) are found in normal subjects

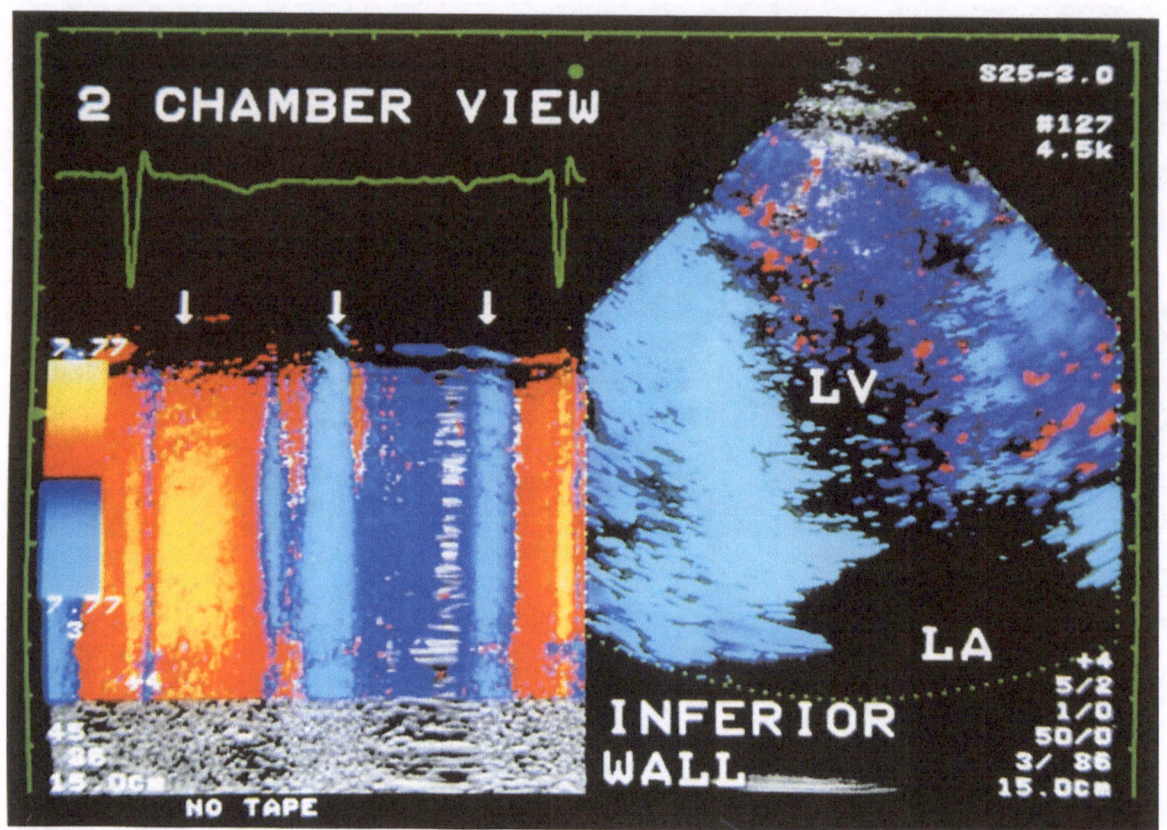

Fig. 13.2. TDE B-mode of the inferior wall (right) from the apical two-chamber view during diastole (colored in blue). On the left panel, the M-mode TDE image is shown. Again, systole is represented by a red band, and diastole by a blue one. As with other projections, the same velocity interfaces are seen within systole and diastole

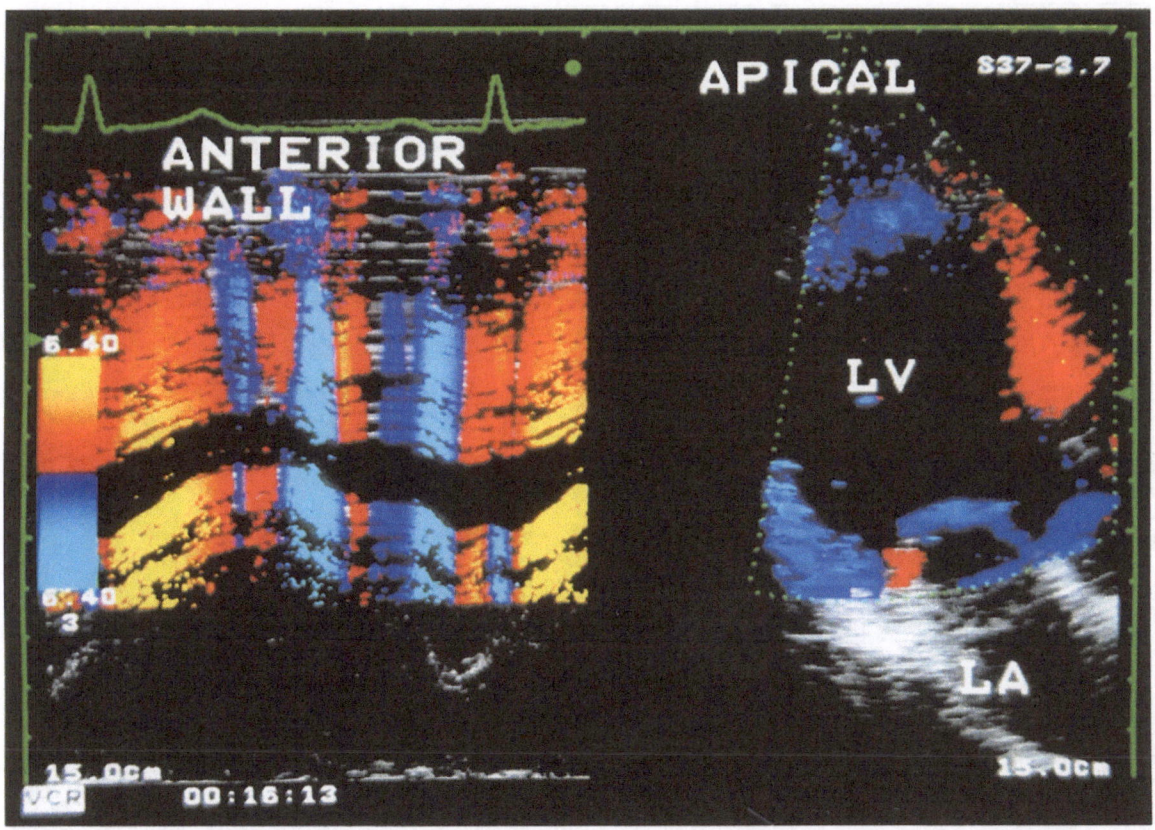

Fig. 13.3. TDE B-mode image (right) of left ventricle from the five-chamber apical view during diastole. On the left side the TDE M-mode of the anterior wall is shown. Notice the consistent velocity pattern obtained from the different cardiac segments. Again, systole is represented by a red band indicating velocity toward the transducer. Diastole is represented by a blue band, indicating velocity away from the transducer. Higher velocities within systole and diastole are displayed as yellow-red and white-blue, respectively

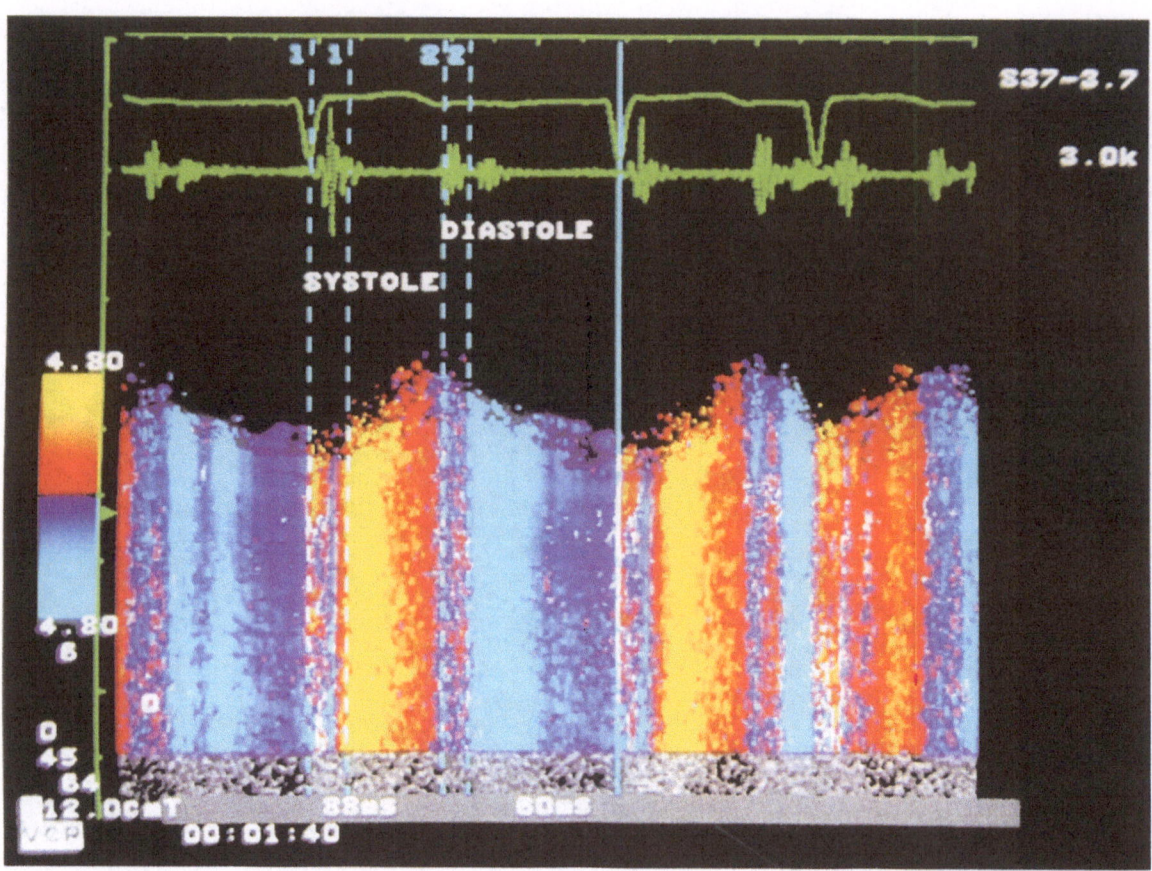

Fig. 13.4. M-mode TDE image of the septum from the four-chamber apical view in a patient with atrial fibrillation. The color velocity pattern in patients with atrial fibrillation is characterized by loss of the last high velocity phase during diastole. As shown in the figure, systolic and early diastolic velocity phases did not change significantly from beat to beat. Major differences from one cardiac cycle to the next are only seen during the second slow phase of diastole. Both observations support the idea that these velocity phases may be related to atrial contraction (last high velocity phase in diastole) and diastasis (last slow velocity phase)

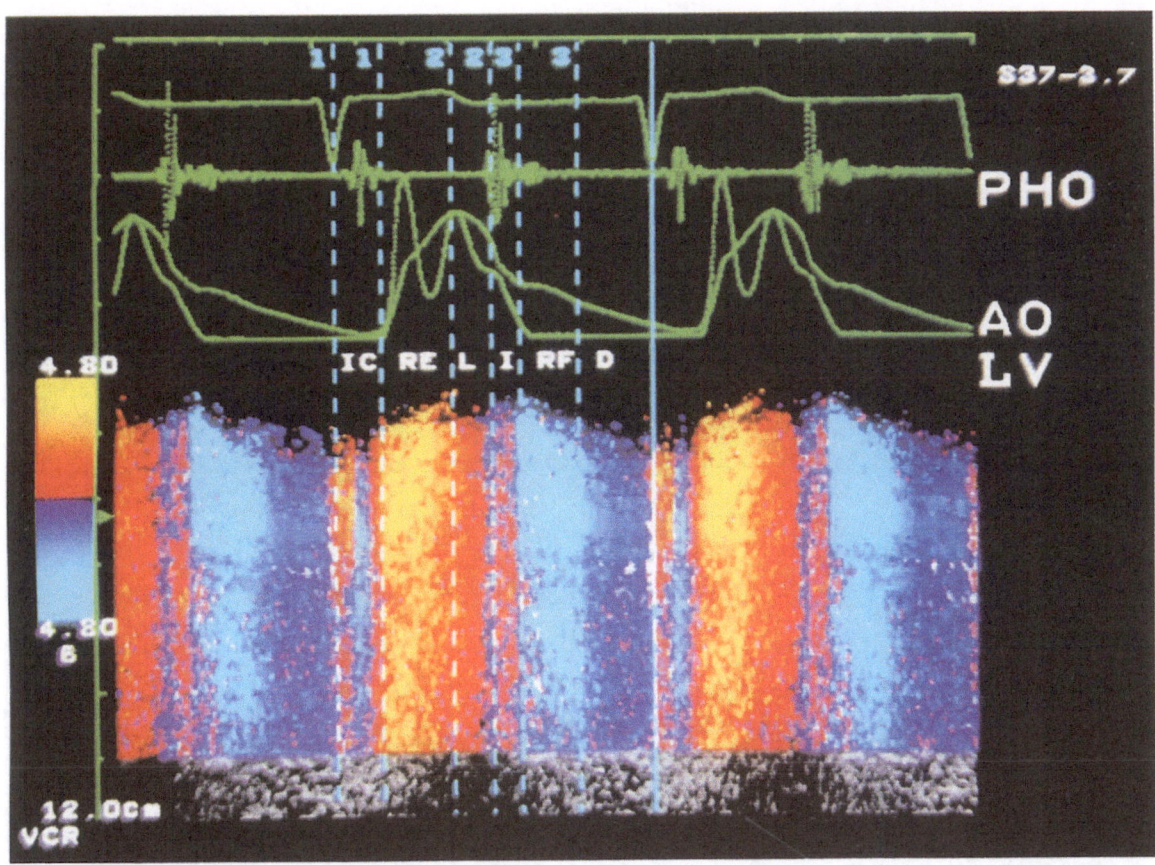

Fig. 13.5. Simultaneous recordings of TDE images of the septum, left ventricular and aortic pressure. Following the opening of the aortic valve, the upstroke of the aortic volume (rapid ejection) is marked by a transition of high velocity (yellow-red). This phase is followed by a lower velocity period (red) that corresponds to the late ejection phase after the peak of the aortic pressure. (Ao = aortic pressure, D = diastasis, I = isovolumic relaxation, IC = isovolumic contraction, L = late ejection, LV = left ventricular pressure, Pro = phonocardiogram, RE = rapid ejection, RF = rapid filling)

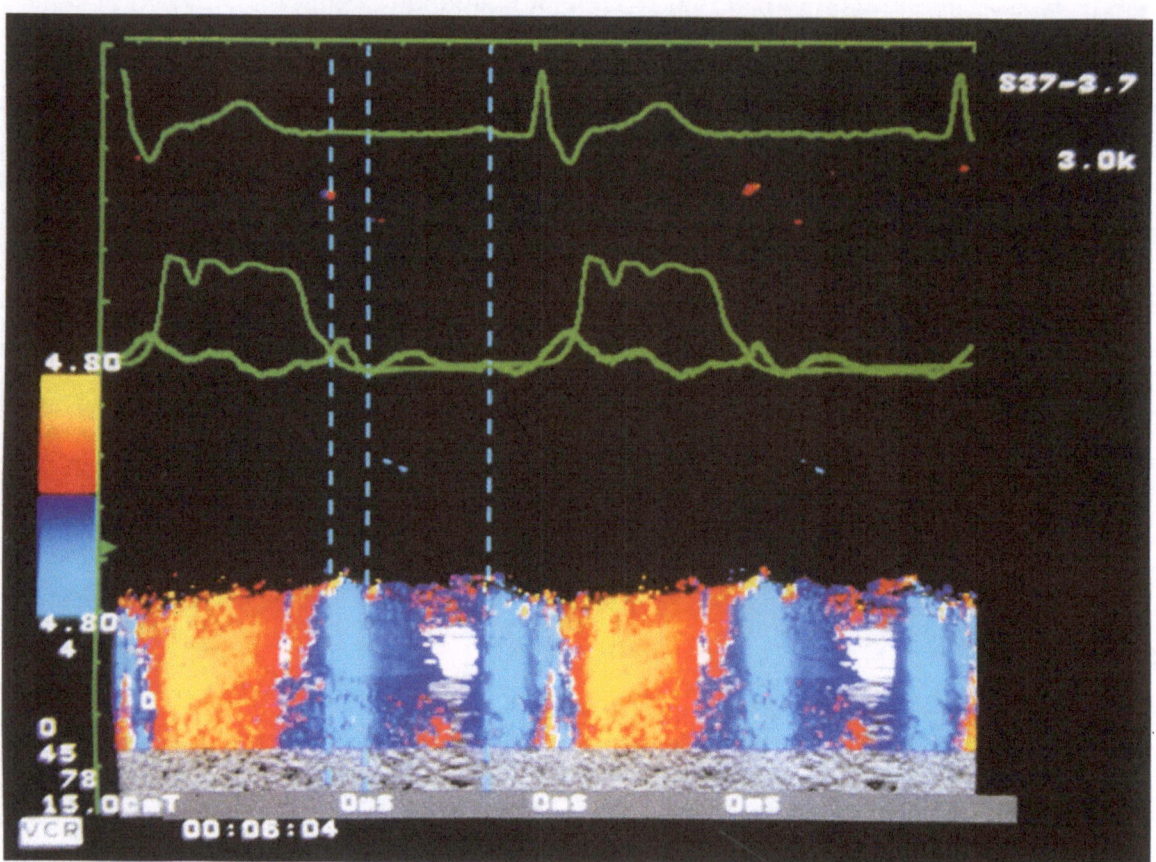

Fig. 13.6. Simultaneous recordings of TDE images of the septum, left ventricular and left atrial pressure. Rapid filling commences when left atrial pressure exceeds left ventricular pressure, and this corresponds to a transition to high myocardial velocities (white-blue). As left atrial and left ventricular pressures equalize, diastasis commences, and myocardial velocities become dark blue. Atrial contraction following the P wave is showed in TDE M-mode by an increase in myocardial velocities (white-blue). (AC = atrial contraction, Diast = diastasis, IR = isovolumic relaxation, LA = left atrial pressure, LV = left ventricular pressure, R = rapid filling)

Chapter 14 **Miscellaneous**

F. Schön

The images presented in this chapter comprise Tissue Doppler Echocardiography findings not yet covered by the previous chapters. The following pathological findings are presented:

- Muscular Dystrophy
- Acromegaly
- Large VSD with Eisenmenger, spontaneous echo-contrast
- Large VSD with Eisenmenger, echo-contrast agent
- Myxoma of the right atrium
- Valvular and congenital heart disease: Mitral stenosis, aortic stenosis and aortic insuffiency, common ventricle.

References

1. Csanady M, Gaspar L, Hogye M et al. (1983) The heart in acromegaly: An echocardiographic study. Int J Cardiol 2:349
2. McGuffin WL, Sherman BM, Roth J et al. (1974) Acromegaly and cardiovascular disorders. Ann Intern Med 81:11
3. Sanyal SK, Johnson WW, Thapar MK, Pitner SE (1978) An ultrastructural basis for the electrocardiographic alterations associated with Duchenne's progressive muscular dystrophy. Circulation 57: 1122

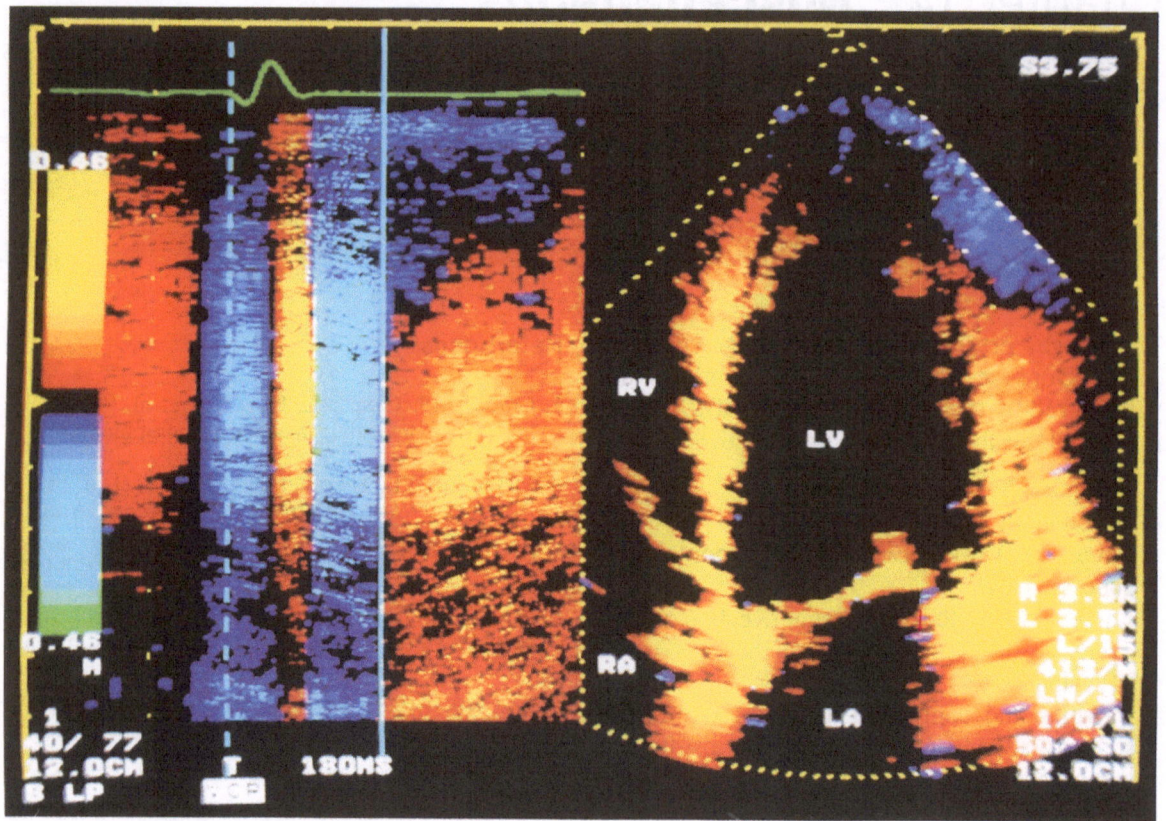

Fig. 14.1. Muscular Dystrophy. Legend see Fig. 14.2, page 143

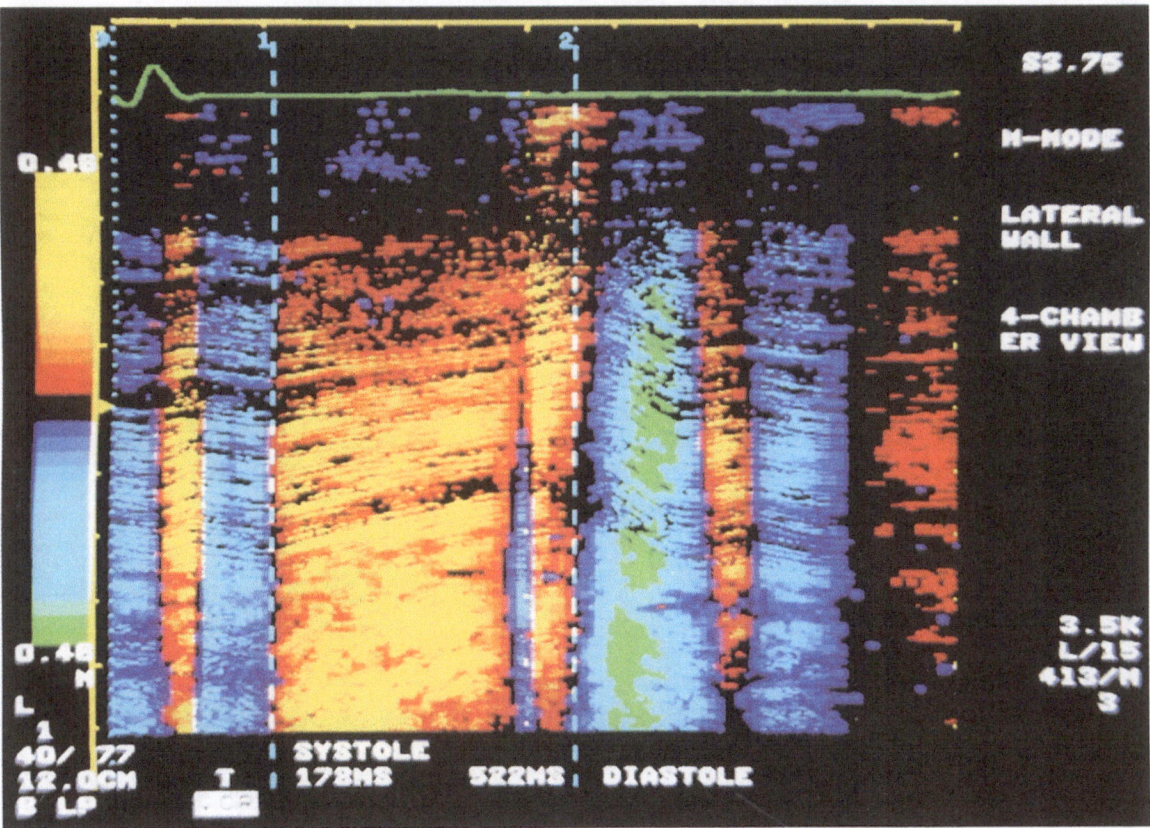

Fig. 14.1, Fig. 14.2. Muscular Dystrophy. Two-dimensional TDE image of the apical four-chamber view (Fig. 14.1) and M-Mode recording of the postero-lateral left ventricular wall (Fig. 14.2). Recordings were performed using a 3.75 MHz transducer. Only the TDE color information is visible without the normally underlying two-dimensional (2D) gray-scale image. As has been described in the chapter covering cardiac amyloidosis, systolic time intervals are prolonged in this patient. Measurement of the time interval of systolic electrical activation, the time between Q-wave and onset of systolic movement clearly reveals an almost tripled time period of 178 ms versus 66 ± 15 ms in the control group. Heart rate is approx. 60 min^{-1} in this patient.

Color reversal indicating the beginning of diastole is delayed. Time between Q-wave and color reversal is 522 ms. The calculated systolic time is 344 ms (normal). Consequently, systole is prolonged at the cost of diastole. Regional myocardial fibrosis, especially in the postero-basal and lateral LV leading to altered electromechanical coupling, has been described [3]

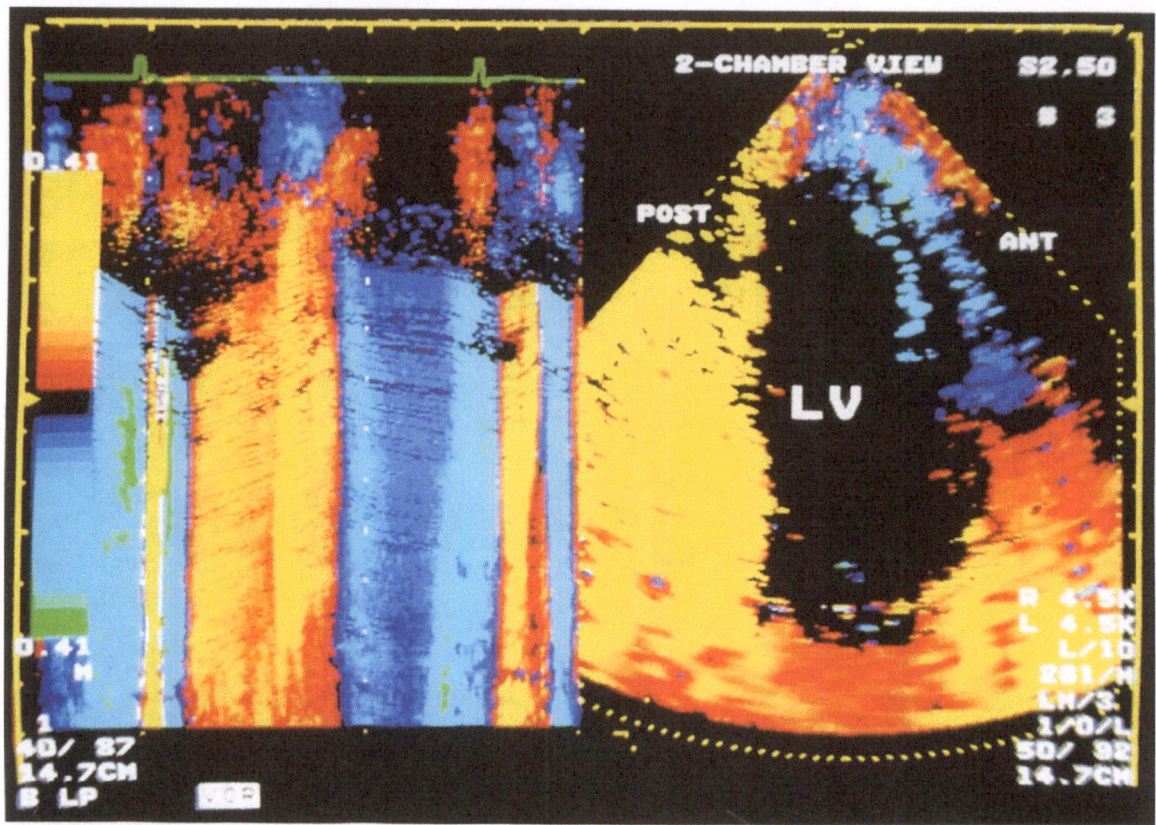

Fig. 14.3. Acromegaly. Two-dimensional TDE image of the apical two-chamber view and M-Mode recording of the posterior left ventricular wall. Recordings were performed using a 2.5 MHz transducer. Only the TDE color information is visible without the normally underlying 2D gray-scale image. Acromegaly is related to an increased secretion of growth hormone by the anterior pituitary gland. Clinical signs and symptoms of acromegaly related to the cardiovascular system are: cardiac enlargement, hypertension, premature coronary disease, congestive heart failure, arrhythmias and intraventricular conduction defects [1, 2]. The M-Mode registration of the posterior wall shows a normal contraction pattern. Systolic movement is coded red and yellow. Diastolic movement is coded by blue and green

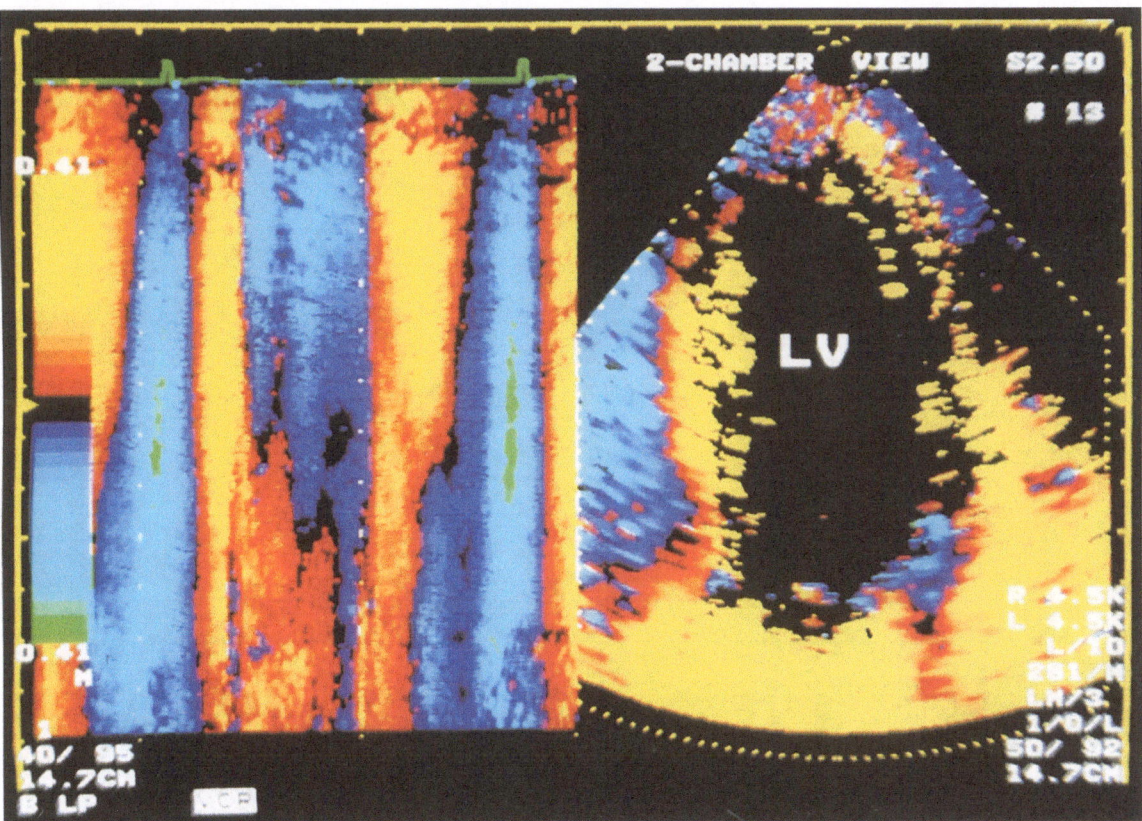

Fig. 14.4. Acromegaly. Two-dimensional TDE image of the apical two-chamber view and M-Mode recording of the anterior left ventricular wall. Recordings were perfomed using a 2.5 MHz transducer. Only the TDE color information is visible without the normally underlying 2D gray-scale image. The recording of the anterior wall shows an altered contraction pattern. During systole the basal myocardium is contracting normally, but velocity is diminished, as indicated by the red color. At the same time the apical anterior wall is coded blue. The following yellow phase during diastole expresses a rapid inward movement. In late-diastole again an outward movement can be observed, which is compatible with the diastolic left ventricular filling

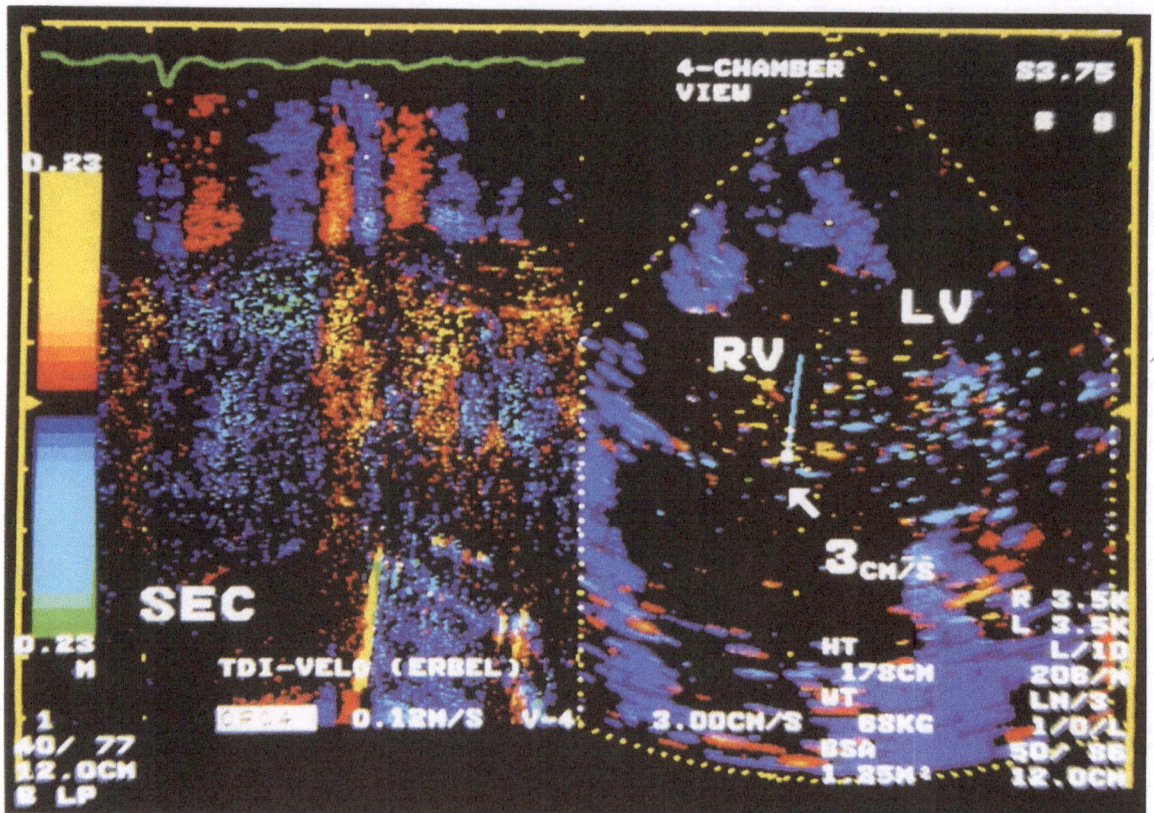

Fig. 14.5. Large VSD, spontaneous echo-contrast. Two-dimensional TDE image of the apical four-chamber view and M-Mode recording of the right ventricular cavity. Recordings were performed using a 3.75 MHz transducer. Only the TDE color information is visible without the normally underlying gray-scale image. Noise-like colored dots can be identified in the 2D and M-Mode section of this image. The dots represent spontaneous echo contrast (SEC) which was observable in the gray-scale imaging mode (standard 2D) as well. The M-Mode registration indicates movement of the SEC away from the transducer during systole and movement towards the transducer during diastole. Velocity in the center 3 cm/s

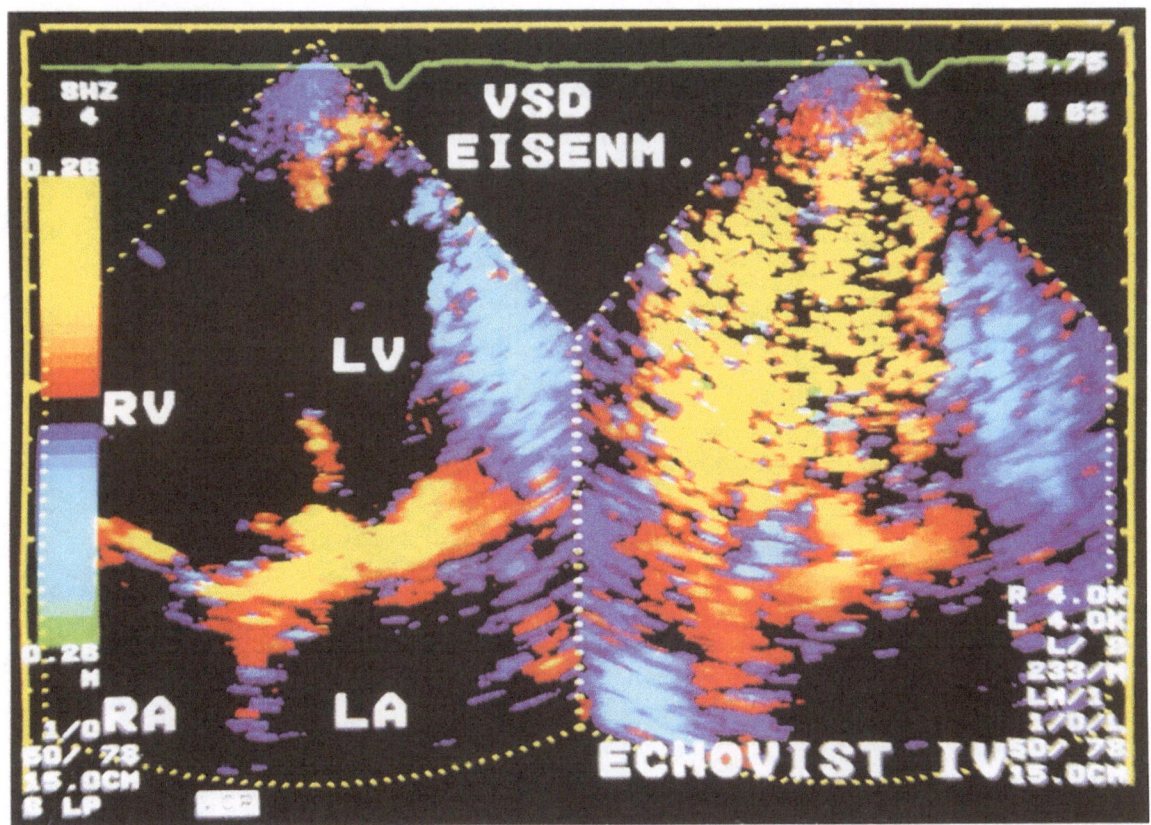

Fig. 14.6. Large VSD, echo-contrast agent.
Two-dimensional TDE split image of the apical
four-chamber view. Recordings were performed
using a 3.75 MHz transducer. Only the TDE color
information is visible without the normally underlying gray-scale image.

The images were taken from the same patient as
described before. The section on the right side
demonstrates the effect of echo-contrast agent
(Echovist) during diastole

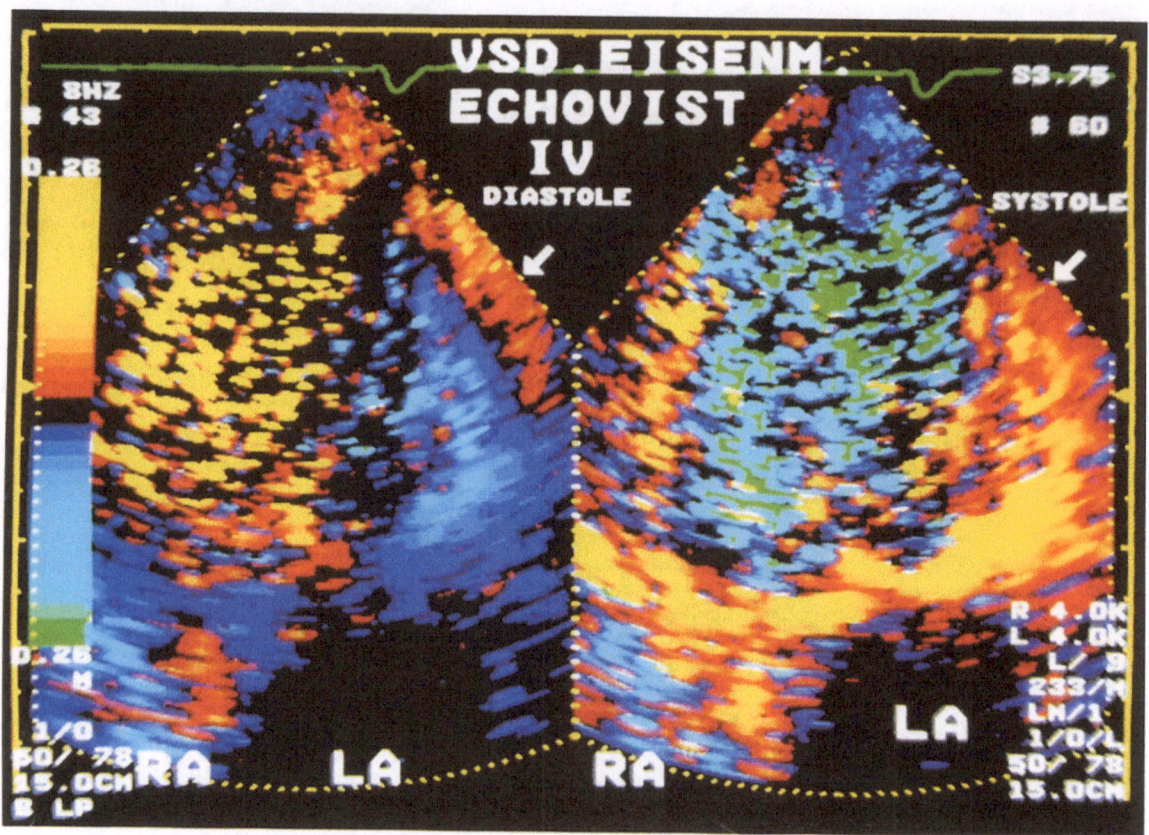

Fig. 14.7. Large VSD, echo-contrast agent.
Two-dimensional TDE split image of the apical four-chamber view. Recordings were performed using a 3.75 MHz transducer. Only the TDE color information is visible without the normally underlying gray-scale image. The left-hand section shows the appearance of the echo-contrast agent during diastole, red and yellow color indicating flow towards the transducer. The right-hand section shows the echo-contrast agent during systole, blue and green colors indicating flow away from the transducer.

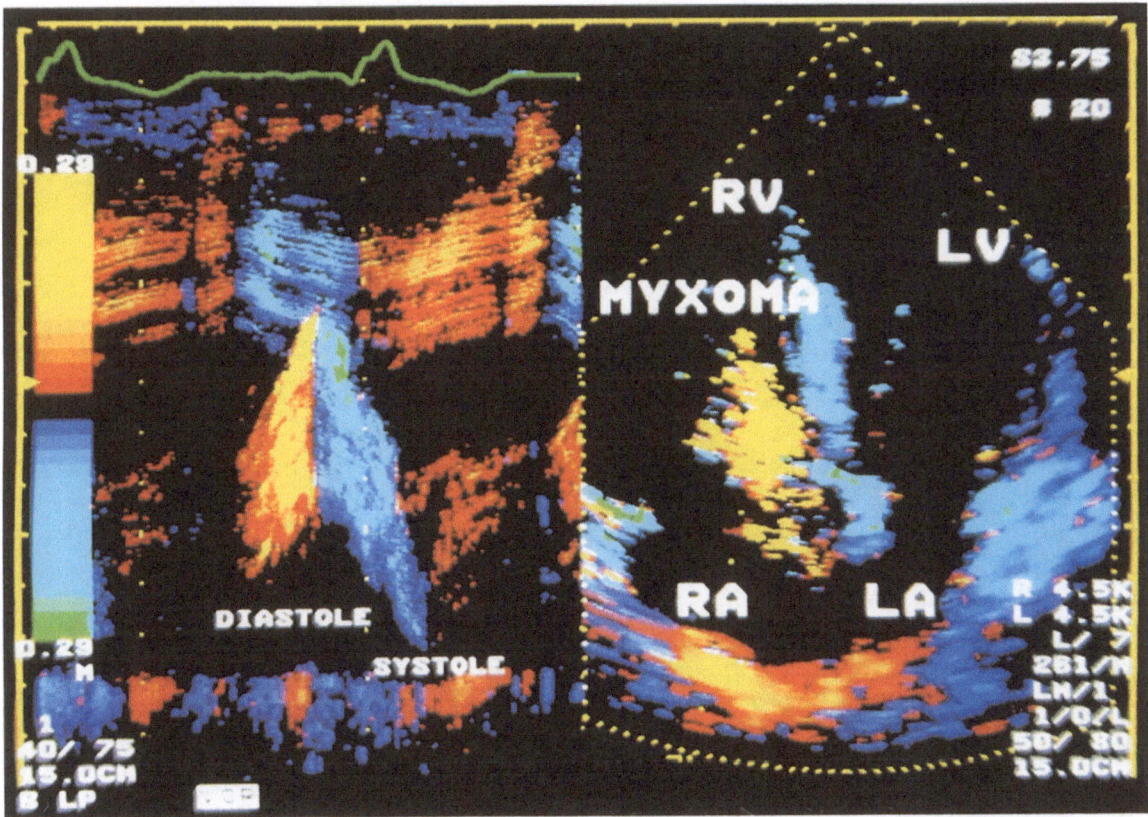

Fig. 14.8. RA Myxoma. Two-dimensional TDE image of the apical four-chamber view. Recordings were performed using a 3.75 MHz transducer. Only the TDE color information is visible without normally underlying 2D gray-scale image. This image demonstrates the presence of a right atrial myxoma. In the two-dimensional image section the yellow colored area originating in the right atrium and protruding into the right ventricular cavity resembles the myxoma. The yellow color indicates that this image was taken in the diastolic phase, the myxoma moves towards the transducer. It is clearly visible in the M-Mode section that the myxoma falls back into the right atrium during late diastole, indicated by the blue color

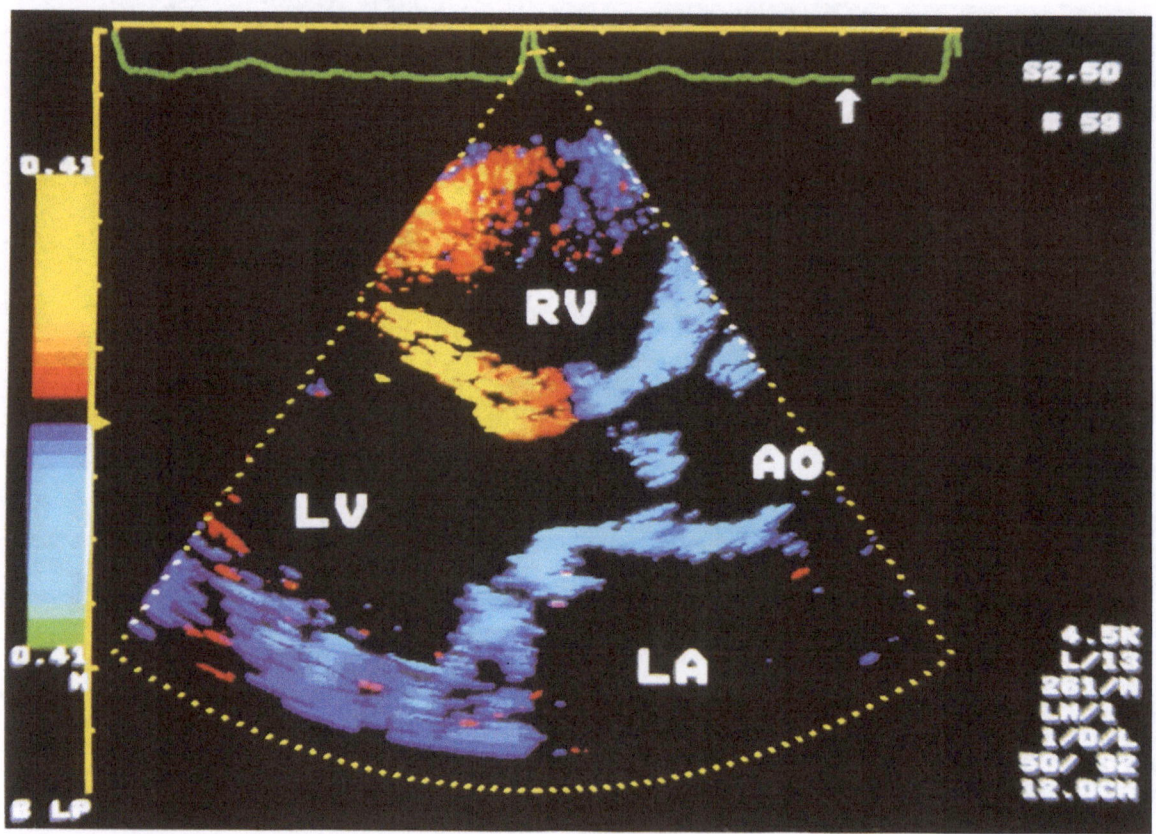

Fig. 14.9. Mitral stenosis. Parasternal long axis view using a 2.5 MHz transducer. Late diastolic frame before the P-wave on the ECG. Machine settings are: non-color-coded velocities up to 0.15 cm/s, red or dark blue coded velocities up to 0.63 cm/s, yellow coded forward velocities above 0.63 cm/s, light blue coded backward velocities from 0.63 cm/s up to 2.1 cm/s, and green coded backward velocities above 2.1 cm/s. Typical diastolic movement directions of the cardiac tissue: forward movement of the interventricular septum and backward movement of the posterior wall and aortic root. However, the velocities of the left ventricular walls are relatively high, with the corresponding color-coding. There is an abnormal pattern of TDE velocities in mitral stenosis at the late-diastole before atrial contraction. At this phase no velocities or very low velocities are observed in healthy subjects. In mitral stenosis the left ventricular filling is prolonged and left ventricular wall velocities remain high. Note good definition of mitral leaflets separation using tissue Doppler. (AO = aorta, LA = left atrium, LV = left ventricle, RV = right ventricle)

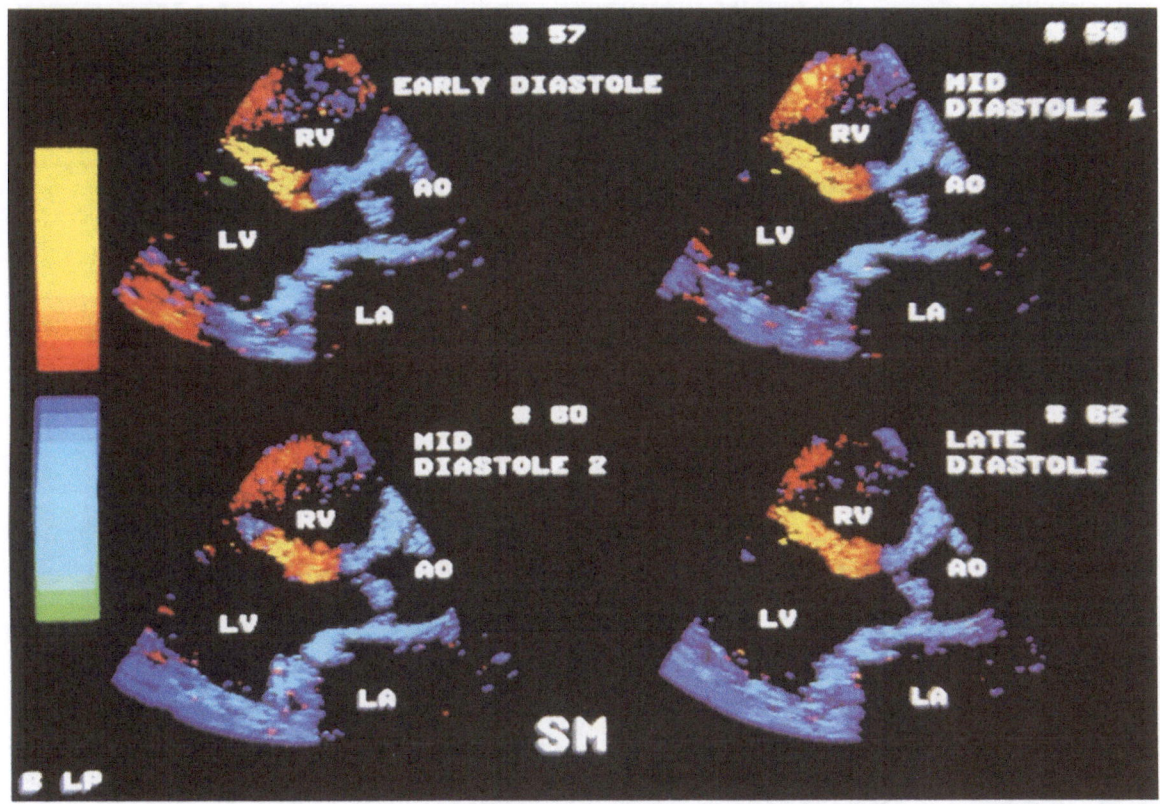

Fig. 14.10. Mitral stenosis. Parasternal long axis view using a 2.5 MHz transducer. Machine settings are the same as in Fig. 14.1. Four frames illustrating TDE velocities during early diastole (*upper left*), mid-diastole (*upper right* and *below left*), and during late diastole (*below right*). The left ventricular wall velocities are relatively high (still higher than 0.63 cm/s) in contrast to velocity pattern in healthy subjects. The aortic root is moving away from the transducer during diastole. Good delineation of the mitral leaflets separation in all presented frames. (AO = aorta, LA = left atrium, LV = left ventricle, RV = right ventricle)

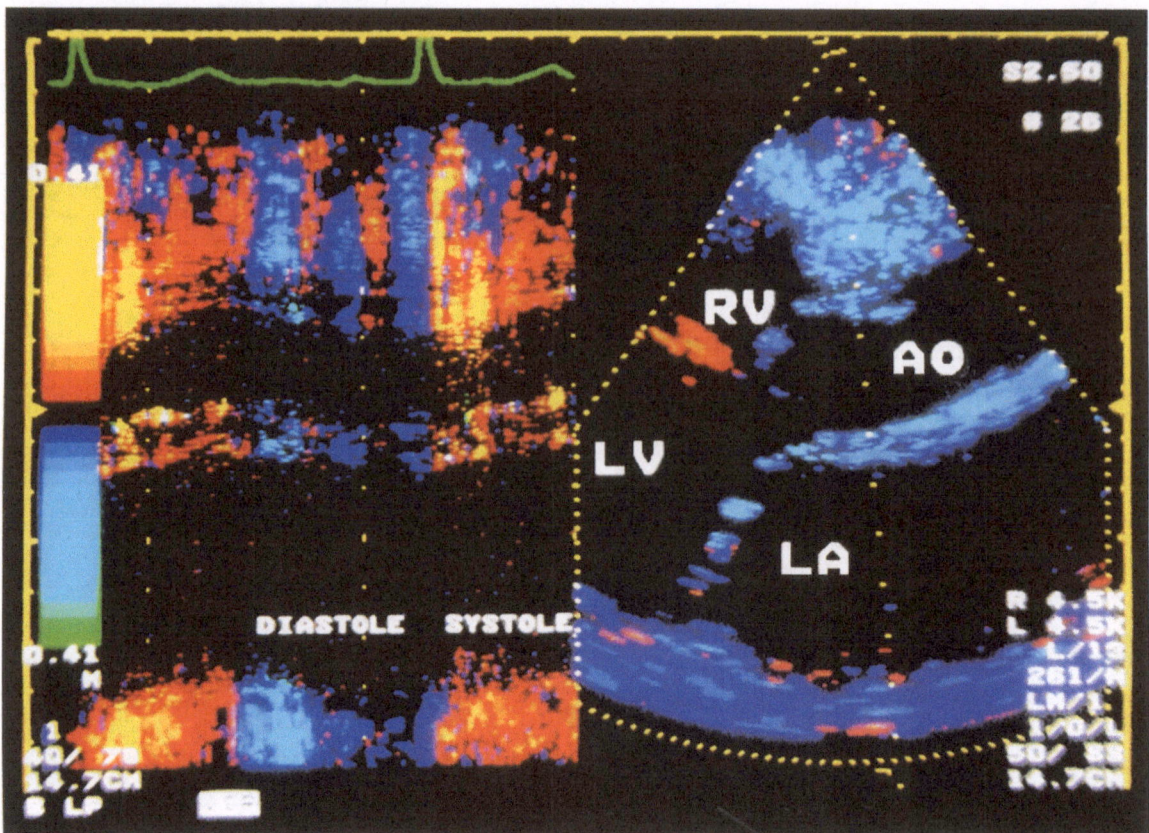

Fig. 14.11. Mitral stenosis. Parasternal long axis view using a 2.5 MHz transducer. Machine settings are the same as in Fig. 14.1. Two-dimensional diastolic frame and M-mode registration through the aortic root and posterior wall of the left atrium. Disturbances of the left atrial function. Both aortic root and posterior wall of the left atrium are moving toward the transducer during systole and away from the transducer during diastole. The velocities of both structures are similar and correspond with the whole cardiac motion. There is no change in the antero-posterior diameter of the left atrium. There is also no mechanical response to the electrical activation of the P-wave on the ECG. During diastole the posterior wall of the left atrium moves away from the transducer with peak velocity during early diastole. In healthy subjects the aortic root shows a backward velocity and the posterior wall of the left atrium a forward velocity in the parasternal long axis view after P-wave on the ECG. (AO = aorta, LA = left atrium, LV = left ventricle, RV = right ventricle)

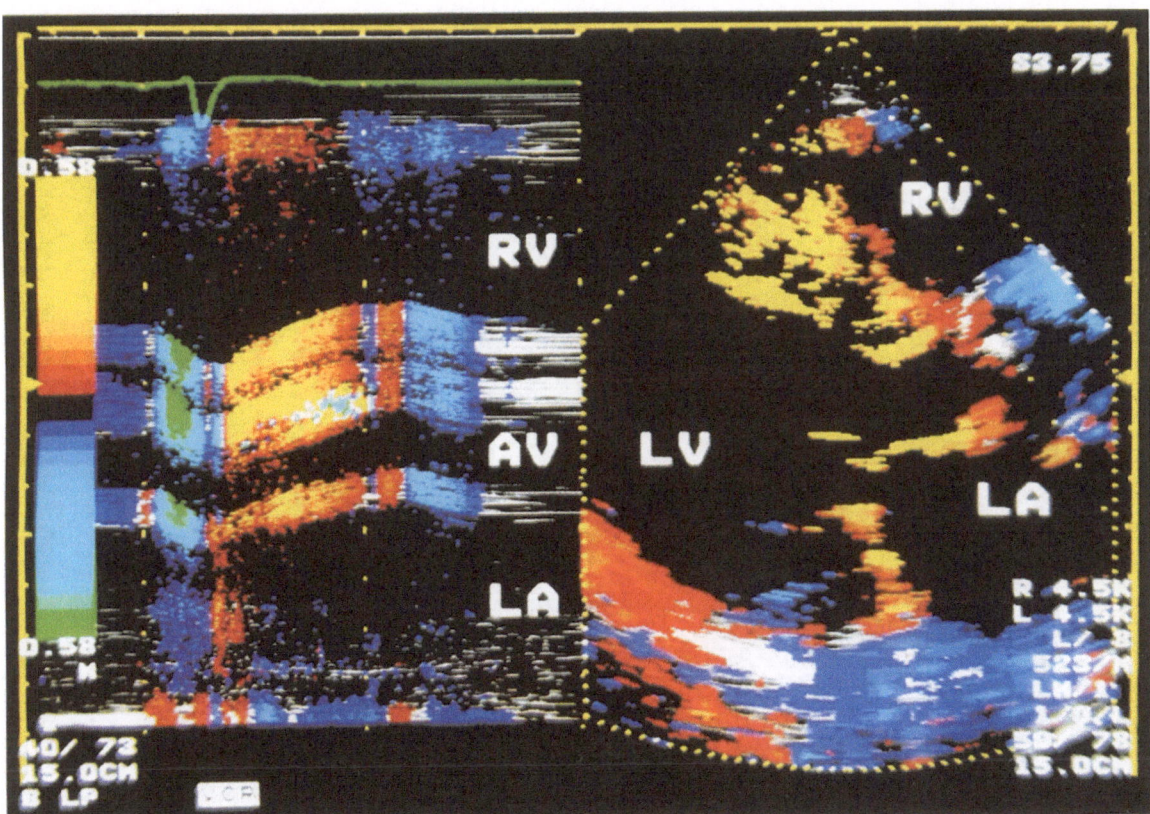

Fig. 14.12. Aortic stenosis and aortic insufficiency. Parasternal long axis view and M-mode recording of the aortic valve using a 3.75 MHz transducer. Machine settings are: non-color-coded velocities up to 0.22 cm/s, red or dark blue coded velocities up to 0.9 cm/s, yellow or light blue coded velocities above 0.9 cm/s, and green coded backward velocities above 3.0 cm/s. During systole the aortic root is moving toward the transducer. The separation of the aortic leaflets is diminished. Systolic fluttering of the aortic leaflets. The aortic root is moving away from the transducer in the early and late-diastolic phase. The velocities during mid-diastole are lower than 0.22 cm/s and the aortic root is not color coded. The highest velocities indicated by green occur in late diastole after the P-wave on the ECG. (AV = aortic valve, LA = left atrium, LV = left ventricle, RV = right ventricle)

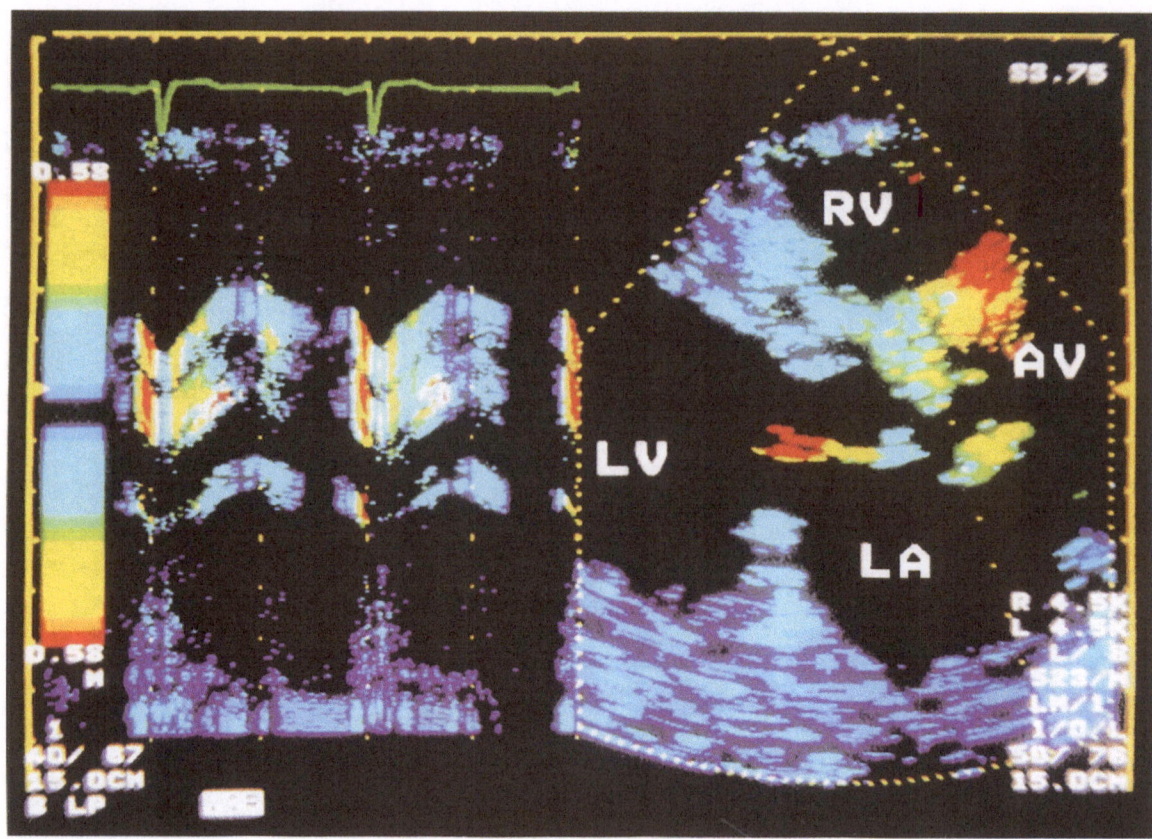

Fig. 14.13. Aortic stenosis and aortic insufficiency. Parasternal long axis view and M-mode recording of the aortic valve using a 3.75 MHz transducer. Different color coding scale used with the same machine settings as in Fig. 14.12. Actual color scale allows comparison of velocities independent of its direction. Non-color-coded velocities are up to 0.9 cm/s, blue coded velocities from 0.9 cm/s to 1.6 cm/s, green coded velocities from 1.6 cm/s to 2.0 cm/s, yellow coded velocities from 2.0 cm/s to 3.2 cm/s, and red coded velocities above 3.2 cm/s. The peak systolic and diastolic velocities are clearly delineated. The peak systolic velocity occurs in early systole and is yellow coded. Peak diastolic velocity occurs in late diastole after P-wave on the ECG and is red coded. The peak diastolic velocity is higher than the peak systolic velocity. The velocity of the aortic leaflets during systolic fluttering exceeds 3.2 cm/s (red coded). (AV = aortic valve, LA = left atrium, LV = left ventricle, RV = right ventricle)

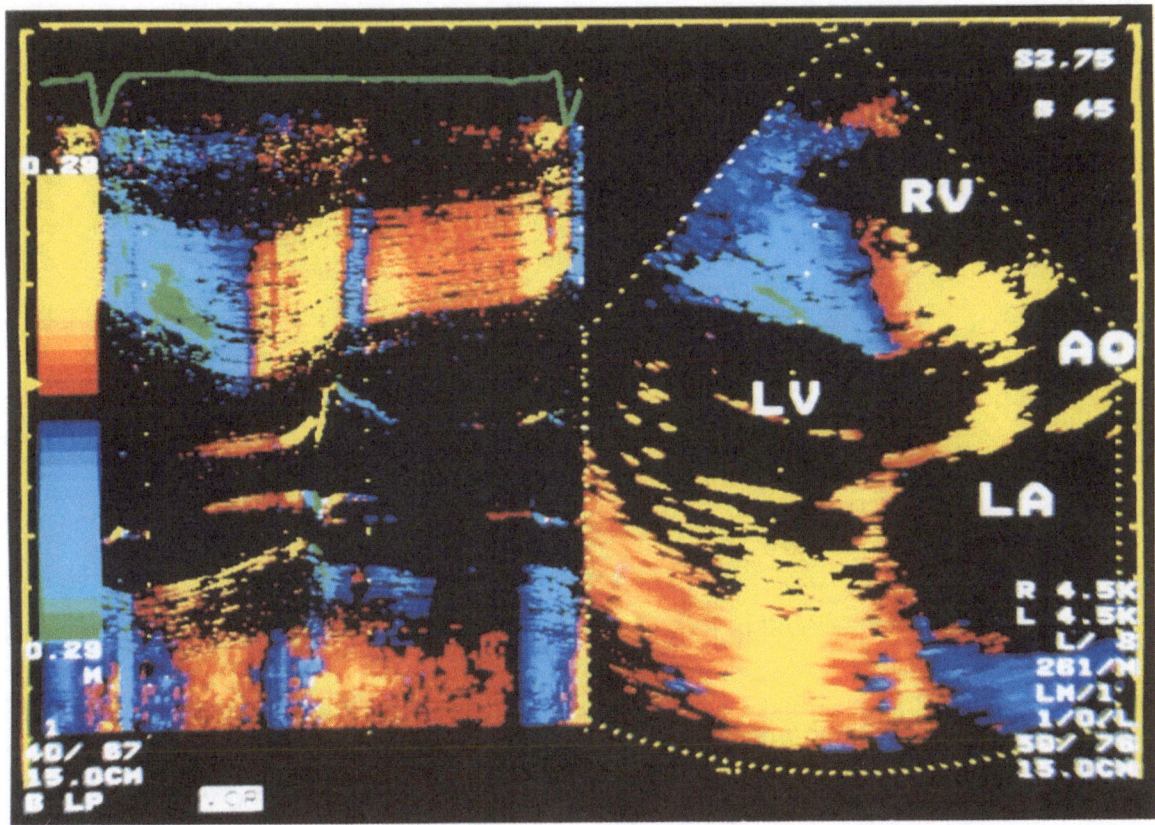

Fig. 14.14. Aortic stenosis and aortic insufficiency. Parasternal long axis view and M-mode recording of the left ventricle using a 3.75 MHz transducer. Machine settings are: non-color-coded velocities up to 0.11 cm/s, red or dark blue coded velocities up to 0.45 cm/s, yellow coded forward velocities above 0.45 cm/s, ligh blue coded backward velocities from 0.45 cm/s up to 1.5 cm/s, and green coded backwards velocities above 1.5 cm/s. The interventricular septum is moving away from the transducer during systole and toward the transducer during diastole. However, a different pattern of interventricular septal movement during diastole is observed with three velocity peaks: early diastolic, mid-diastolic in the opposite direction, and late diastolic phase after the P-wave on the ECG. Long passive filling phase in mid-late diastole with interventricular septum velocities above 0.4 cm/s and relatively low velocities during early diastole as a result of left ventricular compliance disturbance. Note increased interventricular septum thickness. (AO = aorta, LA = left atrium, LV = left ventricle, RV = right ventricle)

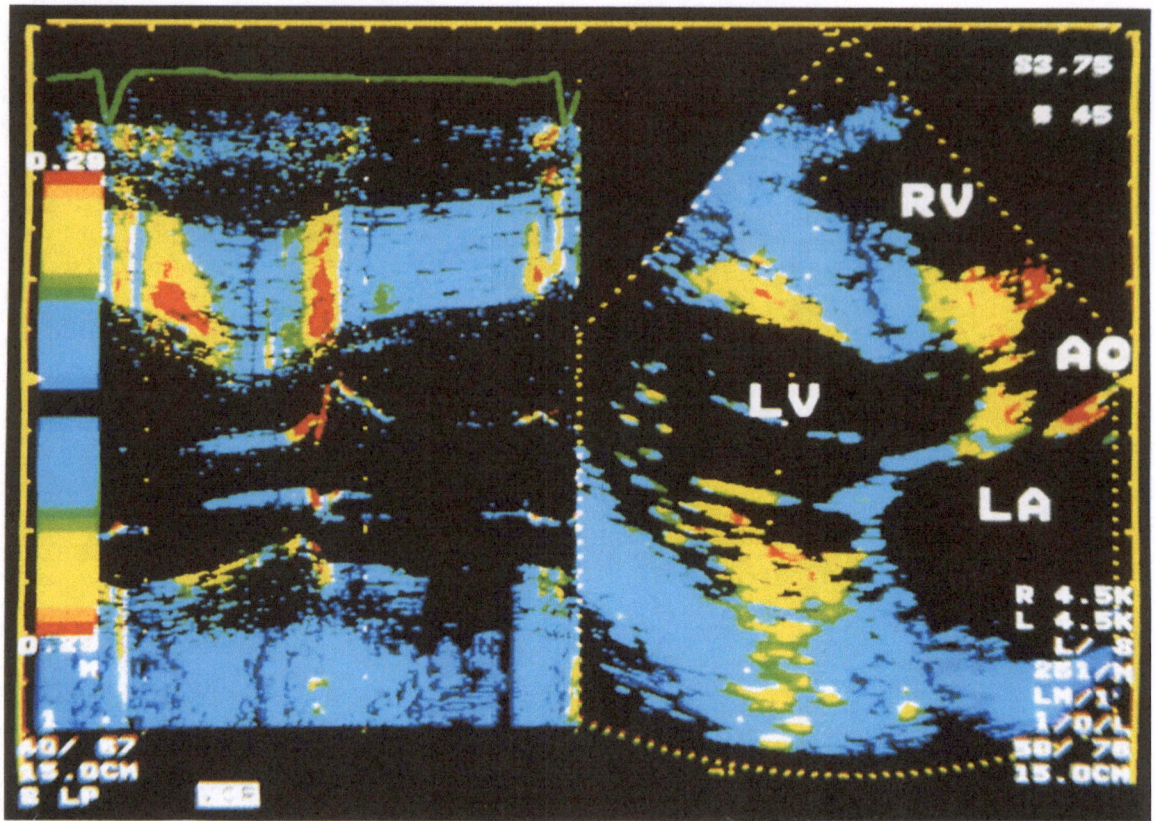

Fig. 14.15. Aortic stenosis and aortic insufficiency. The same frame as in Fig. 14.14 using another color-coding scale. The velocity values are color-coded independent of velocity directions: blue above 0.11 cm/s, green above 0.8 cm/s, yellow above 1.0 cm/s, and red above 1.6 cm/s. The highest wall velocities are recorded over the interventricular septum during mid-systole and early diastole. Different velocities across the wall are visible at the same time (Transmural velocity gradient). The velocities of the left ventricular layers are higher than those of the right ventricular layers related to the myocardial thickening during systole and thinning during diastole. It is also seen on the two dimensional systolic image. (AO = aorta, LA = left atrium, LV = left ventricle, RV = right ventricle)

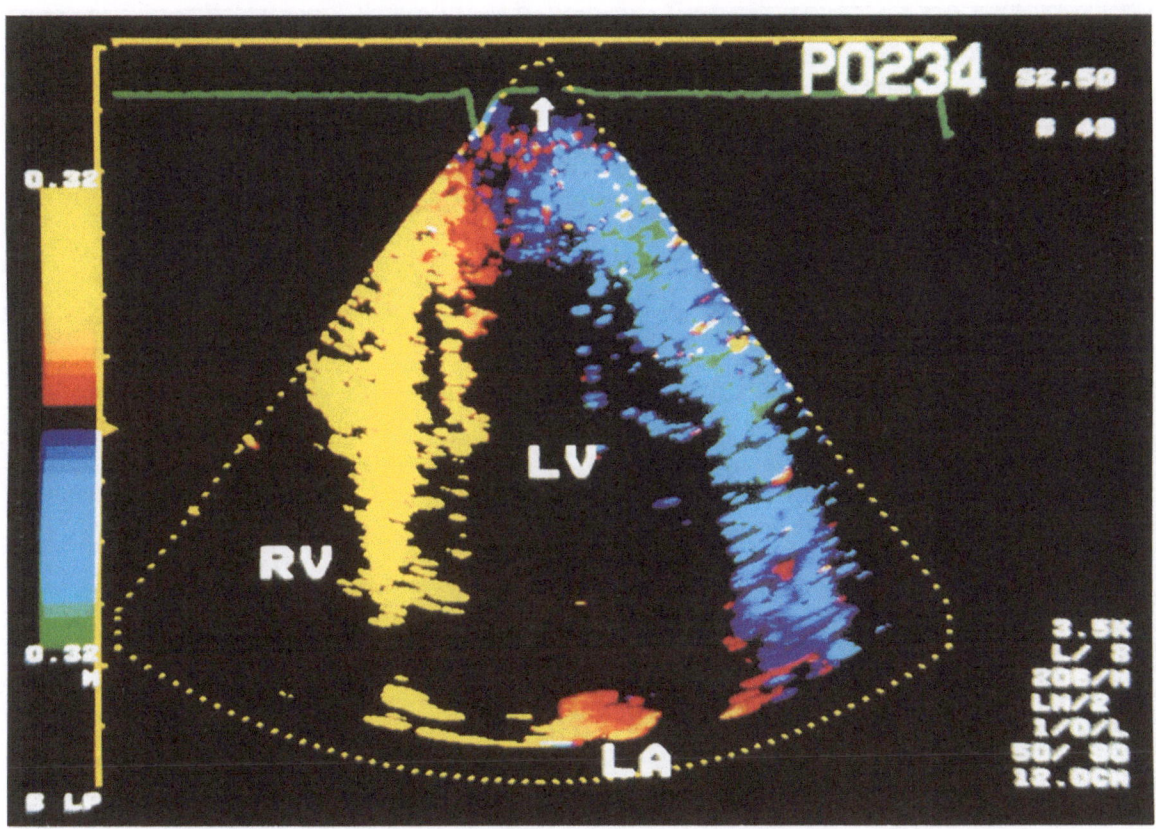

Fig. 14.16. Aortic stenosis and aortic insufficiency. Legend see Fig. 14.17, page 158

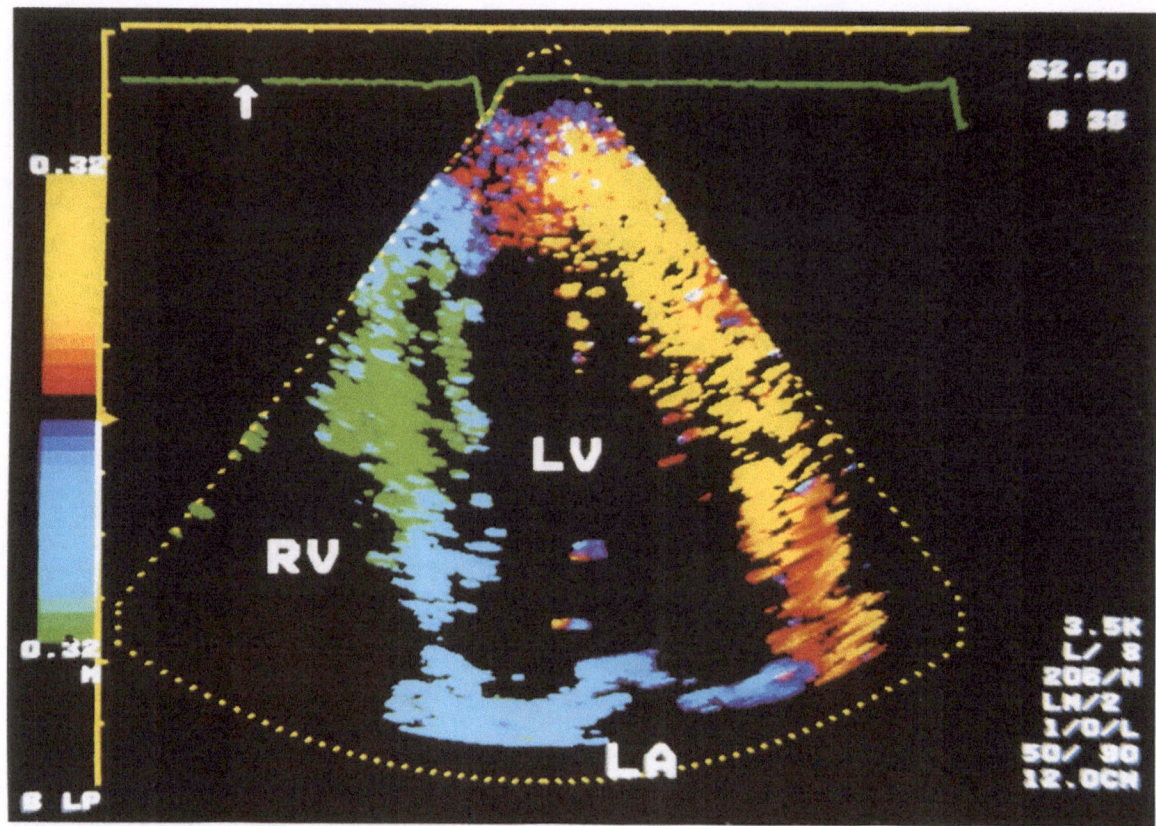

Fig. 14.17. Aortic stenosis and aortic insuffi-ciency. Wall motion abnormalities. Apical four-chamber view using a 2.5 MHz transducer. Systolic (Fig. 14.16) and diastolic frame (Fig. 14.17). Machine settings are: non-color-coded velocities up to 0.12 cm/s, red or dark blue coded velocities up to 0.5 cm/s, yellow coded forward velocities above 0.5 cm/s, light blue coded backward velocities from 0.5 cm/s up to 1.6 cm/s and green coded backward velocities above 1.6 cm/s. The interventricular septum is moving toward the transducer during systole and away from the transducer during diastole with corresponding color coding. In contrast, the lateral wall of the left ventricle is moving in the opposite direction: away from the transducer during systole and toward the transducer during diastole as an abnormal finding LV asynchrony. In healthy subjects both left ventricular walls are moving toward the transducer during systole and away from the transducer during diastole. (LA = left atrium, LV = left ventricle, RV = right ventricle)

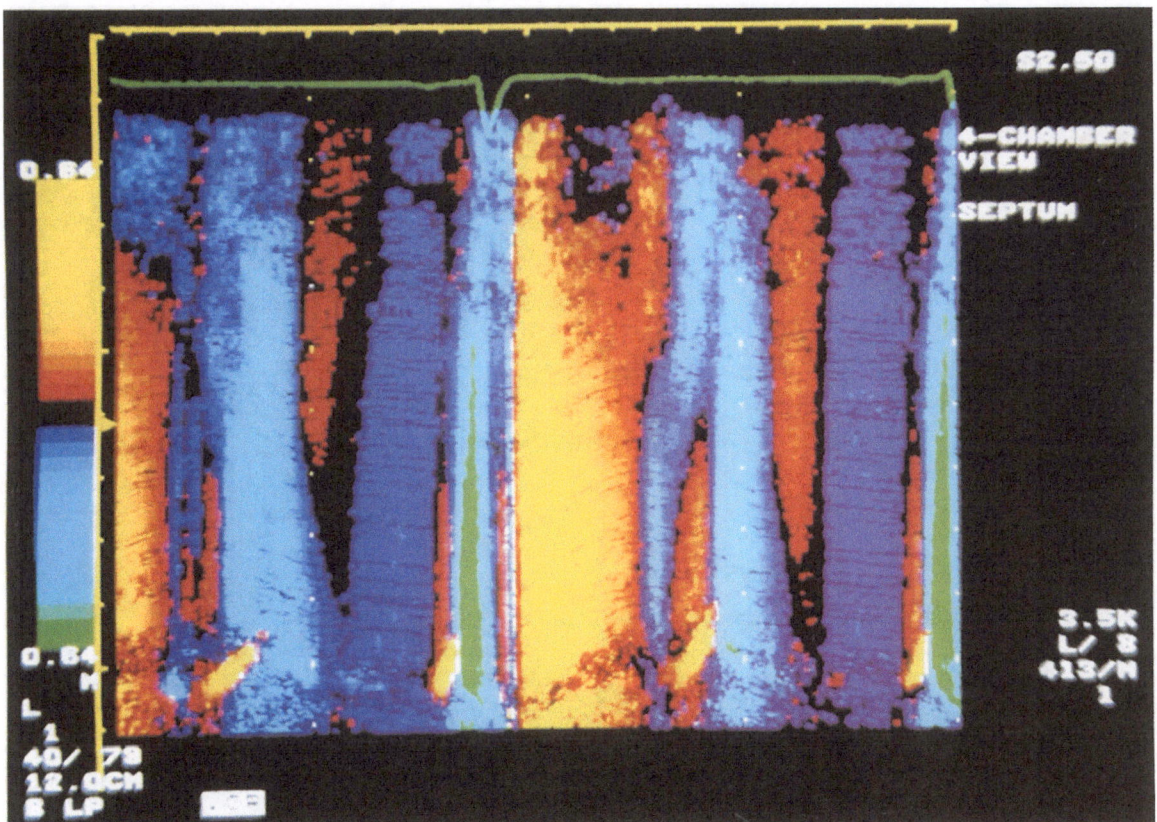

Fig. 14.18. Aortic stenosis and aortic insufficiency. M-mode tissue Doppler echocardiographic image of the interventricular septum from the apical four-chamber view using a 2.5 MHz transducer. Machine settings are: non-color-coded velocities up to 0.24 cm/s, red or dark blue coded velocities up to 1.2 cm/s, yellow coded forward velocities above 1.2 cm/s, light blue coded backward velocities from 1.2 cm/s up to 3.3 cm/s, and green coded backward velocities above 3.3 cm/s. After the Q-wave on the ECG the interventricular septum is moving toward the transducer. At end-systole short backward motion occurs, probably related to the whole cardiac movement in the chest. After early diastolic ventricular expansion the mid-diastolic forward motion and end-diastolic backward motion are recorded. After the P-wave on the ECG the highest backward velocities are presented by the green pattern. Note reproducibility of tissue Doppler recordings

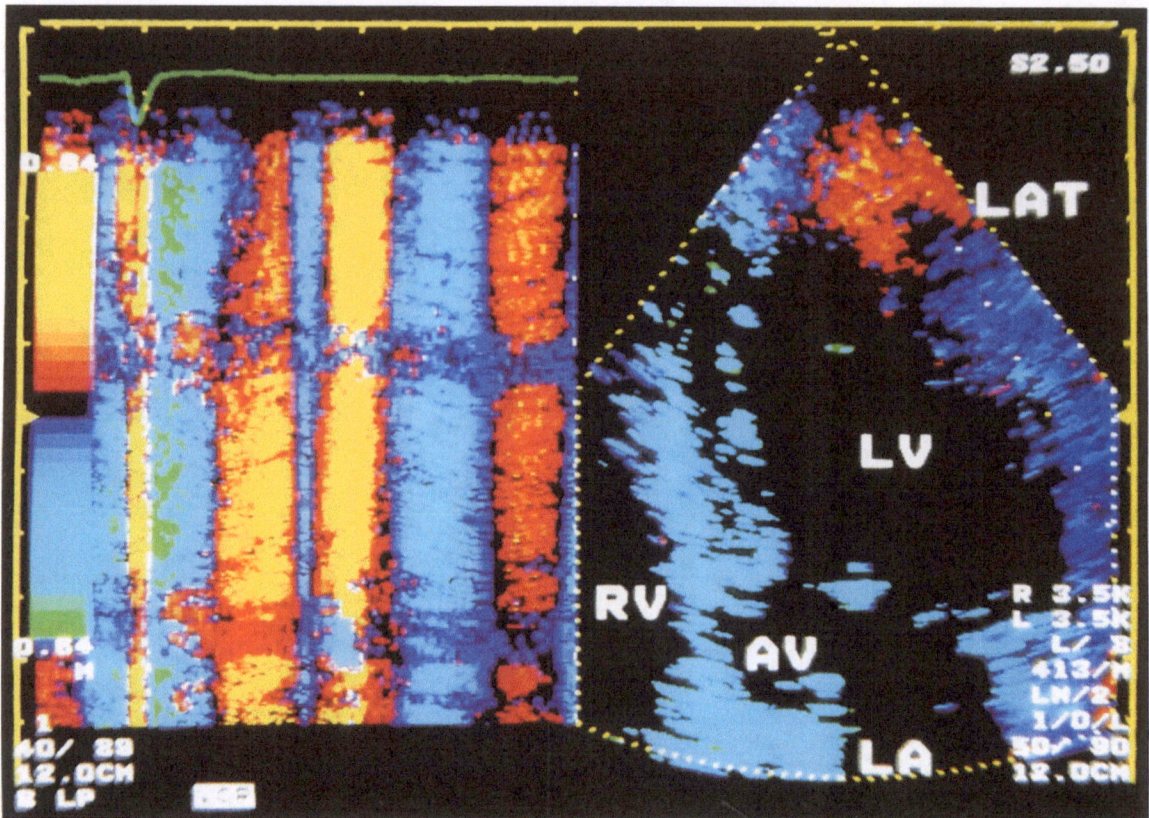

Fig. 14.19. Aortic stenosis and aortic insufficiency. Abnormal velocity pattern of the lateral wall. Apical four-chamber view using a 2.5 MHz transducer. Diastolic frame on the two-dimensional image. M-mode tissue Doppler echocardiographic recording of the lateral left ventricular wall. Machine settings are: non-color-coded velocities up to 0.12 cm/s, red or dark blue coded velocities up to 0.6 cm/s, yellow coded forwards velocities above 0.6 cm/s, light blue coded backwards velocities from 0.6 cm/s up to 1.6 cm/s, and green coded backward velocities above 1.6 cm/s. After the Q-wave on the ECG the lateral left ventricular wall is moving in abnormal direction for this projection: away from the transducer. Subsequently, two phases of forward velocities are recorded: at mid systole and at early diastole. Typical diastolic backward motion occurs in mid diastole, as an abnormal finding. The velocities of this mid-diastolic backward motion are lower (indicated by blue) than the backward velocities during early systole (indicated by green). (AV = aortic valve, LA = left atrium, LAT = left ventricular lateral wall, LV = left ventricle, RV = right ventricle)

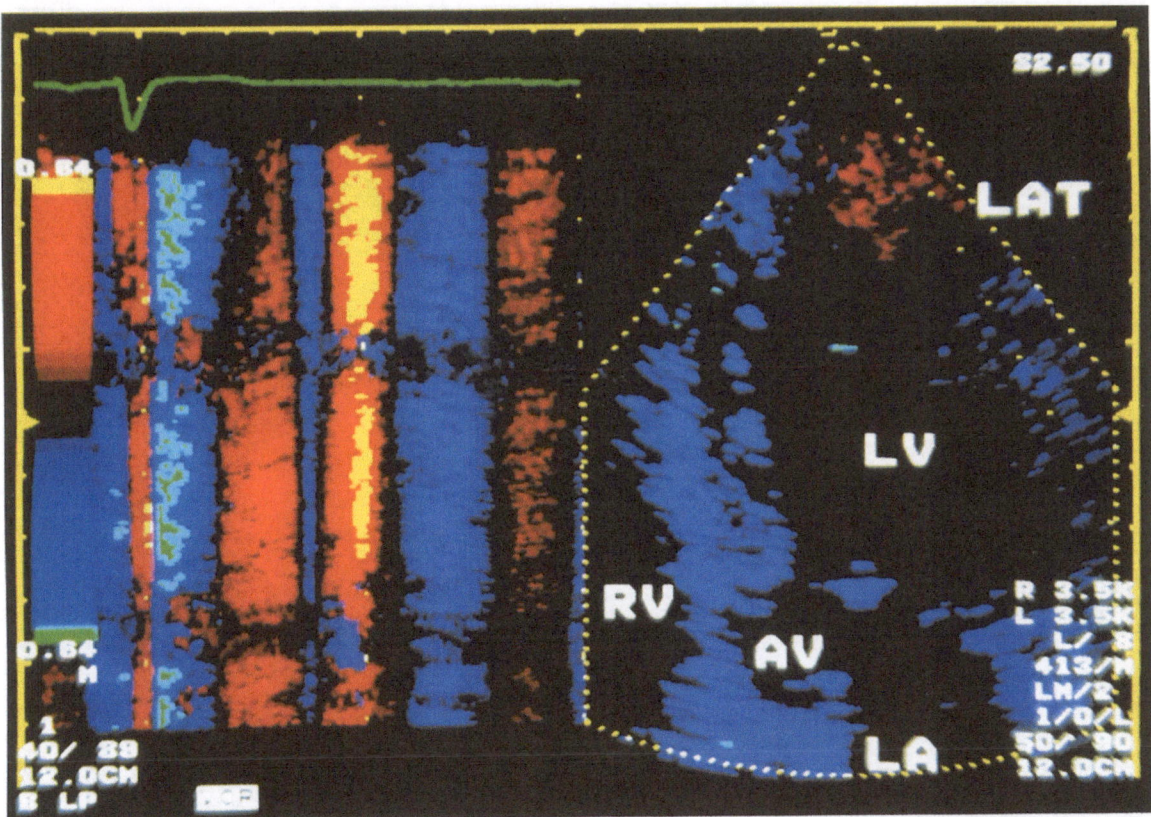

Fig. 14.20. Aortic stenosis and aortic insufficiency. Abnormal velocity pattern of the lateral wall. M-mode tissue Doppler echocardiographic recording of the lateral left ventricular wall in the same patient as shown in Fig. 14.19 using another color scale. Non-color-coded velocities are set up to 0.24 cm/s, red or blue (depending on direction) coded velocities from 0.24 cm/s to 3.72 cm/s, yellow or green coded velocities above 3.72 cm/s. Using this machine setting the peak forward and backward velocities are better visualized. The peak forward velocity occurs during mid-diastole, and peak backward velocity during early systole as an abnormal finding. (AV = aortic valve, LA = left atrium, LAT = left ventricular lateral wall, LV = left ventricle, RV = right ventricle)

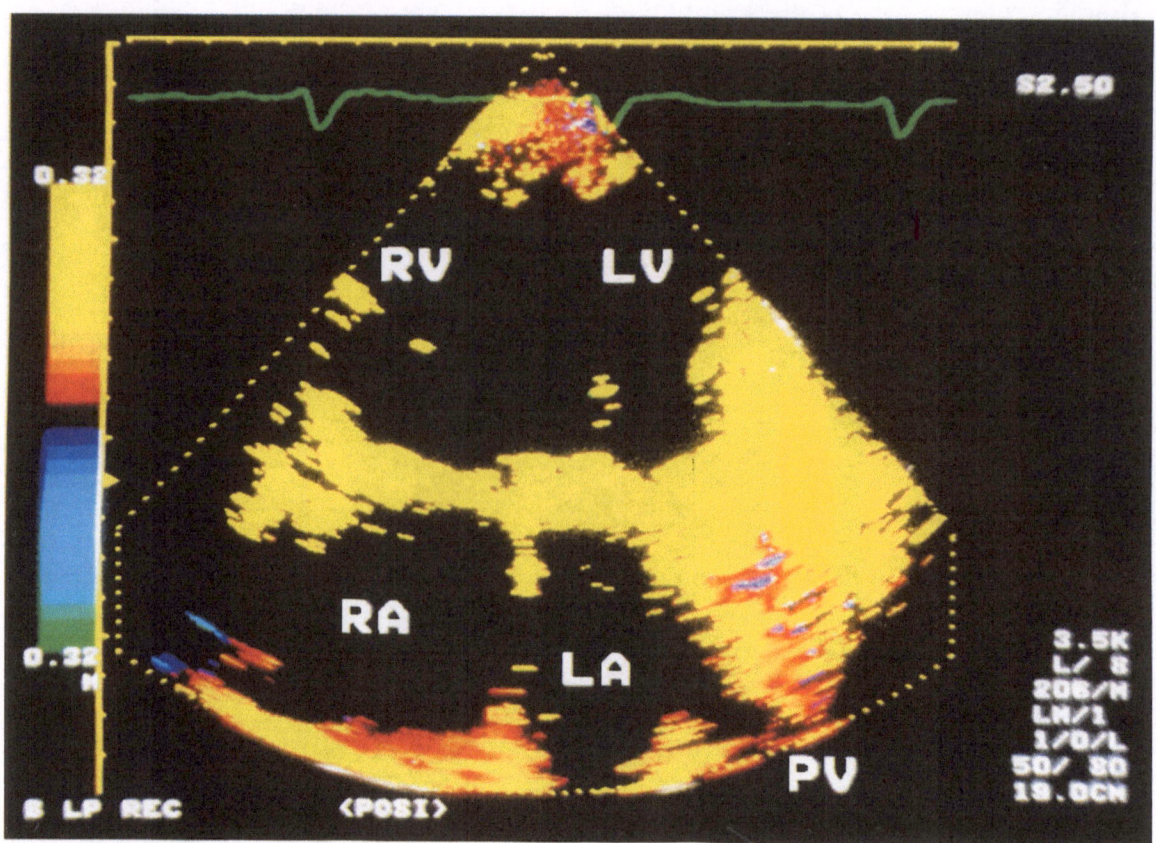

Fig. 14.21. Common ventricle. Apical view using a 2.5 MHz transducer. Systolic frame. Machine settings are: non-color-coded velocities up to 0.12 cm/s and red coded velocities up to 0.6 cm/s, yellow coded velocities above 0.6 cm/s. All visualized cardiac structures are moving toward the transducer with velocities above 0.6 cm/s. Good delineation of the pulmonary vein. (LA = left atrium, LV = left part of the common ventricle, PV = pulmonary vein, RA = right atrium, RV = right part of the common ventricle)

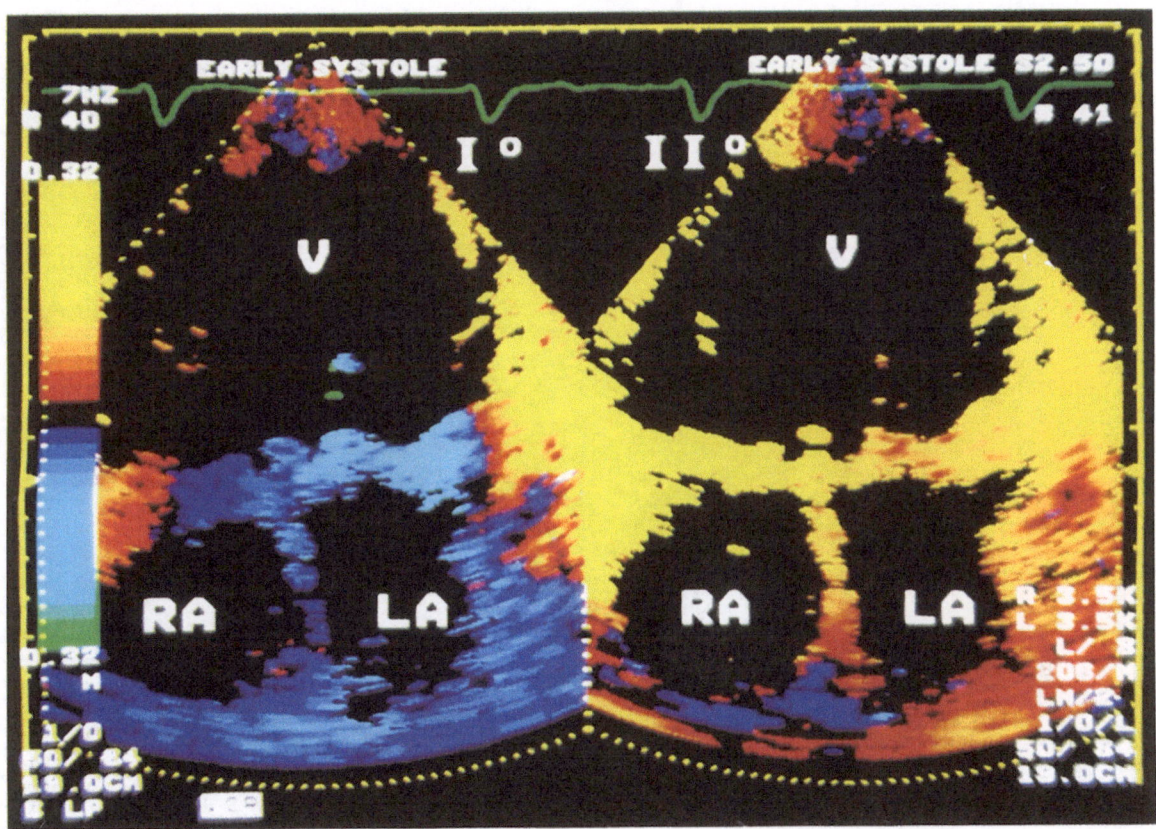

Fig. 14.22. Common ventricle. Apical view using a 2.5 MHz transducer. Early systolic frames. Machine settings are the same as in Fig. 14.21. Ventricular walls are moving first toward the transducer after the Q-wave on the ECG (left). In the next frame forward motion of the remaining cardiac structures is visible and partially related to the systolic motion of the heart toward the apex. (LA = left atrium, RA = right atrium, V = common ventricle)

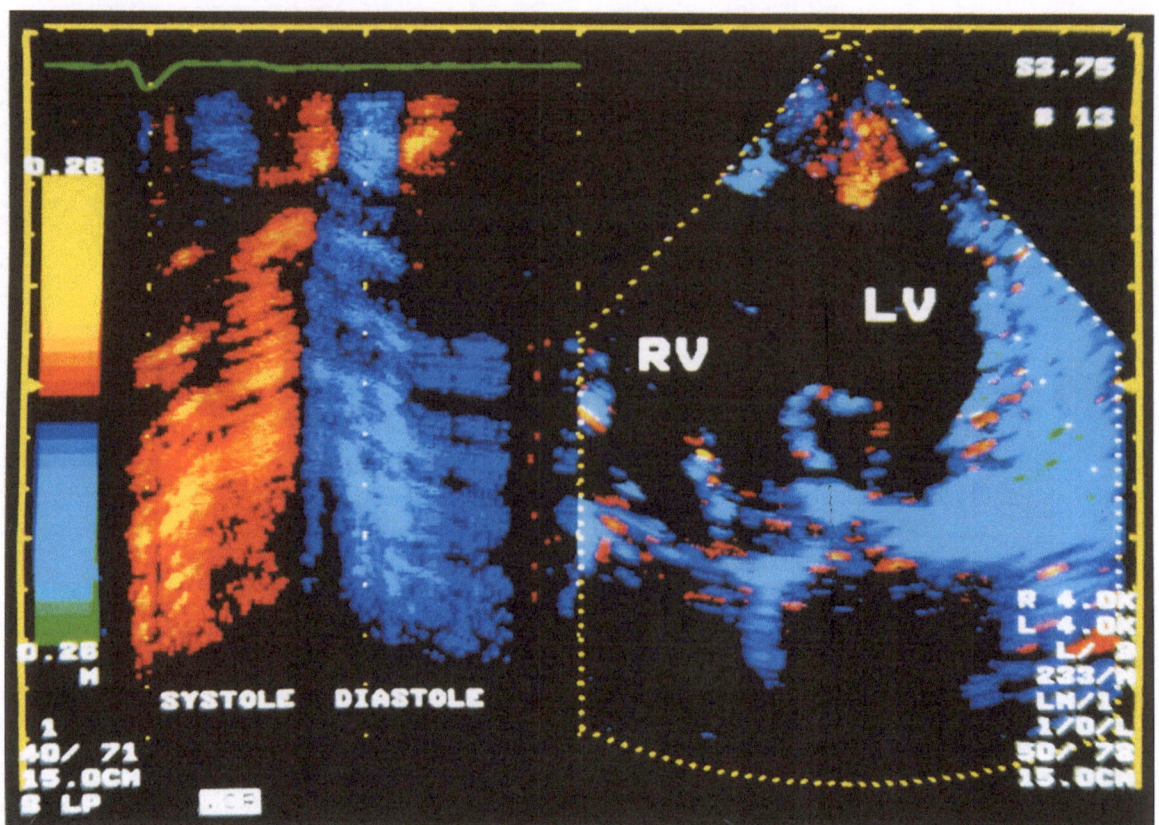

Fig. 14.23. Common ventricle. Apical view using a 3.75 MHz transducer with M-mode recording of the lateral wall. Early diastolic frame on the two-dimensional image. Machine settings are: non-color-coded velocities up to 0.39 cm/s, red or dark blue coded velocities up to 1.6 cm/s, yellow or light blue coded velocities above 1.6 cm/s. During systole the lateral wall is moving toward the transducer with two peaks during early and end-systole. The start of systolic velocity occurs 56 ms after the Q-wave on the ECG. During diastole the lateral wall is moving away from the transducer with the peak velocity in mid diastole 210 ms after color reversal. (LV = left part of the common ventricle, RV = right part of the common ventricle)

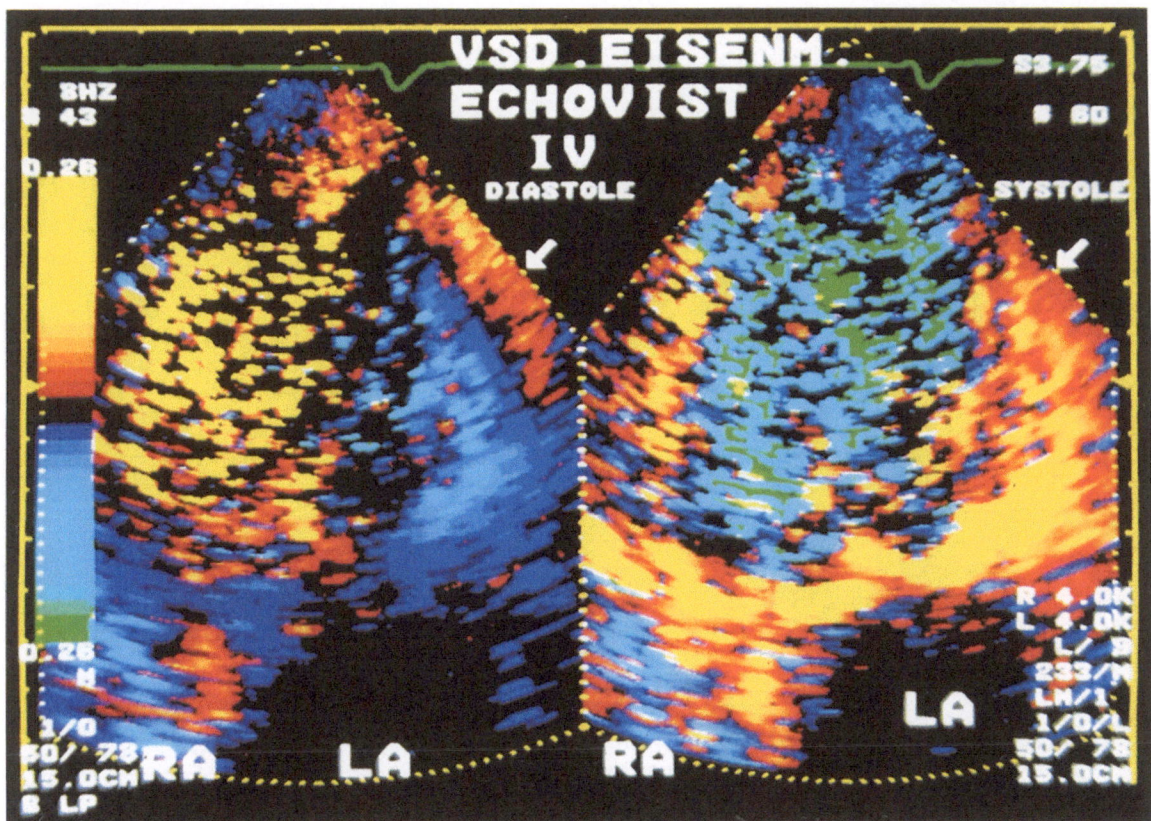

Fig. 14.24. Common ventricle. Apical view using a 3.75 MHz transducer. Early diastolic (*left*) and systolic frame (*right*) after intravenous application of Echovist. Machine settings are the same as in Fig. 14.23. The received ultrasound signal from air-bubbles is strong enough to produce the tissue Doppler signal. The air-bubbles are moving toward the transducer during diastole and away from the transducer during systole with corresponding color coding. The velocity direction of the ventricular walls is still opposite to that of the air-bubbles. Good delineation of the endocardium. (LA = left atrium, RA = right atrium)

Perspectives

R. Erbel

TDE has only recently been introduced in clinical cardiology, and we are now able to appraise initial experience and results. The ability to study on-line velocity without complicated operating procedures will be a valuable addition to the armamentarium for assessing cardiovascular hemodynamics by ultrasound. The study of ventricular synchrony, regional diastolic function, regional systolic and diastolic time intervals, abnormal contraction patterns in arrhythmias, aortic compliance and hysteresis, as well as structure identification are important topics for future research. The usefulness of TDE in studying the effect of cardiomyoplasty has already been shown (G. R. Sutherland).

We are convinced that cardiovascular ultrasound is entering a new era and that TDE will play an important role in the future. It is to be hoped that the technique will be added to all existing types of ultrasound machines.

Subject Index